AF615527

Interdisciplinary Dentofacial Therapy

Interdisciplinary Dentofacial Therapy

A Comprehensive Approach to Optimal Patient Care

Richard D. Roblee, DDS, MS

Clinical Assistant Professor
Department of Restorative Sciences and
Department of Orthodontics
Baylor College of Dentistry
Dallas, Texas

Private Practice
Fayetteville, Arkansas

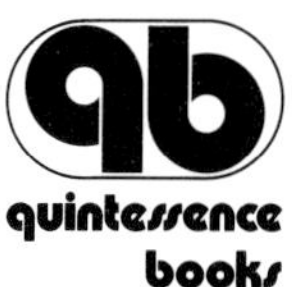

Quintessence Publishing Co, Inc

Chicago, Berlin, London, Tokyo, São Paulo, Moscow, and Warsaw

Dedication

To my wife Julie and our children Anna, James, and Thomas; without their love, support, and sacrifice, this project could not have been completed.

Library of Congress Cataloging-in-Publication Data

Roblee, Richard D. (Richard David), 1957–
Interdisciplinary dentofacial therapy: a comprehensive approach to optimal patient care / Richard D. Roblee.
p. cm.
Includes bibliographical references.
ISBN 0-86715-188-9 (hardcover)
1. Dental therapeutics—Planning. 2. Orthodontics. I. Title.
[DNLM: 1. Orthodontics. 2. Orthodontics, Corrective.
3. Malocclusion—therapy. 4. Maxillofacial Injuries—therapy. WU 400 R6661 1994]
RK318.R63 1994
617.6'43—dc20
DNLM/DLC
for Library of Congress 94-200093
CIP

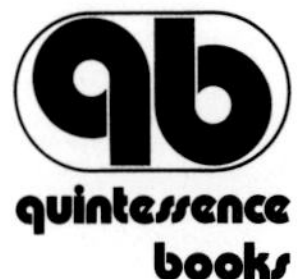

Editor: Adam Haus
Cover: Jennifer Sabella
Production: Timothy M. Robbins
Printing and binding: Toppan Printing Co (S) Pte, Ltd, Singapore
Printed in Singapore

Contents

Contributors

Edward P. Allen, DDS, PhD

Clinical Professor
Department of Periodontics
Baylor College of Dentistry

Private Practice, Dallas, Texas

Periodontal Therapy, Periodontal Plastic Surgery

Thomas G. Wilson, Jr, DDS

Clinical Associate Professor
University of Texas at San Antonio Dental School

Private Practice, Dallas, Texas

Periodontal Therapy, Supportive Periodontal Treatment, Implantology

Scott L. Bolding, DDS, MS

Clinical Assistant Professor
Department of Oral and Maxillofacial Surgery
Baylor College of Dentistry

Private Practice, Dallas, Texas

Adjunctive Facial Cosmetic Surgery

Larry M. Wolford, DDS

Clinical Professor
Department of Oral and Maxillofacial Surgery
Baylor College of Dentistry

Private Practice, Dallas, Texas

Orthognathic Surgery

Foreword

When I was asked to write the foreword for this text, I accepted with enthusiasm for two reasons. First, because I have admired the author's dedication to learning and sharing his quest for quality patient care, and second, because interdisciplinary diagnosis and treatment planning has received too little attention in the literature or in practice. Dr Roblee's comparison between interdisciplinary and multidisciplinary therapy is right on the mark, and we can hope that this text will encourage more general dentists and specialists alike to recognize the difference.

Interdisciplinary treatment planning has been at the center of my own focus for many years, and in 1979 led to t founding of the Center for Advanced Dental Study with a multidisciplinary faculty who agreed to practice together in an academic environment and serve as "an interdisciplinary think tank." This forum seems to be an appropriate place to share some of the most important tenets that have evolved. The three most important requirements for successful interdisciplinary treatment planning are:

1. An accurate starting point
2. A clearly visualized end point, and
3. A treatment "quarterback" who is responsible for coordinating the treatment process.

It appears that the most violated requirement in treatment planning is failure to adequately evaluate the starting point before determining the sequence of treatment.

To have an accurate starting point, every problem to long term health must be recognized. It should be axiomatic that periodontal health, infection control, and resolution of intracapsular TMJ disorders should be sequenced before final correction of dentofacial disorders takes place; but planning the complete process to a visualized end point should come first.

To have an accurate starting point, the correct maxillomandibular relationship must be recorded with properly mounted casts in centric relation. This rule has proven to be uncompromising because unless the condylar axis is correct jaw closure is unknown, and all occlusal planning becomes guesswork. It seems inconsistent to plan alignment of the teeth by any means without knowing what the precisely correct maxillomandibular relationship is.

With properly mounted casts, treatment planning can follow a logical path for determining the best alignment of the teeth in harmony with the maxillomandibular relationship. In addition to mounted casts, cephalometric analysis can be sued to determine if the mandible or the maxilla or both are in disharmony with the cranial base. The best choice or choices for treatment can then be determined. Cephalograms must be corrected to a centrically related condylar axis, or severe errors can occur in determination of treatment objective.

There are five treatment choices to select from. Determining the best choice is accomplished most logically by making corrections on the mounted diagnostic casts. It has become a popular truism that good treatment planning revolves around an articulator. It is through making necessary corrections on the casts that the best type of treatment is selected, and the end point of treatment is visualized. The five treatment choices are considered in sequence. The are:

1. Reductive reshaping of teeth. (Equilibration)
2. Repositioning of teeth within their alveolar process. (Orthodontics)
3. Additive reshaping of teeth. (Restorative)
4. Repositioning of entire segments of dento-alveolar process without changing the skeletal base. (Orthopedically or Surgically)
5. Repositioning the skeletal base in relation to the cranium. (Orthopedically or Surgically)

On mounted casts, it is clear how much advantage can be gained by equilibration. Model surgery can be done to reposition teeth or move entire segments. Diagnostic waxups can be used to visualize a restorative endpoint. It is through this process that an interdisciplinary dialogue becomes definitive and helpful. All specialists involved become a part of the total process, with a three-dimensional model of the treatment objective agreed upon before treatment is initiated.

The "quarterback" who coordinates the treatment planning and sequencing should be the therapist who is responsible for the final phase of treatment. Thus, if it is the restorative dentist who must create the final result, it should be the restorative dentist who directs the total process in collaboration with whatever specialists are needed to aid in achieving a restorable situation.

One more critical tenet should not be overlooked. The final result of interdisciplinary therapy will depend on a through understanding of all the factors which are critical to the harmony and ultimate equilibrium of the masticatory system. Results will fall short if the occlusion is not in harmony with the temporomandibular joints; if the teeth are not in harmony with the neutral zone; or if the anterior guidance is not in harmony with the envelope of function, lip-closure path, and phonetics. Understanding of the total masticatory system should be a neverending goal of every member of the interdisciplinary team.

As dental practitioners involved in the different specialties, we have much to learn from each other. I applaud Dr Roblee for his major contribution toward bringing specialty thinking into a more congruent and logical team approach for better patient care. I feel certain that this text, and the future editions that are sure to follow, will stimulate dialogue among specialists and will help to set new and better standards for interdisciplinary therapy.

Peter E. Dawson, DDS

Preface

Modern science and technology are making exciting and sweeping advances in all aspects of dentistry and medicine at an ever increasing rate. As a result, it is more and more difficult to stay abreast of one area of dentistry, much less all the various disciplines. One of the largest problems in our profession today is not advancing the science of dentistry, but optimally utilizing the science that already exists.

The concept of Interdisciplinary Dentofacial Therapy (IDT) was developed to maximize treatment results by optimally synergizing the knowledge, skills, and experience of all the disciplines in dentistry and its associated fields, while minimizing the frustrating and problematic shortcomings typically associated with working as a team. There are many excellent references that coordinate two disciplines (such as periodontics and restorative dentistry, orthodontics and orthognathics, orthodontics and periodontics, etc), but no source until this text has presented total and equal integration of all disciplines. This book was written to serve as a comprehensive reference for an interdisciplinary team. It presents the needed philosophy and methodology to enable a group of professionals, with individual practices and highly varied expertise, to blend as a cohesive team and consistently provide their patients with the highest level of care.

Everyone readily agrees that the benefits of IDT over traditional approaches are vast, not only to providers, but also (and especially) to patients. However, the justifiable arguments against the concept of IDT in the past have usually been associated with difficulty, confusion, and problems among team members when using a multidisciplinary approach toward dental therapy. This book helps overcome those previous shortcomings by presenting a detailed model for interdisciplinary teams that can be effectively utilized in any individual or group practice; in private, hospital, and university settings; and in urban, rural, and long-distance treatment situations.

For IDT to be consistently successful, two important elements must be present. The first of these elements is *regimental sequencing* to ensure that every procedure is performed in the order closest to ideal throughout the entire interdisciplinary process. The second critical element is *extensive communication* between providers to optimize all aspects of IDT. The philosophy and methodology needed to establish these necessary elements in an interdisciplinary team are outlined in this work through the most comprehensive IDT flowcharts and timetables ever presented. Also described are several different levels of interdisciplinary communication utilizing every modality from verbal interaction to paperless electronic files.

Another important purpose of this book is to give information and "clinical pearls" about all the various aspects of IDT. This information is not given in detail, with the intent of educating different team members on how to perform in their areas of expertise, but rather the material is presented in an overview to educate individual team members on what the rest of the team members can do to help them help their patients. An exhaustive bibliography has also been included if more detailed information about a certain topic is desired.

Extensive numbers of clinical cases and examples have been included to illustrate the concepts, benefits, and dramatic results of IDT. It is intended that these clinical examples also be used in "picture book" fashion by the interdisciplinary team to assist in the dentofacial counseling and motivation of their patients.

Lastly and most importantly, it must be pointed out that although there are many benefits to the provider, the greatest benefactor of the IDT concept is the patient. IDT gives the patient consistent access to an enhanced quality of life that only the highest level of dentofacial care and our great profession can provide. I sincerely hope that this text will enable my colleagues to raise their level of patient care and, at the same time, experience the same enormous benefits and professional satisfaction that I enjoy while practicing IDT.

Richard D. Roblee, DDS, MS

Acknowledgments

Like the practice of Interdisciplinary Dentofacial Therapy (IDT), this book required a comprehensive team effort to complete with optimal results. The concept of IDT is the summation of many individuals' work in dentistry, most of whom are referenced throughout this text. I would like to thank each one of them for their contribution to the dental profession. I also want to recognize many other people who have had a more direct influence on this book and on me.

Many sincere thanks go out to the contributors already listed. They are all international experts in their particular fields and this book could not have been as complete without their invaluable help.

Additional thanks to Dr Peter Dawson for taking time from his busy schedule to share his wisdom and experience in the Foreword to this book.

In addition to the main contributors, I need to acknowledge additional experts who, among others, reviewed the text and made valuable contributions.

Dr Larry White *(Orthodontist)*
Dr Ronald Woody *(Prosthodontist)*
Dr Gerry Glickman *(Endodontist)*
Dr John Bain *(Restorative Dentist)*
Dr Richard Ceen *(Orthodontist)*
Dr Larry Cloetta *(Prosthodontist)*
Dr Robert Waugh *(Orthodontist)*

Special recognition must go to all the members of my IDT team and study group. Their patience, cooperation, and support were crucial to the development of the material in this book. I also want to recognize Dr Robert Waugh for reviewing the text and, more importantly, for establishing an outstanding IDT network in Athens and Winder, Georgia. He helped test the concepts in this book and provided valuable insight and ideas to the IDT philosophy.

Thanks to my fabulous staff whose hard work and dedication helped give me the support and time needed to write this book, as well as give me a testing ground for my ideas. Individual recognition must be given to Nona Boatright, Laurie Normand, and Shirley Fitzpatrick for typing and proofing the manuscript.

Lastly, I would like to thank some very special people who indirectly had a strong influence on this book and the concept of IDT through the profound impact they have made on my dental career. They are my wife, Julie; my parents, Bill and Marge Roblee; my second parents, Jimmy and Gaye Cypert; my mentor, Dr Jesse Bullard; and my first associate, Dr Frank Higginbottom.

1

Present Status of the Dental Profession

There has never been a more exciting time to be part of the dental profession. Dentistry, with its multiple disciplines and in conjunction with modern science and technology, is making enormous advances, seemingly on a daily basis. Today, dentistry is helping people in ways never before thought possible. The profession is no longer just concerned about controlling oral pathology; it is now striving to enhance the overall quality of life for patients.

The various dental disciplines have been making advances in their ability to improve the overall well-being of their patients. Through tremendous breakthroughs, such as fluorides and sealants, preventive dentistry has changed the way most of us practice. The profession is shifting more and more to a preventive approach to dental caries and periodontal disease. Today, nearly fifty percent of all elementary school children in the United States have yet to have their first cavity. This dramatic shift in the caries rate has allowed dentistry to change from a "drill and fill" profession to one that is continuously striving to find new and exciting ways to help patients.

An excellent example of this change is the explosion of new esthetic dental materials and techniques. The interest and excitement surrounding esthetic dentistry has added a new dimension to the profession. New widespread public awareness has created a demand for superior esthetic results, and is a primary motivating factor for patients seeking dental care. One of the many positive byproducts of esthetic dentistry is that some of the materials that were once developed for esthetic enhancement have now been improved to a point where they are being chosen for their outstanding mechanical properties. The introduction of the enamel acid-etch technique and composite-resin bonding has revolutionized the practice of restorative dentistry; it has also impacted orthodontics, periodontics, and endodontics. New esthetic materials and techniques are being developed on a continuing basis. The most exciting aspect of the advent of esthetic dentistry, in the wake of the new preventive procedures is that dental providers and their staffs can now enjoy the luxury of doing what their patients actually want rather than just need.

The reliability of endosseous osseointegrated implants now allows the dentist to esthetically and optimally restore function and stability in many partial and fully edentulous patients who previously only had the option of a removable prosthesis. Even in traditional fixed prosthodontics, enhancements in materials and techniques allow the restorative dentist or prosthodontist to restore broken-down and missing teeth with unsurpassed esthetics, precision, and tissue health.

Through an increased understanding of the disease process associated with endodontic problems, as well as improvements in the materials and techniques, endodontists are now salvaging teeth previously given a "hopeless" prognosis. In addition, advancements in the restoration of endodontically-treated teeth are ever increasing the predictability of restoring and maintaining severely broken-down teeth.

Recent discoveries now enable periodontists to more predictably treat and control most periodontal diseases. In fact, new discoveries are allowing the rebuilding of previously diseased or altered hard and soft periodontal tissues through grafting, ridge augmentation, bone regeneration, and soft tissue procedures.

An increased understanding of the physiology associated with hard and soft tissues during tooth movement, in conjunction with many sweeping advances in orthodontic appliances, has changed orthodontics from primarily a specialty which deals with adolescent patients to one that can help improve the dental health and overall well-being of dentulous patients in virtually any age group. Even the stigma associated with adults wearing orthodontic appliances has been nearly eliminated with the development of tooth-colored brackets and lingual approaches. The orthodontist, often in conjunction with other dentists, can now treat complex dental malocclusions with unsurpassed precision and efficiency, while minimizing the deleterious side effects previously associated with orthodontic tooth movement.

Tremendous advancements have also been made in oral and maxillofacial surgical procedures. Complex skeletal jaw dysplasias can now be managed with unprecedented sophistication, predictability, and stability. These advancements give the oral and maxillofacial surgeon the opportunity to restore or improve facial esthetics in addition to restoring or improving oral function. This enhancement of facial esthetics can have a very positive affect on patients by elevating their self-image[1] as well as improving the social perception of them by others.[2]

Through all of this progress, dentistry has developed the capacity to treat complex dentofacial problems with results that have unprecedented predictability, function, stability, longevity, and esthetics. One of the major problems dentistry faces today is that its various disciplines are becoming so sophisticated that it is virtually impossible for a dental professional to stay abreast of all areas. To optimally treat patients by today's standards, the different dental disciplines and their medical counterparts are increasingly having to rely on one another. Open communication and proper coordination of therapy between the various disciplines are two of the most important and too-frequently overlooked ingredients necessary for performing optimal dental and dentofacial therapy.

The purpose of this text is to provide information and structure to each member of the dental team, thus facilitating dental and dentofacial therapy and improving the chances of consistently obtaining optimal results.

References

1. Flanary CM, Barnwell GM, Van Sickels JE, Littlefield JH, Rugh AL. Impact of orthognathic surgery on normal and abnormal personality dimension: A 2-year follow-up study of 61 patients. Am J Orthod Dentofacial Orthop 1990;98: 313–322.
2. Cash TF, Horton CE. Esthetic surgery: effects of rhinoplasty on social perception of patients by others. Plast Reconstr Surg 1985;76:543–548.

2

Interdisciplinary Dentofacial Therapy (IDT)

Dental and dentofacial therapies are performed at various levels of sophistication with proportionally various degrees of success. All these levels can be divided into three major types of therapy. They are *(1)* unidisciplinary therapy, *(2)* multidisciplinary therapy and *(3)* interdisciplinary therapy.

Unidisciplinary Therapy

Unidisciplinary therapy encompasses diagnostic procedures, treatment planning, therapy, and maintenance care accomplished entirely by one dental provider. It is the natural tendency of a sole provider to characterize a patient's dental and dentofacial problems in terms of the dentist's own background and interests. In fact, some dentists develop treatment plans according to their own capabilities, rather than by what the patient actually needs and by the treatment options the profession can provide. This approach to patient care will frequently lead to compromised results that may produce more problems than it solves.

If the full scope of therapy is not addressed or understood, dentists may be guilty of providing unidisciplinary therapy by trying to solve complex dental and dentofacial problems using only restorative means. These attempts often fail to address the esthetic, stability, functional, and periodontal aspects, because the providers are actually treating symptoms rather than the underlying problems (Fig 2-1).

Another example of unidisciplinary therapy is a sole provider attempting to provide comprehensive therapy encompassing one or more of the different dental specialties. The major shortcoming of this "isolationist" attitude is that it is exceptionally difficult to become an expert in one dental specialty, much less two or more of them. This type of unidisciplinary therapy can be the most damaging, because the lack of knowledge in one discipline means a lack

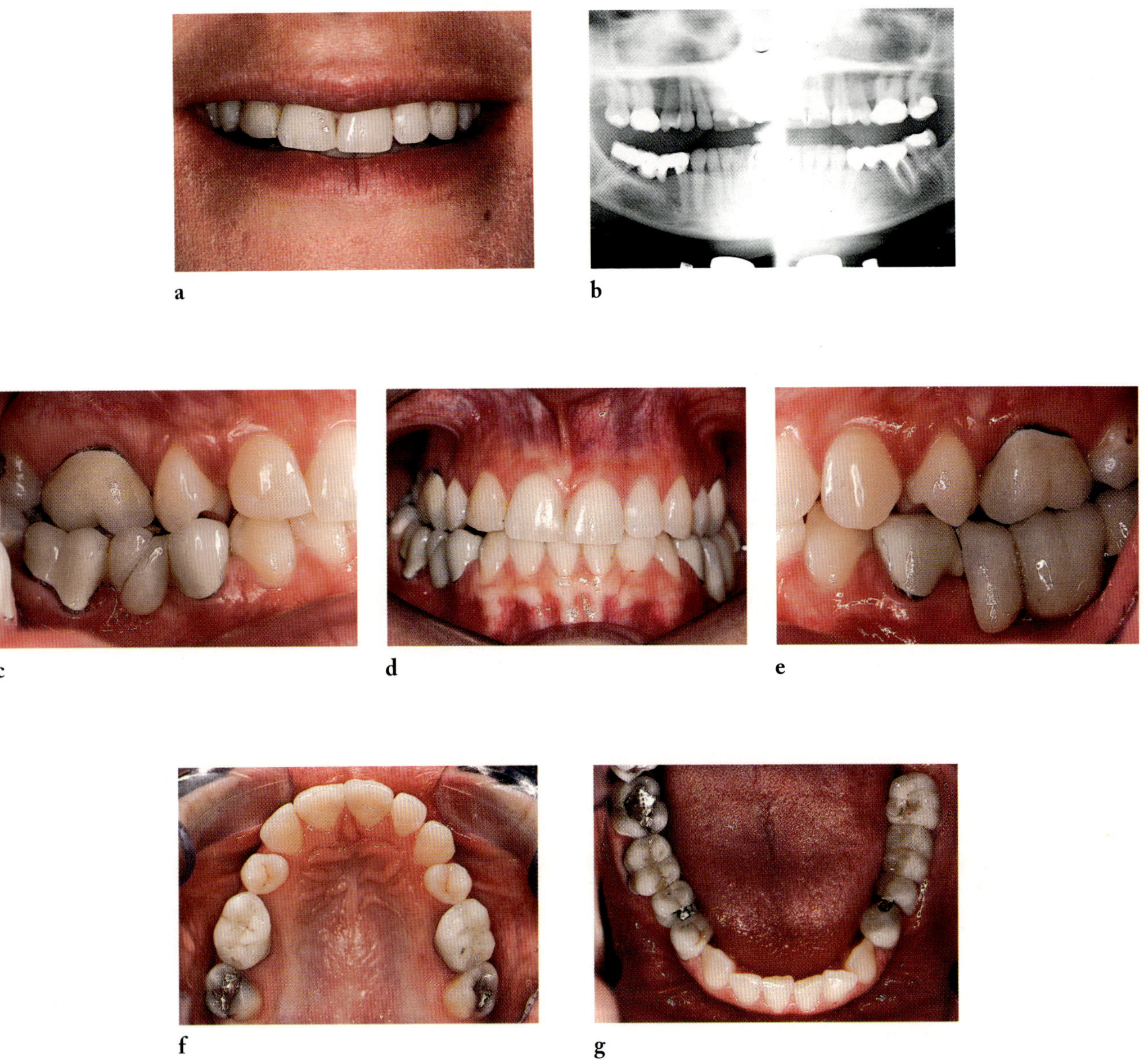

Fig 2-1 a to g Unidisciplinary therapy was recently performed on this patient to restoratively compensate for dental and skeletal malrelationships. Posttherapy photographs and panoramic radiographs illustrate the compromised results. The patient has a transverse skeletal discrepancy and is missing several teeth, with adjacent teeth tipped and shifted into the extraction sites. The restorative dentist worked extremely hard to produce this compromised result, never presenting the option of interdisciplinary therapy to optimally correct the underlying dental, periodontal, and skeletal problems. The shortcomings of performing unidisciplinary therapy in complicated cases such as this include that compromises made during therapy can lead to less-than-optimal esthetics and long-term problems with occlusion, stability, and periodontal health. To optimally correct this patient's dentofacial problems, interdisciplinary therapy would have to be performed, in addition to replacing all the restorations placed as part of unidisciplinary therapy. This patient was very distressed when she found, after her unidisciplinary therapy was already completed, that a more satisfactory interdisciplinary treatment option existed. The effect to the provider in this case is that he had to work much harder to get this compromised unidisciplinary result than if he would have done optimal restorative therapy as part of an interdisciplinary team. He is now left with an unhappy patient and a potential long-term dental and periodontal maintenance problem. Unidisciplinary therapy like this does occasionally have to be performed, but the patient (not the provider) should make an intelligent, informed decision about their best choice after they have been educated about their dentofacial problems and potential treatment options.

of knowledge of its potentially damaging side effects. This treatment philosophy frequently leads to an incomplete diagnosis and treatment plan, and thus to compromised results, which can make a subsequent optimal dentofacial correction more difficult and occasionally impossible.

These unidisciplinary trends in our profession have many different sources. First, many dental schools inadvertently train their students to think in this fashion. To compound these problems, the success of preventive dentistry has led many general dentists to feel compelled financially into performing procedures that were in the past performed primarily by specialists. The uninformed patient will frequently promote this unidisciplinary therapy with a desire to have all procedures done by one person in one location. Unidisciplinary therapy has many significant shortcomings that usually do not promote optimal care and frequently lead to problems.

Many specialists are also guilty of treating from a unidisciplinary point of view. Just as in a general or a restorative practice, this point of view can lead to incomplete diagnostics, improper treatment planning, and compromised results. The problem is that a single provider views and treats all problems in terms of his or her own specialized expertise and skills. This shortsightedness can lead to incomplete and less than optimal results, with secondary problems from esthetic, functional, stability, and periodontal standpoints (Fig 2-2).

In complex dentofacial problems, diagnostic procedures have to be comprehensive, encompassing all the different perspectives of the dental disciplines. Only through this process can the problems be analyzed from many specialized viewpoints which will lead to an unbiased overall evaluation. Only then can an ideal treatment plan be formulated that will lead to optimal dentofacial results.

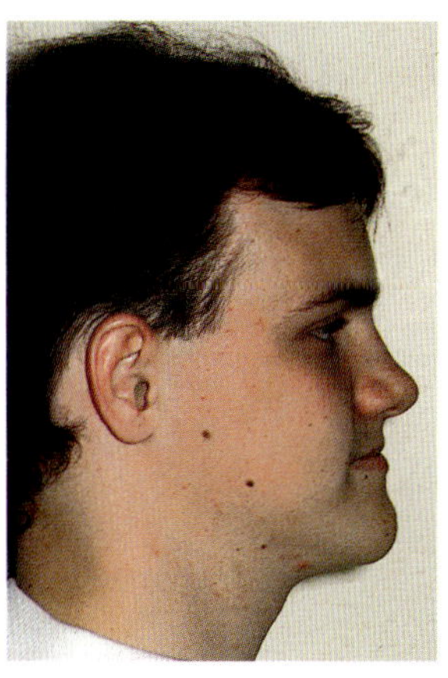

a

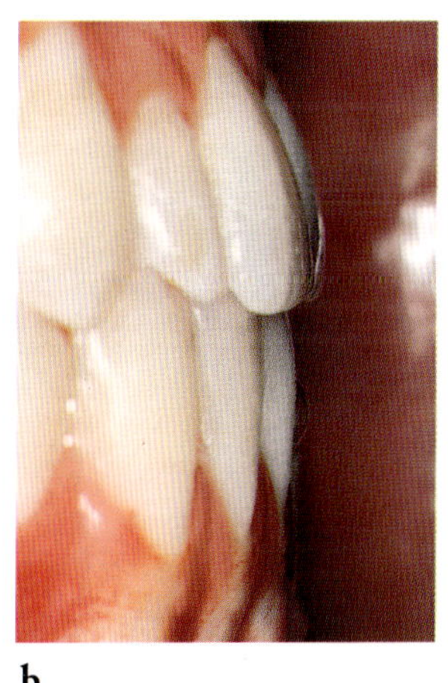

b

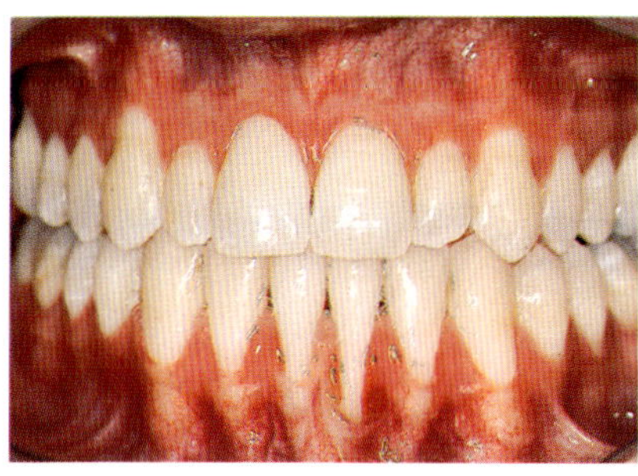

c

Fig 2-2 Unidisciplinary compromised therapy is frequently performed by all the various disciplines in dentistry.

a Postorthodontic lateral facial view of 16-year-old male with a prognathic mandible.

b, c Postorthodontic lateral and frontal intraoral views illustrating the relationships of the proclined maxillary incisors and retroclined and extruded mandibular incisors attained to compensate for Class III skeletal discrepancy. Note iatrogentric gingival stripping on the facial aspect of the mandibular incisors that developed as a negative side-effect of this compromised therapy. Both the orthodontist and the patient worked extremely hard to obtain these results, but neither the patient nor his family were presented with the option of orthognathic surgery until they went for a posttreatment second opinion. The various disciplines in dentistry should be used when necessary, or at the very least patients should be fully educated of their dentofacial problems and options, so that they can make intelligent decisions about their treatment needs.

Multidisciplinary Therapy

Multidisciplinary therapy is a major advancement over the unidisciplinary approach. Through multidisciplinary therapy, complex dentofacial problems are treated using the skill and knowledge of specialists in multiple disciplines. These highly specialized perspectives increase the level of care; however, the mulidisciplinary approach has several major shortcomings. Multidisciplinary therapy is characterized by insufficient communication and haphazard organization among the multidisciplinary team members. These problems rarely promote optimal care, and often lead to frustration and failures. One source of the problems associated with multidisciplinary therapy is that the individual team members frequently lack an understanding of where their therapy realistically fits into the comprehensive philosophy of treatment. Often, these team members do not have a general knowledge of the potential or limitations of the other disciplines' therapies and how they relate to their own therapies. Overall, these shortcomings lead to a multidisciplinary team whose members act as separate islands during diagnostics, treatment planning, and therapy with little or no communication or organization between providers.

Multidisciplinary therapy has many negative similarities with unidisciplinary therapy, even though several specialists may be involved. Each team member has "specialty bias" and tries to solve as many of the patient's dentofacial problems as possible through their own perspective, because they usually do not understand the potential of the other disciplines.

An example of multidisciplinary therapy at one of its simplest levels is an adult who has lost several permanent teeth, resulting in severe tipping of the adjacent teeth and making them unrestorable by conventional means. Out of necessity, a restorative dentist or prosthodontist may refer the patient to the orthodontist to have the abutment teeth uprighted in preparation for restorative therapy. There is characteristically little or no communication between the two providers, with the orthodontist frequently making all the decisions pertaining to the final positioning of the abutment teeth. The restorative team member, with an extensive knowledge in fixed prosthodontic procedures, is, however, the best-qualified team member to make these decisions. The frequent result of this type of therapy is an improved tooth relationship that may still have several significant shortcomings from a restorative standpoint, for which the restorative team member will have to make compromises in therapy. In this example, another discipline, such as periodontics, may be totally left out of the treatment because the other providers underestimated its importance; this is a frequent problem in multidisciplinary approaches. In reality, this neglected aspect may be as important as, if not more important than, the represented disciplines for obtaining optimal results.

An example of multidisciplinary therapy at its highest level is a patient with severe dental and dentofacial deformities requiring orthodontic, orthognathic surgical, and restorative correction (Fig 2-3). All too frequently, the orthodontic and surgical disciplines in dentistry diagnose, plan, and treat from their own very focused perspectives, often overlooking or disregarding other equally important perspectives. In this example, the orthodontic and surgical team members finished with an outstanding dentofacial esthetic improvement; however, they totally overlooked any input from a restorative dentist or prosthodontist (who are frequently the most underused members of a multidisciplinary team during diagnostic and treatment-planning procedures). As a result, this patient has undergone dramatic esthetic dentofacial improvements, but she is still a dental cripple, even though her initial chief concern was the lack of proper oral function. In this example, the multidisciplinary team appears to have disregarded their original role as oral health professionals. Through proper planning of the prosthodontic problems and the inclusion of restorative expertise, the providers could have performed the same procedures, with minimal alterations, and yielded a result with optimal dental restorative results, in addition to the outstanding esthetic facial improvement. Due to the lack of proper planning, this patient is now in need of another surgical procedure to allow an acceptable dental reconstruction. The need for a dental team to properly plan treatment and cooperate with one another is becoming increasingly more important as the different disciplines become more advanced and sophisticated; this is especially true with the addition of osseointegrated implants as viable and predictable treatment options (Fig 2-4).

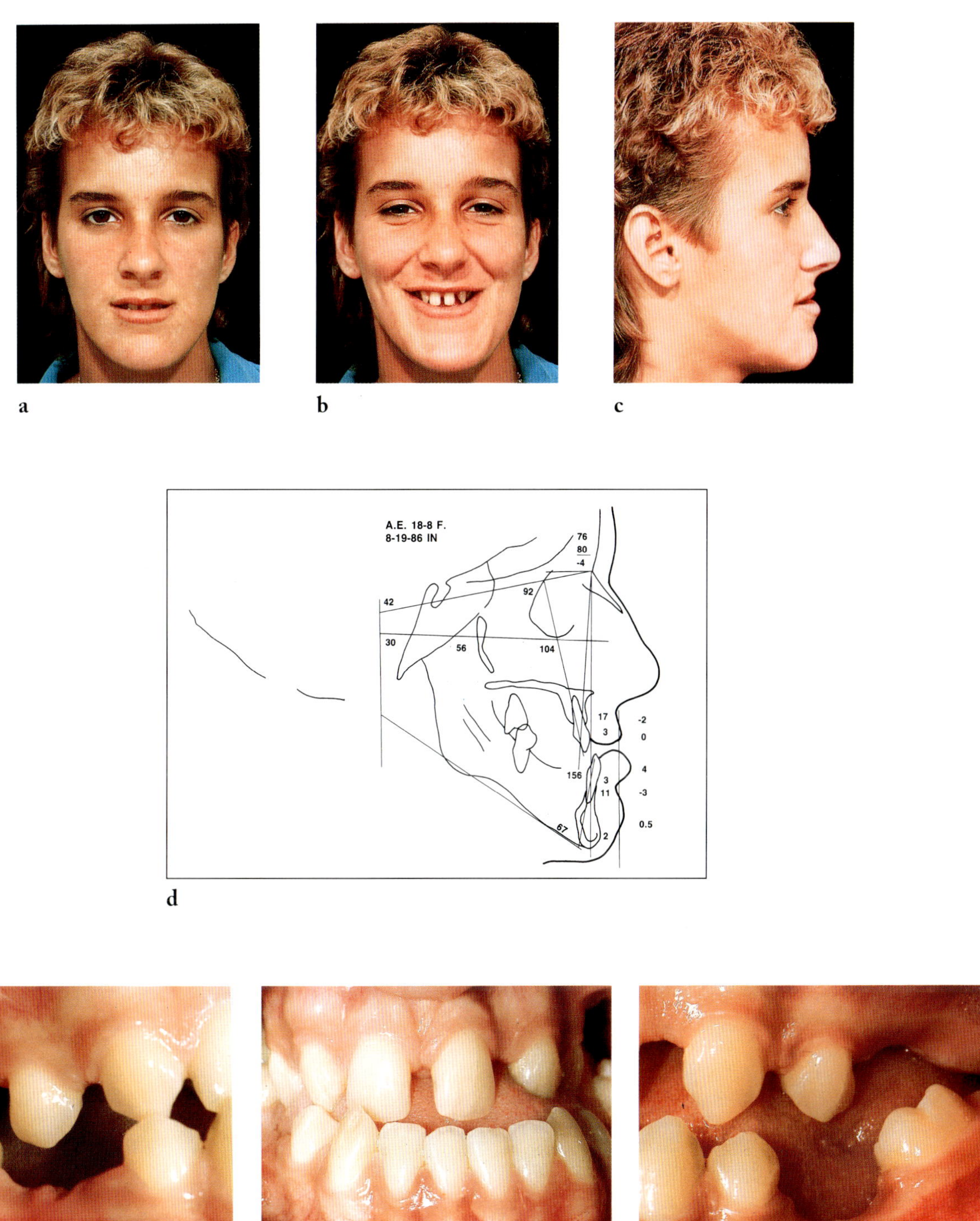

Fig 2-3 Multidisciplinary therapy, with its inherent shortsightedness and lack of proper communication in diagnostic, treatment-planning, and definitive-therapy procedures, were performed on this 18-year-old female.

a to c Initial facial appearance illustrating asymmetries and concave profile.

d Initial cephalometric analysis showing a maxillary deficiency in conjunction with a prognathic mandible.

e to g Initial intraoral appearance showing a partial anodontia and a complete crossbite from narrow maxilla and broad mandible.

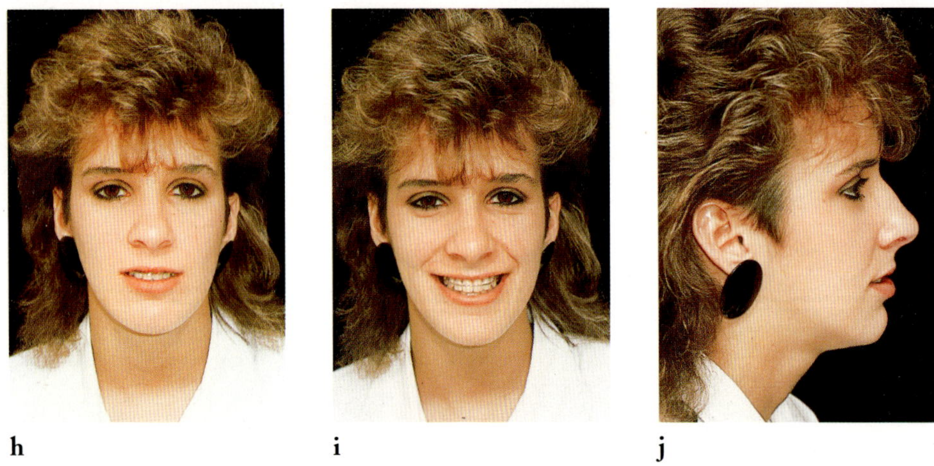

h i j

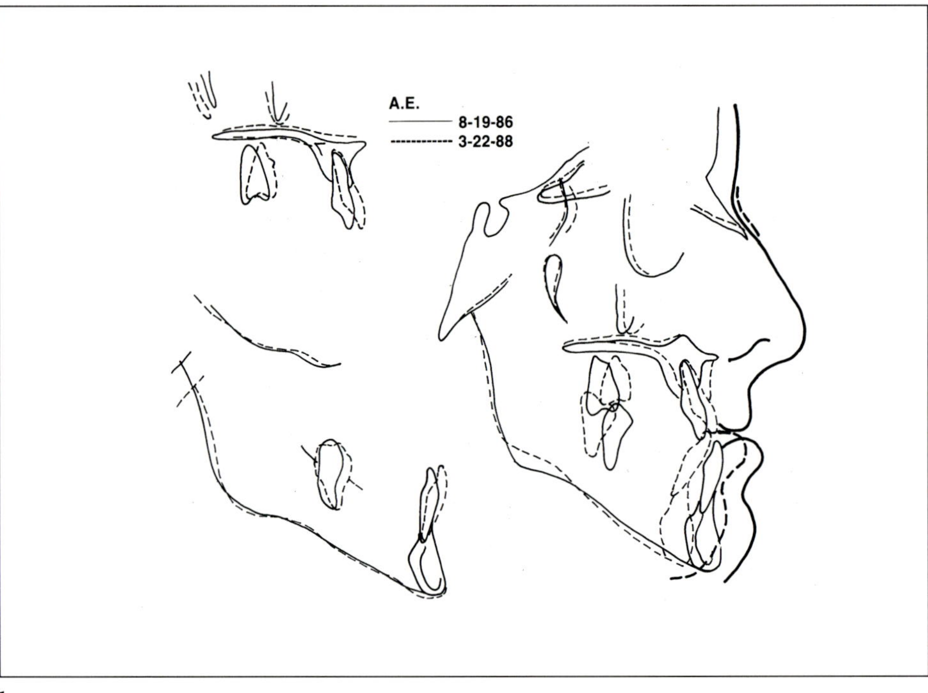

k

Fig 2-3 (continued)

h to j Postorthodontic and postoperative facial result, illustrating significant enhancement of facial harmony. Orthognathic surgical procedures consisted of a three-piece maxilla to expand and advance, and an asymmetrical mandibular setback.

k Cephalometric superimposition depicting orthodontic and surgical changes.

l to n Postorthodontic and postoperative dentoalveolar result with remaining transverse and vertical discrepancies. Another major surgical procedure is indicated on the maxillary arch to enable construction of an acceptable dental prosthesis. With proper interdisciplinary communication and planning, the providers could have made minimal alterations in the original procedures they performed and finished with optimal dental restorative results, in addition to the outstanding esthetic facial improvement. This patient is still severely dentally impaired, even though her initial chief concern was the lack of proper oral function.

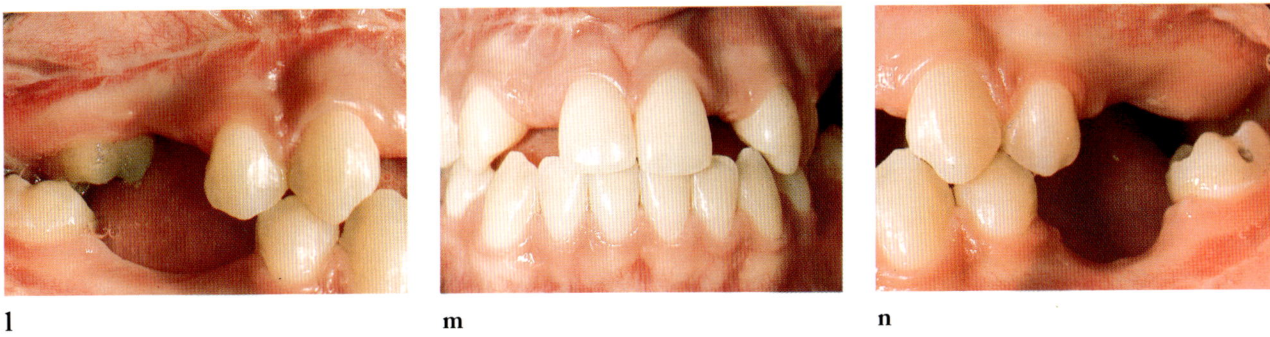

l m n

Fig 2-3 (continued)

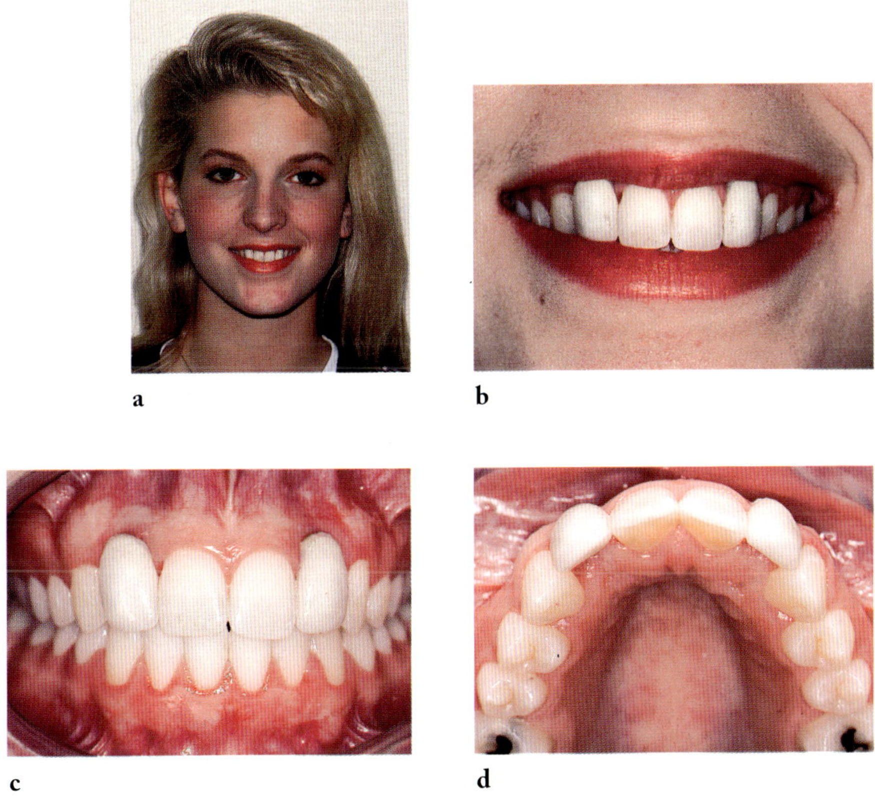

a b c d

Fig 2-4 Multidisciplinary implant therapy. Lack of proper team coordination and communication can be especially damaging when utilizing dental implants.

a, b Postoperative smiling views of a 15-year-old female who received single-tooth dental implants to replace congenitally missing maxillary lateral incisors. Note the disruption of proper harmony and proportionality of the dentition and gingiva caused by the malpositioned implants and implant prosthetics.

c, d Postoperative intraoral views further illustrating poor implant placement and subsequent compromised prosthetic results. The patient saw the implant surgeon first, who immediately placed the endosseous implants without consulting the restorative dentist and/or properly planning the implant placement. The anatomy of the edentulous areas in this case would have been compatible with an ideal implant position. This case could have had ideal results if the implant placement would have been properly planned by the appropriate interdisciplinary team members utilizing the various adjunctive diagnostic procedures available in conjunction with preparatory restorative-type IV therapy. Lack of proper planning in this example led to an embarrassing failure that will be extremely difficult to correct.

Interdisciplinary Therapy

The ultimate utilization of the expertise and skills in the various dental disciplines is called *interdisciplinary dentofacial therapy* (IDT). Its hallmark is the combination of regimental diagnostic, treatment-planning, and therapeutic procedures with extensive communication between the team members. The terms *interdisciplinary* and *multidisciplinary* are similar in that they both involve two or more different disciplines; however, the prefix "inter" signifies working "between" the different disciplines, instead of the disciplines acting as separate entities. Interdisciplinary therapy permits the synergism of each different discipline's specialized expertise and skills into a comprehensive therapy that consistently delivers optimal patient care.

Advantages of an Interdisciplinary Approach

The most obvious advantage of IDT is the consistent attainment of optimal results when treating patients with complex and unique dentofacial problems. Described below are several less-obvious advantages of an interdisciplinary approach over a unidisciplinary or multidisciplinary approach. When combined, these advantages create an environment which is conducive to optimal results. The Case Summary presented with Fig 2-5 exemplifies all these advantages of interdisciplinary dentofacial therapy.

Idealize and Simplify Therapy

A frequent misconception of interdisciplinary therapy is that it makes the individual team member's treatment more complex. In reality, it actually simplifies this treatment by idealizing it. A good example of this is the uprighting of a tipped molar to allow placement of an ideal fixed partial denture. The resulting restorative procedures will be simplified compared to the unidisciplinary approach of utilizing a precision attachment to compensate for the nonparallel abutment teeth. The utilization of different disciplines frequently allows each discipline the luxury of idealizing their therapy and, as a result, simplifying their individual procedures and, of course, improving patient care.

Improve Prognosis

Through the idealization of the different therapies, an interdisciplinary approach improves the overall treatment prognosis. In the previous example, the uprighting of the abutment teeth allowed for optimal tooth preparation, retention, oral hygiene, and distribution of occlusal forces. The result is a better endodontic, periodontic, and restorative prognosis.

Turn Problems into Advantages

Interdisciplinary treatment planning allows the formulation of creative solutions to complex dentofacial problems. Some of these problems, when properly analyzed by the interdisciplinary team, can often be turned into advantages to help solve other more complex problems. If these problems were dealt with through unidisciplinary or multidisciplinary therapy, chances are greater that the creative solutions would not be found and treatment would involve unnecessary compromise. In other words, interdisciplinary therapy can minimize the disadvantages and maximize the advantages of each discipline's therapies.

Prevent Unnecessary Procedures

Another common misconception among unidisciplinary and multidisciplinary providers is the feeling that the involvement of more providers will lead to unnecessary procedures being performed. However, the opposite is true. The more detailed and thorough the diagnostic and treatment-planning procedures are, the more creative and efficient the actual therapy will be. As a result, unnecessary treatment can be eliminated. In some cases, even orthognathic surgical procedures that were initially thought necessary may be deemed as overtreatment through the formulation of creative solutions utilizing the various disciplines.

Shorten Treatment Time

Poor communication during multidisciplinary therapy often leads to extended treatment time. When a team member does not fully understand his or her therapy's relationship with the other team members' therapy, he or she may actually overtreat to unnecessary ideals. Through proper communication and enhanced understanding in interdisciplinary therapy, compromises can frequently be made among the different providers' therapies to shorten the overall treatment time without negatively affecting the overall results. This is called *interdisciplinary compromise* and is a positive aspect of IDT. For example, when uprighting a tipped and rotated molar for a fixed partial denture, it may be possible to significantly shorten treatment time by uprighting the tooth without correcting the rotation. However, this should only be attempted if the restorative dentist and/or periodontist evaluated the supporting structures and determined that the restoration of the molar in that relationship would not compromise periodontal health.

With an interdisciplinary approach, the individual team members' therapies frequently overlap, so that time is not wasted waiting for each procedure to be completed before starting the next. Proper communication and organization between team members leads to consistent, optimal treatment results in the most efficient manner possible.

Enhance Individual Team Members' Results

Through the optimal utilization of the different disciplines, interdisciplinary therapy frequently lets the individual providers idealize their specific aspects of treatment, thus enhancing each provider's results. The compounding effect of the successive therapies lets each provider build upon and enhance the previous provider's result. The net effect is the attainment of optimal results that can make each individual provider's results many times more successful.

Enhance Professional Relationships

The open communication associated with IDT will often overcome the discontentment commonly found between multidisciplinary providers. This open communication encourages each interdisciplinary provider to more fully understand the limitations of the other team members' therapy. Thus, it builds appreciation for the results other team members attain, while reducing unrealistic expectations and disappointment. Also, IDT lets each team member provide their specialized expertise throughout all stages of therapy. This prevents the team member currently treating the patient from making a less-than-ideal treatment decision in an area other than his or her specialty, which might negatively affect another provider's therapy. In the tipped-molar example, the orthodontist should educate the restorative dentist as to the limitations of uprighting the molar, and the restorative dentist should give advice as to the best relationship of the abutment teeth. Interdisciplinary therapy is built on a philosophy of teamwork, in which all members helps one another to best help the patient. This cooperative and educational process strengthens professional relationships, and promotes better teamwork and results in the future.

Increase Patient and Doctor Satisfaction

Through the consistent attainment of optimal results, IDT can lead to the highest levels of patient and provider satisfaction in the therapies performed. In this fashion, interdisciplinary therapy can provide two important assets to a professional practice. First, through the high levels of provider satisfaction, the individual team members will be rewarded psychologically in their role as health professionals, thereby promoting their growth in that role. Second, the attainment of optimal results usually leads to high patient satisfaction, which is necessary for the growth of a provider's practice. IDT can provide the most effective and professional means for internal marketing and promoting a practice.

Case Summary

Patient: H.M. was a 15-year-old white female who presented for orthodontic therapy with poor self image due to an unattractive smile.

Interdisciplinary Problem List

Chief Concern(s)/Motivation/Expectation

- "My teeth are small and far apart."
- Self-motivated for treatment
- Expects a prettier smile

History

- 15-year-old white female
- Poor self-image due to unattractive smile
- Unremarkable medical, temporomandibular, and dental histories

Facial/Skeletal

- Concave profile with insufficient lip support and strong chin button
- Short upper lip
- Excessive incisor exposure with lips at rest
- Excessive gingival display during smile
- Class I skeletal relationship with bimaxillary dentoalveolar retrusion
- Maxillary and mandibular dentoalveolar extrusion of anterior segments

Temporomandibular

- Unremarkable

Occlusion

- Class I dental malrelationship
- Excessive anterior vertical overlap and insufficient anterior horizontal overlap
- Anterior crossbite 12, 32, and 53
- Unstable and traumatic interincisal relationship
- Initial centric contact is on left second molar and mandible shifts 1.5 mm anteriorly into maximum intercuspation position
- Traumatic functional occlusion with severe working and balancing interferences
- No anterior guidance

Periodontal

- Excessive free and attached gingival tissues throughout maxillary arch
- Minimal attached gingival tissues in mandibular anterior region

Dental/Implant

- Generalized microdontia with excess archlength and spacing in both arches
- Peg lateral incisors teeth 12 and 22
- Retroclined maxillary and mandibular incisors
- Retained maxillary primary canines with severe wear
- Defective restoration tooth 31
- Impacted maxillary canines and maxillary right second molar

Diagnosis

- Class I skeletal and dental relationship with bimaxillary dentoalveolar retrusion, vertical maxillary excess and microdontia

Treatment Plan

Interdisciplinary Dentofacial Therapy

- Evaluate for and arrest active carious and periodontal lesions
- Preparatory periodontal surgery to expose impacted teeth 13, 17, and 23
- Comprehensive non-extraction orthodontic therapy
    - Full-mouth orthodontic appliances including second molars
    - Transpalatal arch for transverse support
    - Maxillary intrusion arch to intrude maxillary anteriors and correct excessive anterior vertical overlap
    - Extrude impacted canines
    - Retain primary canines to maintain esthetics until impacted canines are ready to be aligned in arch
    - Level and align arches
    - Phase I periodontal plastic surgery to remove redundant gingival tissues in maxillary arch
    - Procline maxillary and mandibular anteriors to enhance lip support and establish a more stable and functional interincisal relationship
    - Space maxillary and mandibular anteriors to develop potential for proper anterior coupling and allow for most esthetic restorations
    - Gnathologically finish occlusion in Class I molar relationship
    - Phase II periodontal plastic surgery to refine gingival contours
    - Retain dental relationships with maxillary and mandibular bonded lingual retainers
- Restorative procedures
    - Bonded ceramic restorations teeth 11, 12, 13, 21, 22, 23, 31, 32, 33, 41, 42, and 43
- Monitor deficient attached gingival tissue in mandibular anterior region and perform free gingival grafts if necessary
- Maintain regular dental maintenance and hygiene schedule throughout therapy and after completion

Treatment Time

Estimated: 24 to 30 months
Actual: 19½ months

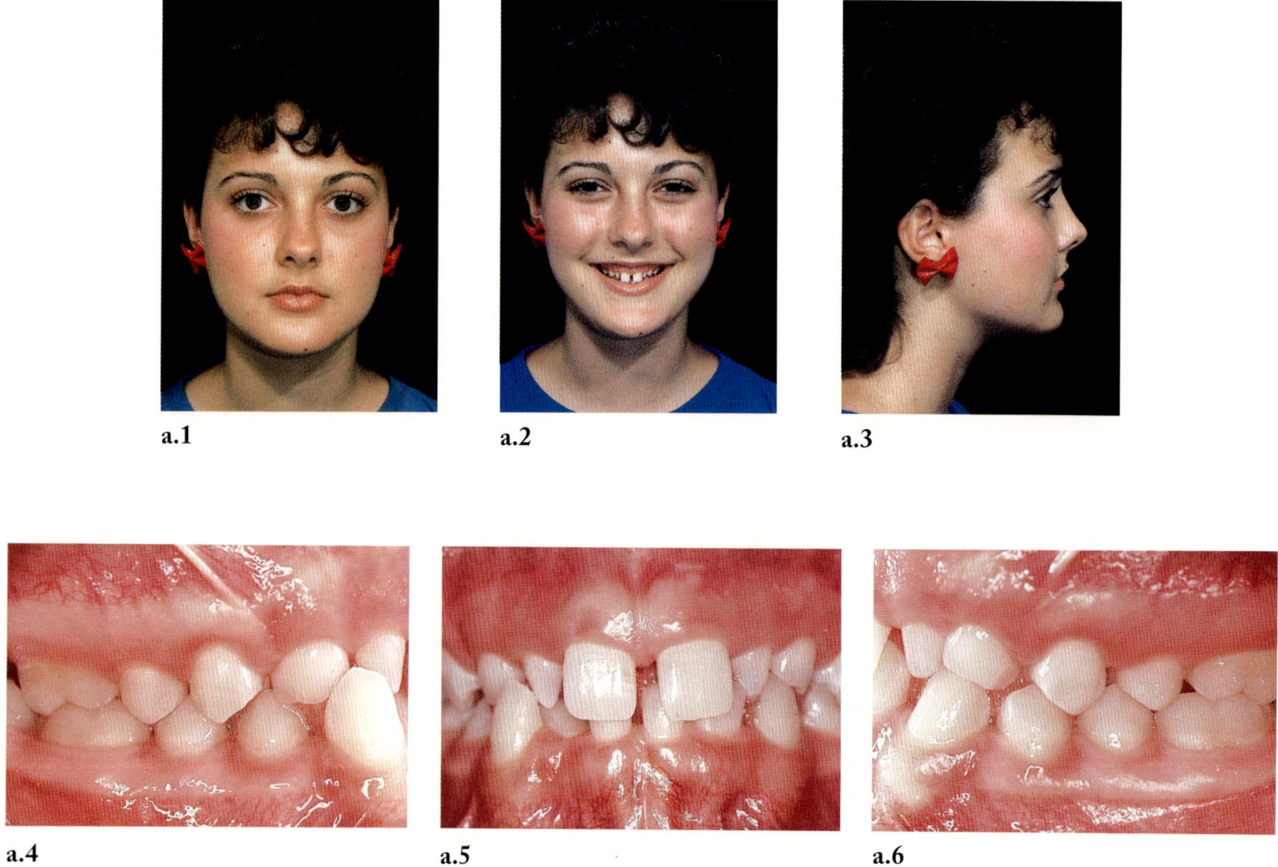

Fig 2-5 This case is presented in detail to introduce the concept of interdisciplinary dentofacial therapy. It will be referred back to throughout this text.

a Pretreatment records (refer to problem list and history for description).

a.1 to a.3 Facial views.

a.4 to a.6 Intraoral views.

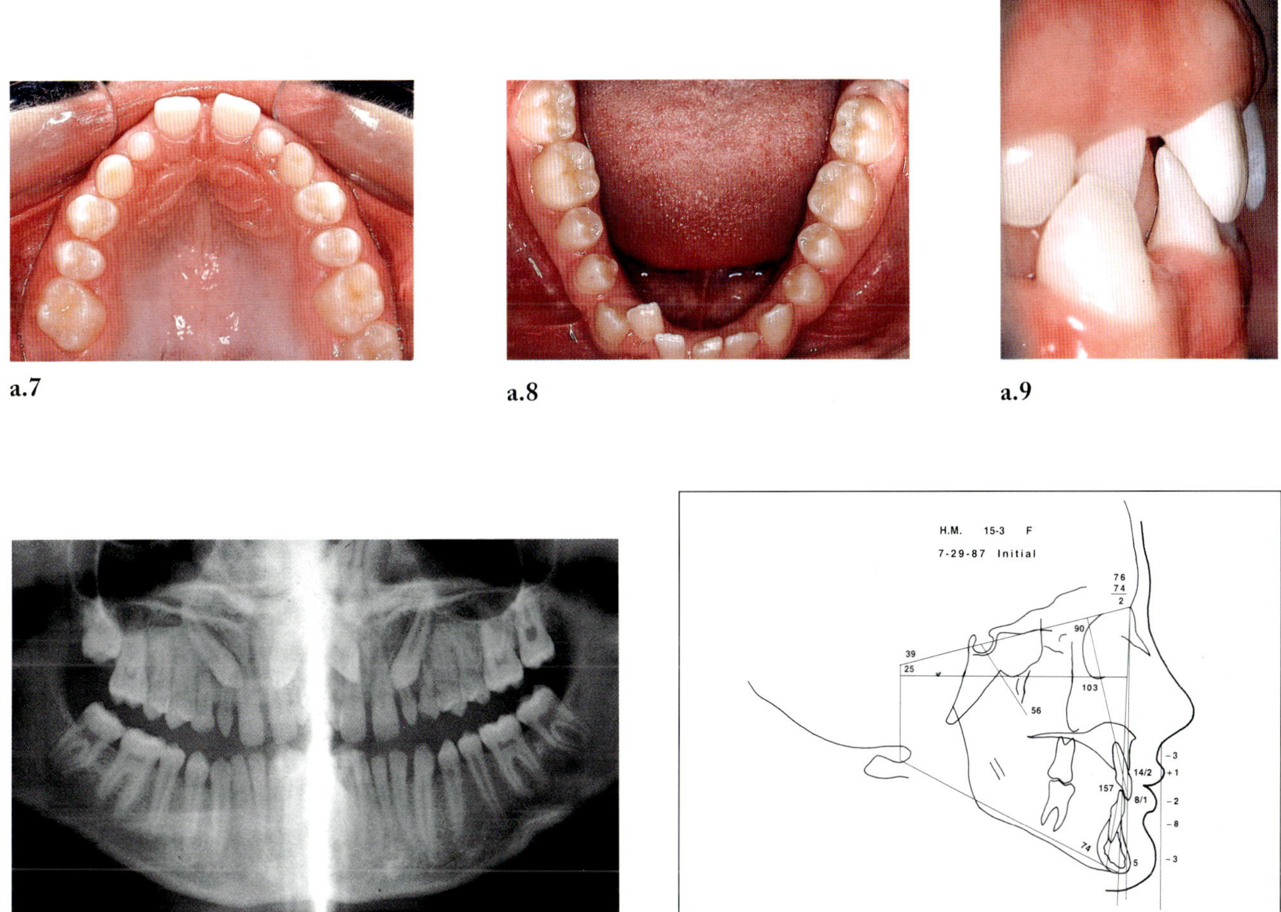

a.7 a.8 a.9

a.10 b

Fig 2-5 (continued)

a.7 to a.9 Intraoral views.

a.10 Panoramic radiograph.

b Pretreatment cephalometric analysis illustrating normal relationships with the exception of bimaxillary dentoalveolar retrusion with insufficient lip support.

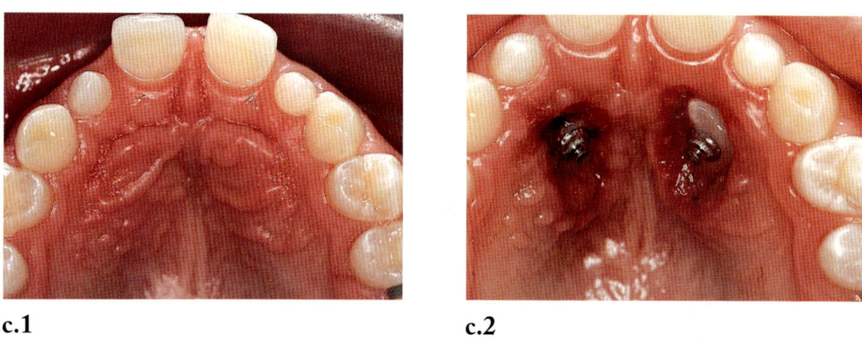

c.1 c.2

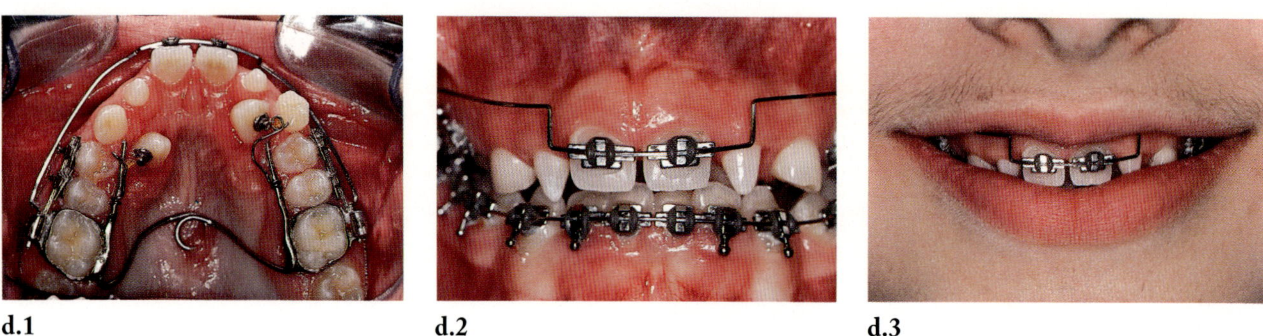

d.1 d.2 d.3

Fig 2-5 (continued)

c Preparatory dentoalveolar surgical therapy to uncover palatally impacted maxillary canines.

c.1 Preoperative occlusal view. Note bulging areas in anterior palate.

c.2 Postoperative occlusal view with orthodontic buttons bonded in place.

d Definitive orthodontic therapy.

d.1 to d.3 Progress photographs made 6 months into definitive orthodontic therapy. Note position of previously impacted maxillary canines and the amount of intrusion of the maxillary central incisors. Creative treatment planning allowed the extrusive forces of the canines to counteract the intrusive forces of the central incisors, thus augmenting the results of each of the individual therapies. The maxillary peg lateral incisors were not included in therapy at this point, minimizing the stresses to their thin roots in an attempt to reduce the possibility of root resorption. The retained maxillary primary canines will be left in place to maintain esthetics until the previously impacted permanent canines are ready to replace them.

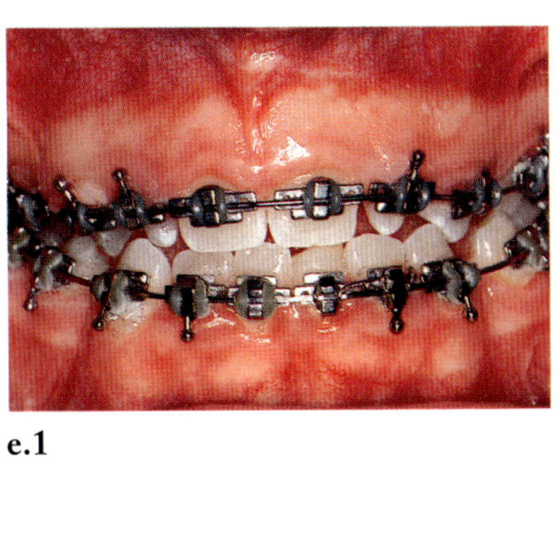

e.1

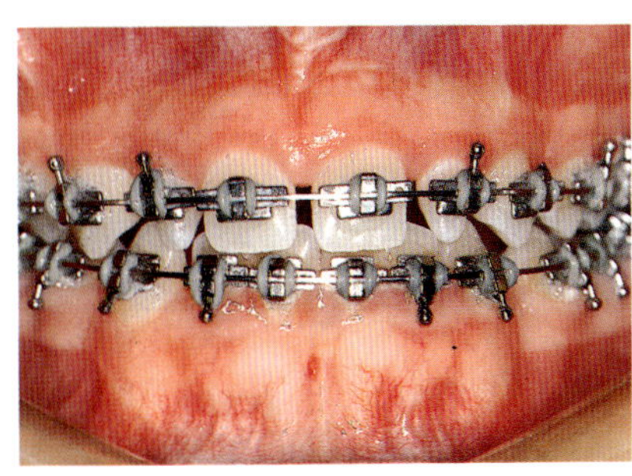

e.2

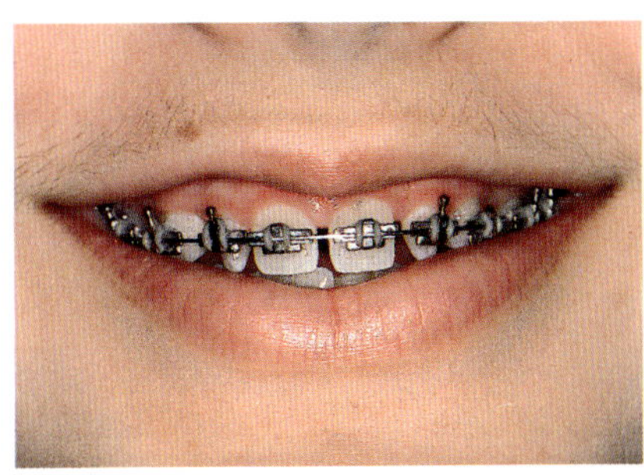

f.1

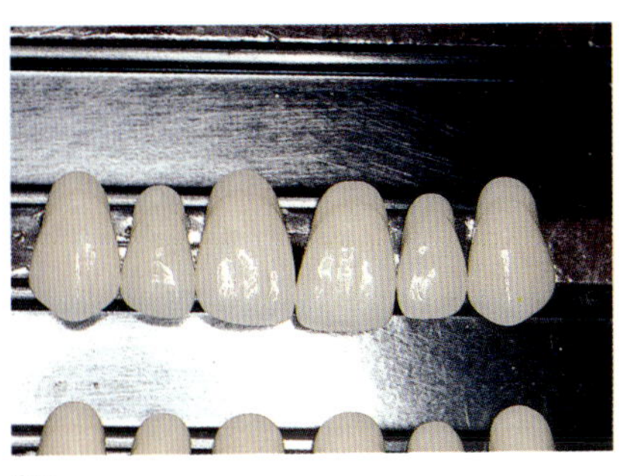

f.2

Fig 2-5 (continued)

e Definitive periodontal therapy.

e.1 Preoperative view 12 months into definitive orthodontic therapy. Note hyperplastic and redundant gingival tissues in maxillary arch after incisor intrusion had been completed.

e.2 Postoperative view 6 weeks after periodontal plastic surgery was performed to reduce gingival tissues in maxillary arch. This procedure was necessary to facilitate the remaining orthodontic therapy and further reduce the patient's "gummy smile." The alignment of the periodontal tissues will be finalized in a Phase II periodontal surgery, after the active tooth movement has been completed.

f Preparatory restorative-type II therapy.

f.1 Smiling view 13 months into definitive orthodontic therapy. Orthodontist is now ready to begin final positioning of the anterior teeth for definitive restorative procedures.

f.2 Restorative member selects a denture tooth mold that closely represents the ideal tooth size and form of the future restorations. This mold gives the orthodontist a three-dimensional object to measure while interproximally and interincisally positioning the anterior teeth to help ensure that optimal restorative procedures can be performed later in definitive therapy.

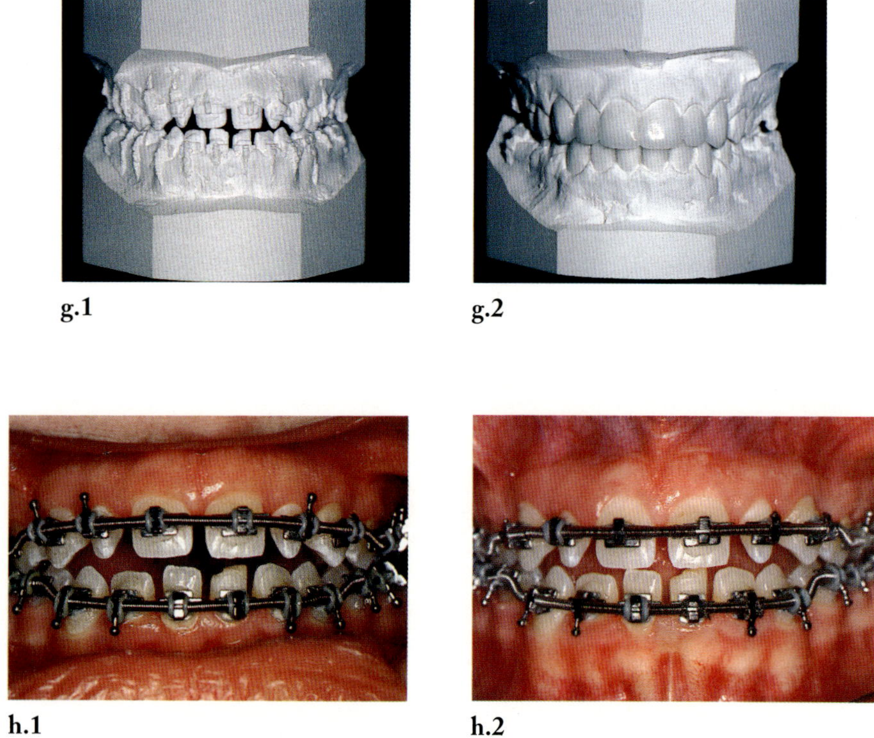

g.1 g.2

h.1 h.2

Fig 2-5 (continued)

g.1 Progress dental casts were made 15 months into definitive orthodontic therapy.

g.2 Orthodontic brackets were removed from the progress dental casts and a diagnostic waxup was performed. This gave the orthodontist the information needed to perform the final prerestorative positioning of the maxillary and mandibular anterior teeth. It also gave the periodontist the optimal dimensions of the second gingival recontouring procedures.

h Definitive periodontal therapy. Phase II periodontal plastic surgery to perfect gingival relationships in the anterior maxilla.

h.1 Preoperative view 16 months into definitive orthodontic therapy.

h.2 Postoperative view 6 weeks after gingival recontouring procedures were performed. If possible, periodontal plastic surgery procedures such as this should be performed after active tooth movement is completed, but prior to orthodontic appliance removal. This will aid in the retention of the new tooth positions by allowing some reorganization of the periodontal ligaments to the new positions.

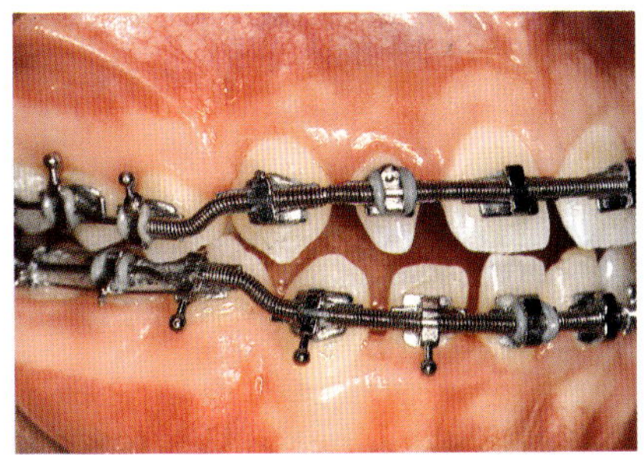
i.1

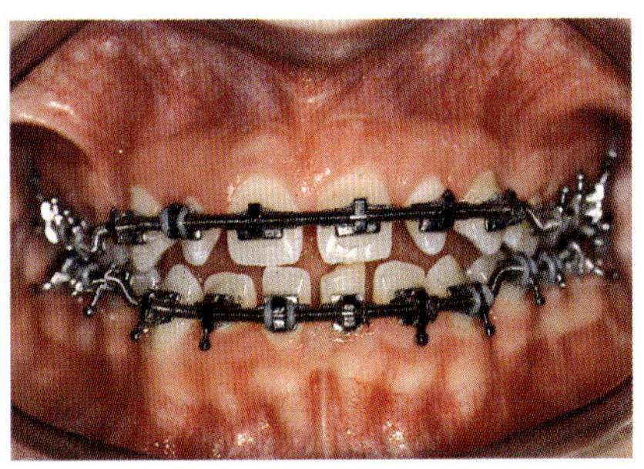
i.2

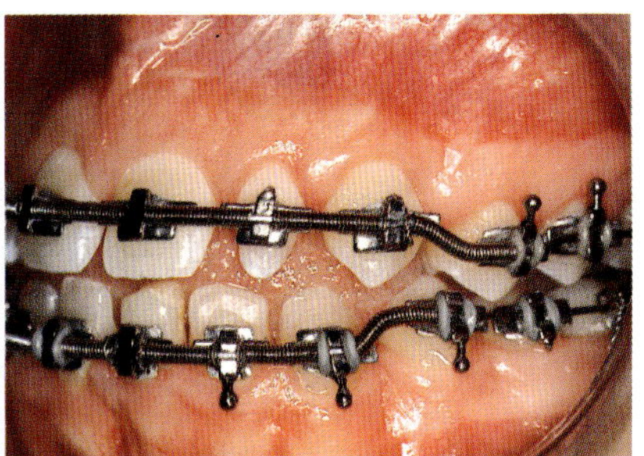
i.3

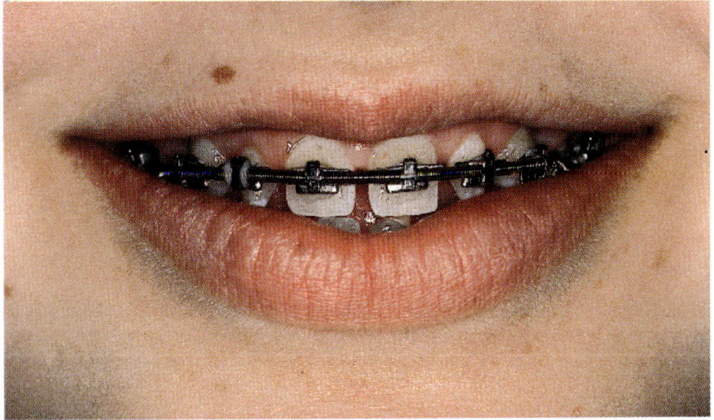
i.4

Fig 2-5 (continued)

i Progress photographs 17 months into definitive orthodontic therapy.

i.1 to i.3 Intraoral views illustrating optimal prerestorative relationships of anterior dentition. Note interproximal and interincisal spacing to allow placement of ideally sized restorations. The posterior occlusion is in an ideal Class I dental relationship.

i.4 Smiling view of final orthodontic and periodontal plastic surgery results, illustrating the amount of reduction of the patient's preoperative excessive gingival exposure.

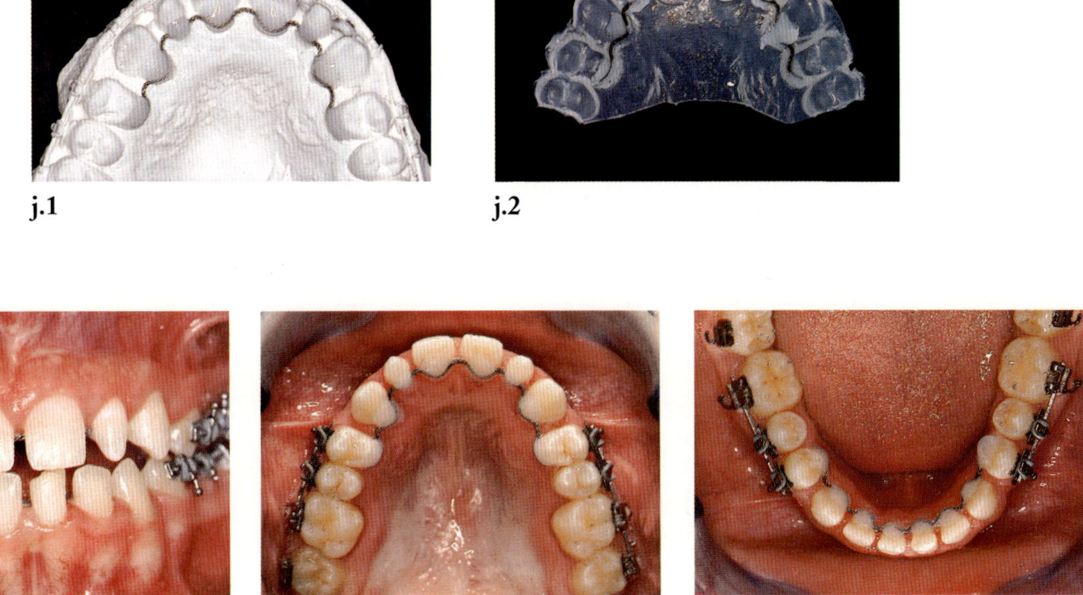

j.1 j.2

j.3 j.4 j.5

Fig 2-5 (continued)

j.1, j.2 Baylor indirect light-cured bonded retainers were constructed for the maxillary and mandibular arches. These retainers were constructed on a dental cast and a transfer tray was made to ideally position the retainer in the mouth.

j.3 to j.5 The indirect lingual retainers were bonded to place and the anterior orthodontic appliances were removed. These retainers will be used to maintain the new dental relationships during and after the definitive restorative therapy. The use of an indirect technique gives the operator greater control and precision during placement, in addition to reducing chair time. Creative retention procedures such as this frequently have to be performed during interdisciplinary dentofacial therapy. Traditional orthodontic retention appliances would probably have been inadequate in this case, and may have interfered with definitive restorative therapy.

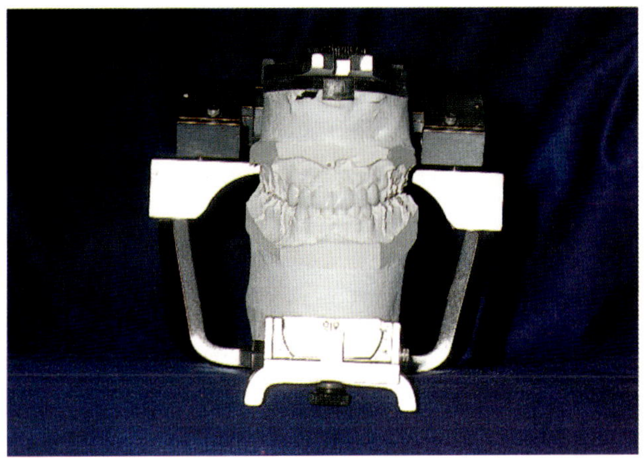
k

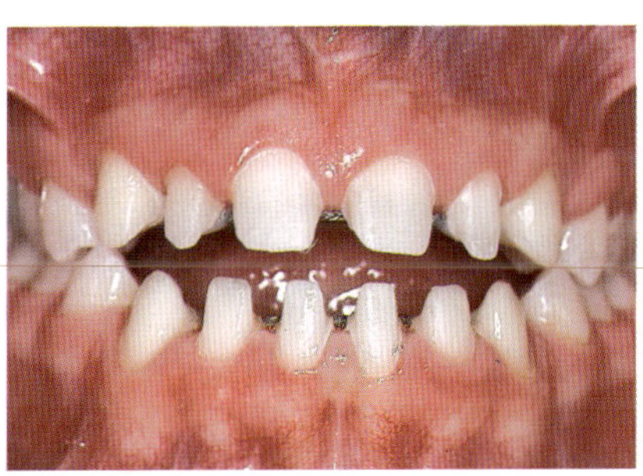
l.1

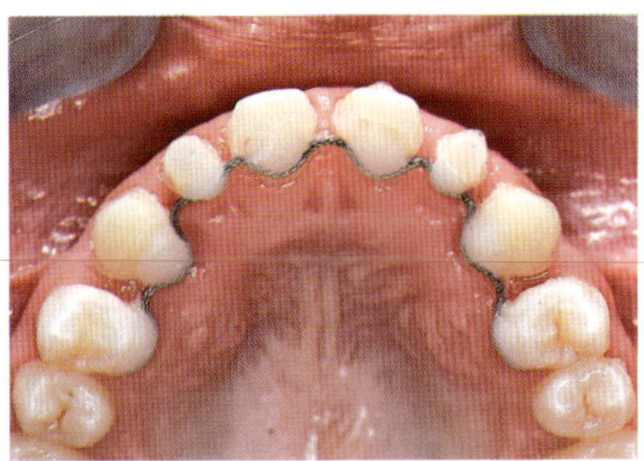
l.2

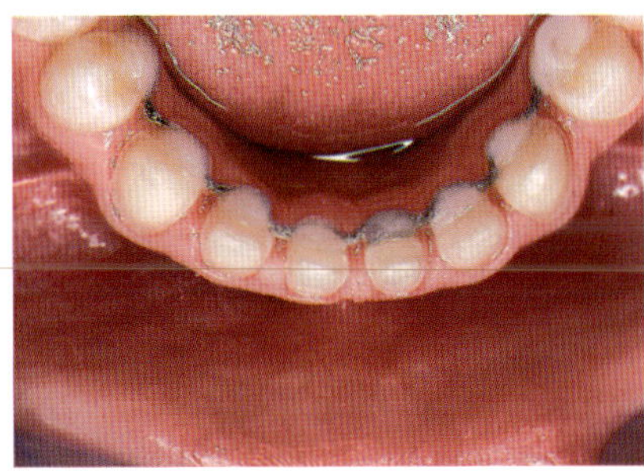
l.3

Fig 2-5 (continued)

k Another diagnostic waxup was performed as an adjunctive diagnostic procedure for the final planning of the bonded porcelain crowns to be placed during definitive restorative therapy. This diagnostic waxup was also used to construct a template for the construction of the provisional restorations.

l Definitive restorative therapy.

l.1 to l.3 Final tooth preparations for all-porcelain restorations. A reverse 7/8s intraenamel preparation was performed which allowed the lingual retainer to be maintained. The gingival margins of the restorations were placed at or above the level of the free gingival margin to promote long-term periodontal health and esthetics.

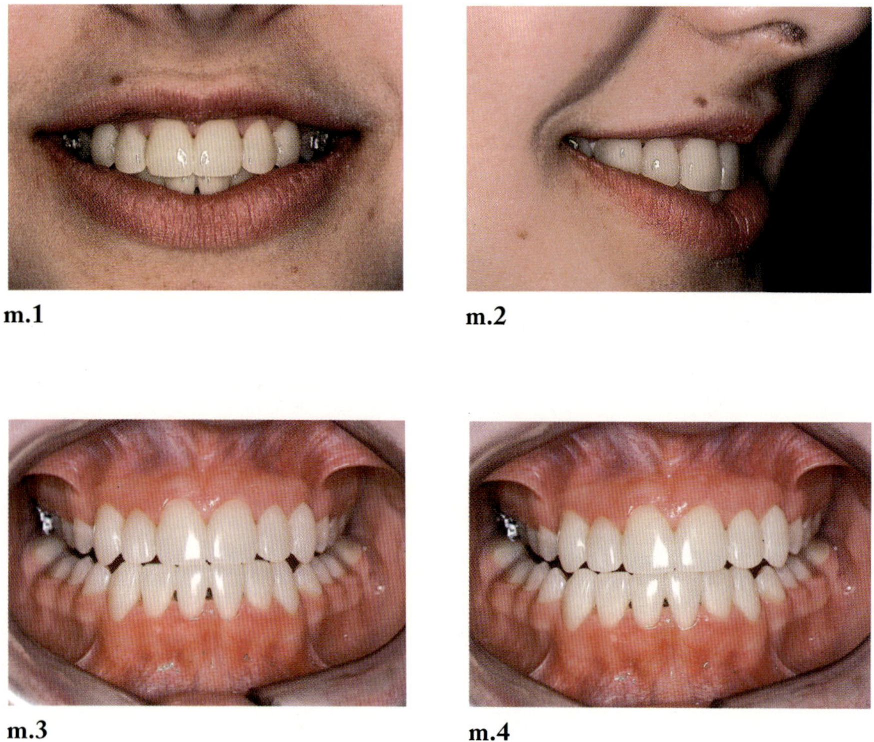

Fig 2-5 (continued)

m Provisional restorations.

m.1, m.2 Frontal and lateral smiling views of provisional restorations, illustrating how they were customized to promote optimal dentofacial esthetics.

m.3, m.4 These provisional restorations were constructed in centric relation. Optimal functional relationships were developed in protrusive *(m.3)* and lateral *(m.4)*excursive movements. Provisional restorations such as these are not only therapeutic but also diagnostic, and were used to precisely communicate the desired size, form, and functional relationships of teeth to the laboratory technician. These restorations also gave the patient a tremendous boost during dentofacial therapy by giving her a preview of the final dental appearance and function. It also gave the patient a chance to communicate her feelings about the planned dental restorations.

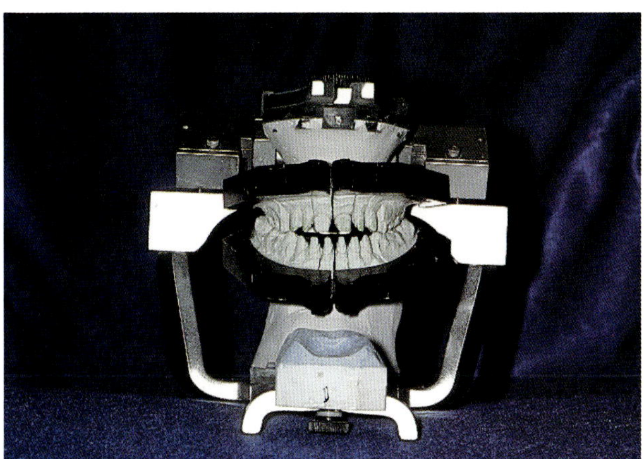

n.1

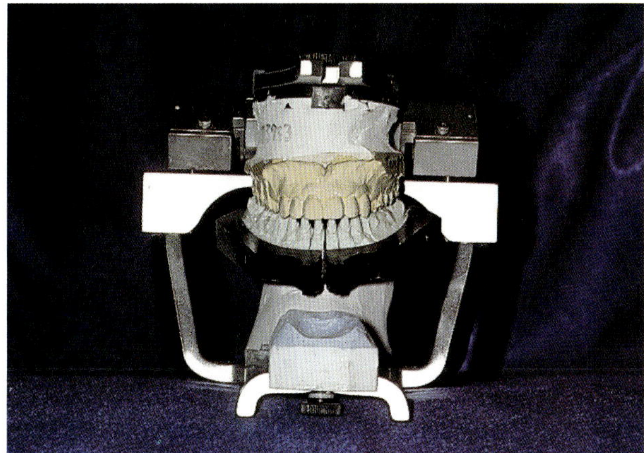

n.2

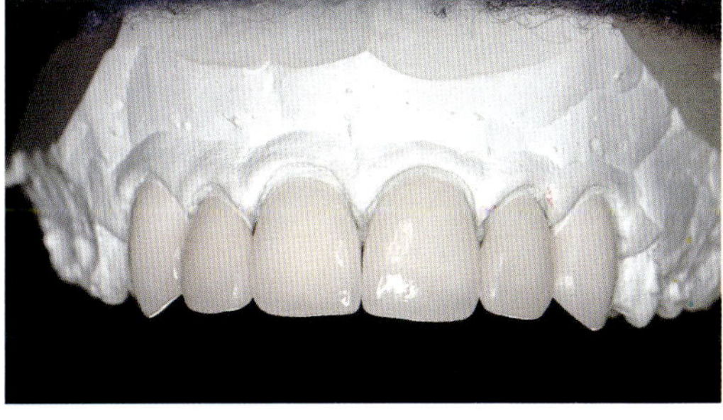

o

Fig 2-5 (continued)

n Restorative laboratory procedures.

n.1 The maxillary and mandibular working casts were mounted in a semiadjustable articulator using a face-bow transfer and an accurate centric relation record.

n.2 The restorative dentist accurately communicated the desired dental size, form, and functional relationships to the laboratory technician by mounting accurate study casts of the provisional restorations to the working casts of the prepared teeth. Thus, the laboratory technician did not have to guess the desired relationships of the dental restorations.

o Final restorations seated on a solid cast of the prepared maxillary teeth. Note the accuracy of the margins on these all-porcelain restorations.

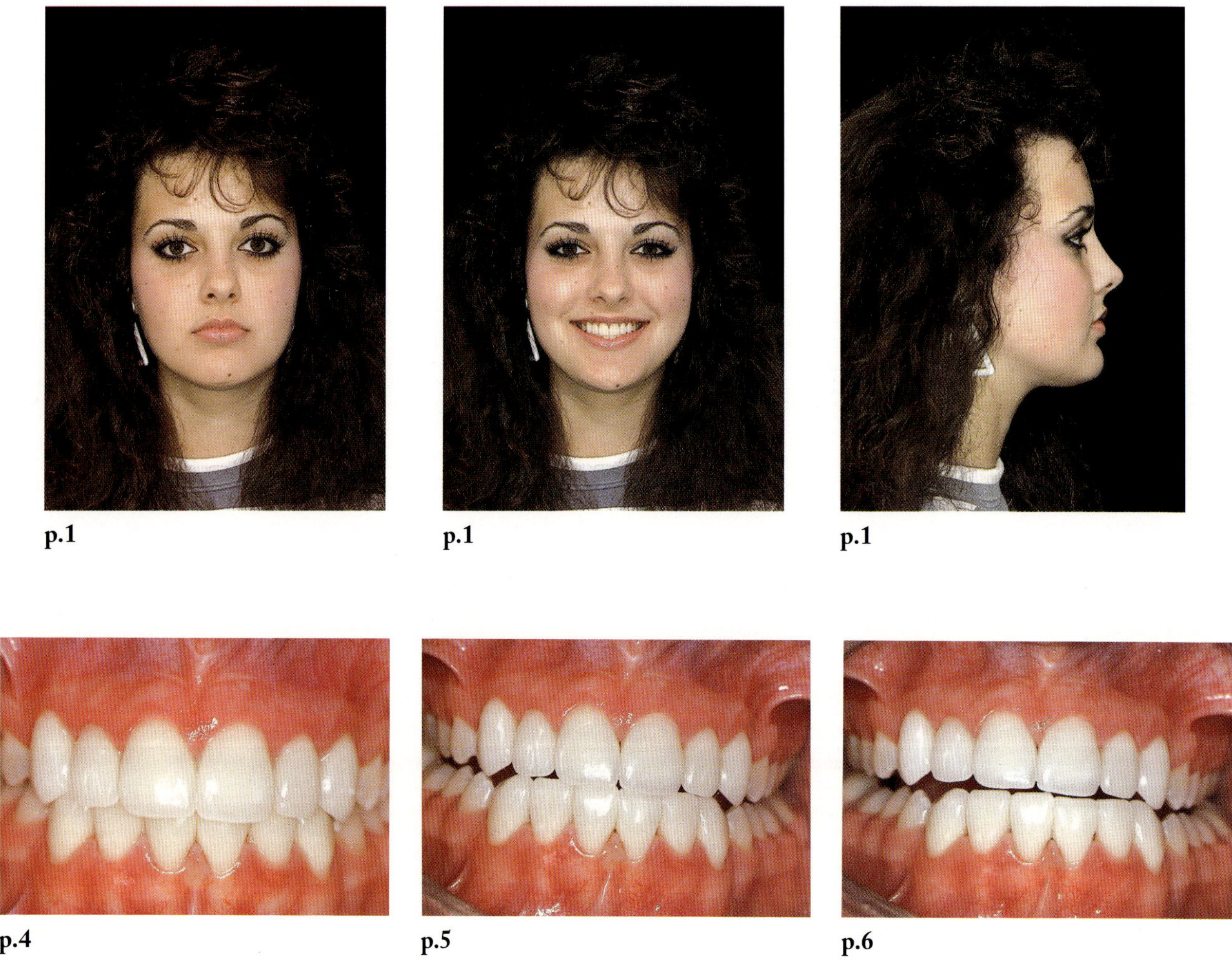

Fig 2-5 (continued)

p Final photographs after completion of interdisciplinary dentofacial therapy.

p.1 to p.3 Final facial photographs illustrating greatly enhanced dentofacial appearance from the frontal relationship and improved lip support in the profile view.

p.4 Final intraoral photograph of completed dental restorations bonded in place with composite resin. Additional periodontal plastic surgical procedures were recommended to augment the insufficient attached tissues of mandibular incisors.

p.5, p.6 Optimal protrusive and lateral functional relationships were developed with the final restorations to promote long-term dental and temporomandibular health.

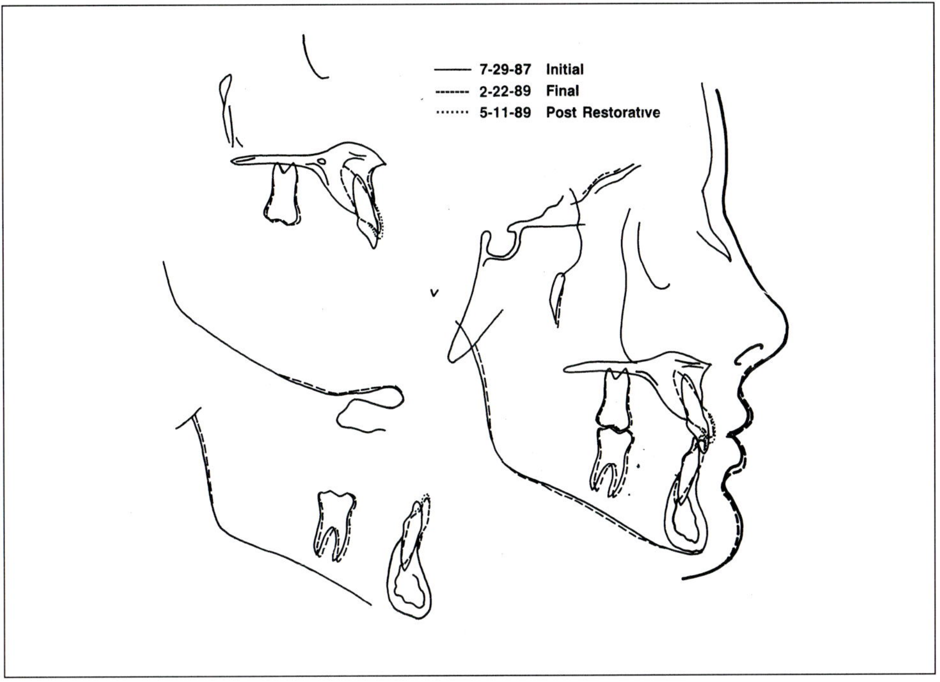

q

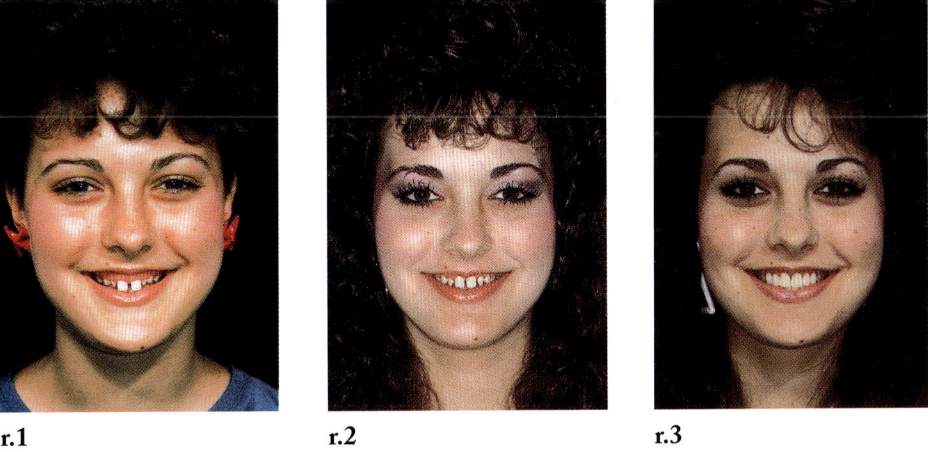

r.1 r.2 r.3

Fig 2-5 (continued)

q Cephalometric superimposition illustrating the soft tissue and dental changes achieved with interdisciplinary dentofacial therapy. Note the amount of intrusion in the maxillary incisors and the increased lip support.

r.1 to r.3 Comparison of smiling facial photographs taken during the initial, postorthodontic and postperiodontic, and postrestorative stages of IDT, illustrating dramatic improvement of the smile.

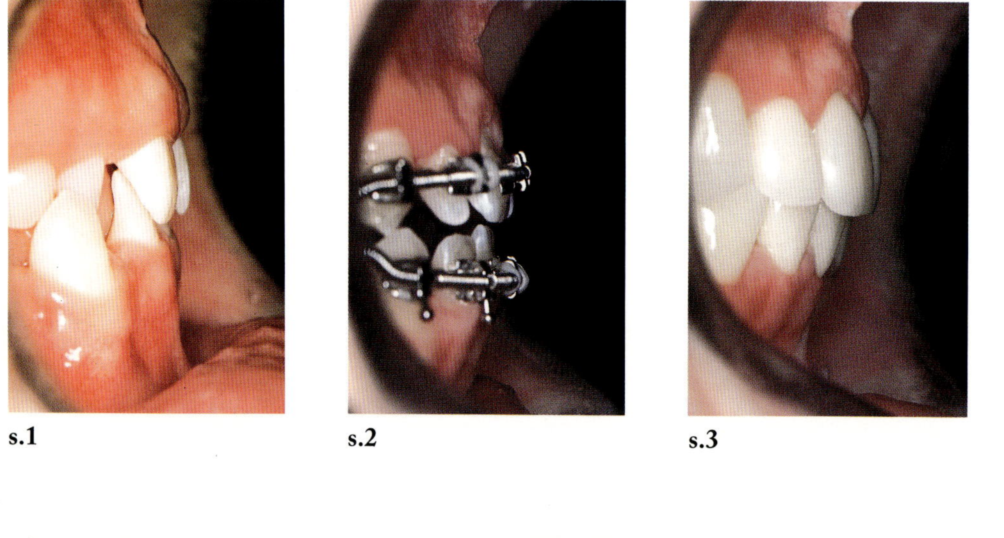

s.1 s.2 s.3

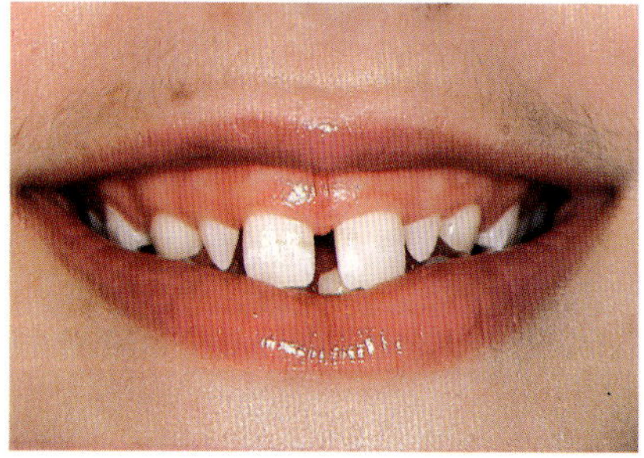

t.1

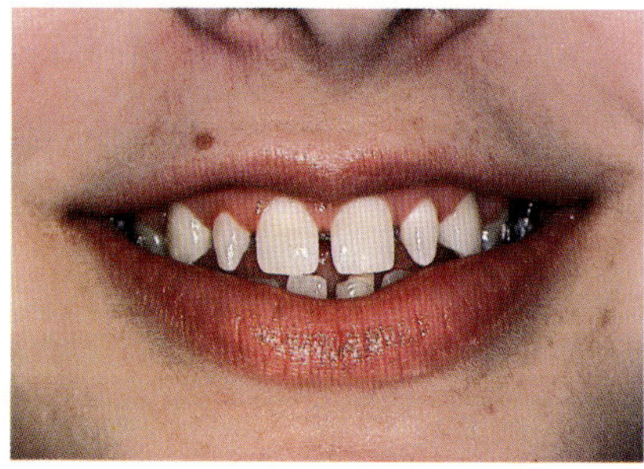

t.2

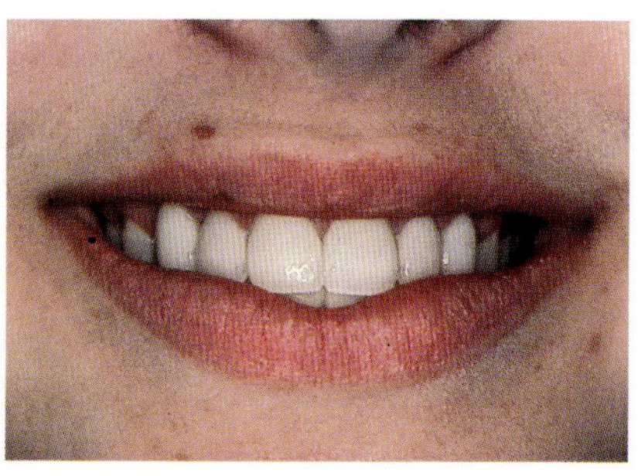

t.3

Fig 2-5 (continued)

s Comparison of lateral photographs of incisal relationships taken during different stages of therapy.

s.1 Initial view of traumatic and unstable interincisal relationship.

s.2 Postorthodontic and postperiodontic view illustrating the ideal interincisal relationship that was set up to allow optimal restorative procedures.

s.3 Final postrestorative view illustrating optimal interincisal relationships for dental stability, functional occlusion, and esthetics.

t Smile comparison of different stages of interdisciplinary dentofacial therapy clearly illustrating how the different team members can help each other produce optimal dentofacial results.

t.1 Initial smile with microdontia and excessive gingival display.

t.2 Postorthodontic and postperiodontal smile illustrating positioning of anterior teeth and reduction of excessive gingival display.

t.3 Postrestorative photograph after final restorations were placed.

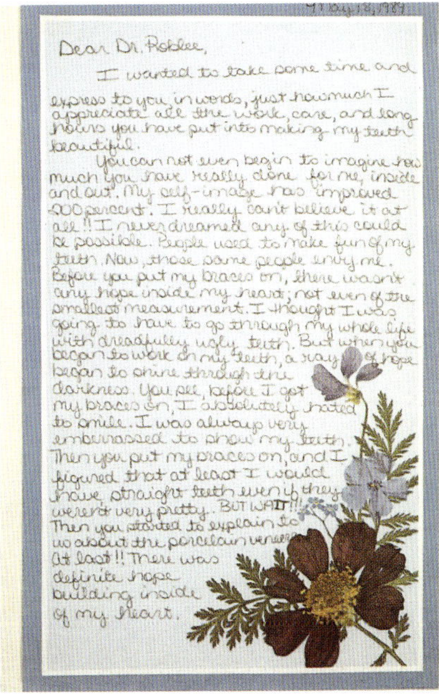

May 18, 1989

Dear Dr. Roblee,

I wanted to take some time and express to you, in words, just how much I appreciate all the work, care, and long hours you have put into making my teeth beautiful.

You can not even begin to imagine how much you have really done for me, inside and out. My self-image has improved 200 percent. I really can't believe it at all!! I never dreamed any of this could be possible. People used to make fun of my teeth. Now, those same people envy me. Before you put my braces on, there wasn't any hope inside my heart; not even of the smallest measurement. I thought I was going to have to go through my whole life with dreadfully ugly teeth. But when you began to work on my teeth, a ray of hope began to shine through the darkness. You see, before I got my braces on, I absolutely hated to smile. I was always very embarrassed to show my teeth. Then you put my braces on, and I figured that at least I would have straight teeth even if they weren't very pretty. BUT WAIT!!! Then you started to explain to us about the porcelain veneers. At last!! There was definite hope building inside of my heart.

u.1

②

I told myself that I didn't care what I had to go through; I was going to have beautiful teeth. Many times since then, I have had to remind myself of what I'd set my face to do. There were many days, weeks, & months when I wanted to give up; but each time you stepped in and encouraged me. You were always there telling me not to give up and that you knew I could do it. BOY!! I don't know what I would have done without your support!! We went through a lot together, but it was worth it! Every single ounce of pain meant that I was one step closer to happiness.

Do you know what else you've done? You have made one of my biggest dreams come true. You made the one dream come true that I didn't think would ever come true. And all because you made it possible! I used to really jealous when I would see girls with pretty teeth because they could smile as big as they wanted. Now, I'm one of those girls! I don't have to be embarrassed of my teeth ever again. And you made it all possible. Thank you sooo very much!!!!

u.2

Fig 2-5 (continued)

u.1, u.2 Letter that patient wrote interdisciplinary team leader expressing her great appreciation of the level of care that she was provided. This exemplifies that interdisciplinary dentofacial therapy, in conjunction with proper dentofacial counseling, can enhance a patient's self-image and overall quality of life.

Periodontist: Edward P. Allen, DDS, PhD/*Orthodontist and Restorative Dentist:* Richard D. Roblee, DDS, MS
Laboratory Technician: Jeffrey Singler, CDT

Discussion

The patient was a 15-year-, 3-month-old female who was seeking interdisciplinary help for her significant dentofacial problems. Through the use of orthodontic, periodontal, and restorative therapy, it was possible to idealize and simplify therapy. None of the procedures performed could have been omitted without negatively compromising and complicating the other procedures. With thorough diagnostic procedures, treatment planning, and proper communication, the team members were able to idealize and therefore simplify their individual therapies, because their shortcomings were compensated for by the other providers. This idealization of the individual therapies also helped to improve the prognosis of the results compared to compromises that may have been made in a unidisciplinary or multidisciplinary approach.

Many creative solutions to complex problems were made in this case that allowed the providers to turn problems into advantages. For example, the forces needed to orthodontically extrude the impacted canines were used to intrude the maxillary anterior teeth and reduce the "gummy smile" (Figs 2-5d.1, 2-5d.2, and 2-5d.3). The correction of these individual problems would have been much less effective if they were addressed separately. Also, the restorative correction of the generalized microdontia enabled the orthodontist and periodontist to correct the problems of insufficient lip support and excessive gingival display.

Interdisciplinary therapy can prevent unnecessary procedures. Initially, the patient appeared to have a severe vertical maxillary excess that would require an orthognathic surgical procedure (impacting the maxilla) to correct. By thorough interdisciplinary diagnostic and treatment-planning procedures, a treatment plan was developed to optimally treat the patient's dentofacial problems without orthognathic surgical procedures. This may not have been true in a multidisciplinary approach.

The coordination of the different therapies and the communication between providers in this case allowed the attainment of optimal results in a short treatment time. If these same results were attempted through a multidisciplinary approach, they most likely would have required a minimum of 30 months, instead of 19½ months, to complete. Even an orthodontic unidisciplinary approach to this case would most likely have taken significantly longer than 19½ months to attain compromised results.

The comprehensive utilization of the different disciplines in this case enhanced the individual team members' results. Neither the orthodontic nor the restorative results could have been as ideal without the other discipline's help. At the same time, the periodontal plastic surgical procedures further enhanced the orthodontic and restorative results. This cooperative effort to properly coordinate and communicate during therapy also concurrently enhanced professional relationships between the providers. If the same treatment plan would have been performed without the thorough coordination and communication of treatment objectives, the orthodontic therapy may have resulted in dental relationships that would require the restorative team member to negatively compromise the restorative procedures to compensate for the shortcomings in dental positions. This would not only have led to less-than-ideal results, but would also have broken down professional relationships; this frequently happens during traditional multidisciplinary therapy.

There is no question that the optimal results obtained in this case led to increased patient and doctor satisfaction with the therapy performed. At the beginning of therapy, the patient was introverted, with little self-esteem and a poor self-image. She gradually transformed during therapy, and by the end of treatment, she was considered extroverted. She had a tremendously improved self-image and level of self-esteem. These results led to far greater patient and doctor satisfaction than just improving or maintaining oral health. Increased satisfaction has a high motivating effect on the patient to refer more friends and family to the providers. At the same time, it motivates the doctors and their staffs to further improve their quality of therapy.

Interdisciplinary Dentofacial Therapy Flowchart

The illustrations and Case Summary in Fig 2-5 are presented in detail to introduce the concept of IDT, and it will be referred to throughout this text. To obtain consistent quality results such as those in this case, dental and dentofacial problems must be analyzed, planned, and treated in a regimental fashion to ensure that all necessary expertise has been included and that no problems or potential solutions have been overlooked. The interdisciplinary dentofacial therapy flowchart was developed to facilitate the interdisciplinary team in providing consistent optimal results. In this flowchart, interdisciplinary dentofacial therapy is divided into five distinct stages (Fig 2-6). The first stage is the preliminary therapy necessary to get the patient into the interdisciplinary process. The remaining four stages consist of the four phases of actual IDT. These four phases are *(1)* diagnostics, *(2)* treatment planning, *(3)* definitive therapy, and *(4)* maintenance.

The remaining portions of this book will deal with the mechanics and philosophy of optimal interdisciplinary dentofacial therapy, using the flowcharts as a framework. There is a chapter dedicated to each of the five stages of the flowchart. A generalized overview will be given so that all interdisciplinary team members will be able to use this text as a reference. This same treatment philosophy and flowchart can be modified and adapted to facilitate any dental and dentofacial therapy, no matter how simple or complex. In fact, it is suggested that even apparently simple problems being treated by one provider be analyzed in this fashion to make sure that no less obvious and potentially more important problems or solutions are overlooked.

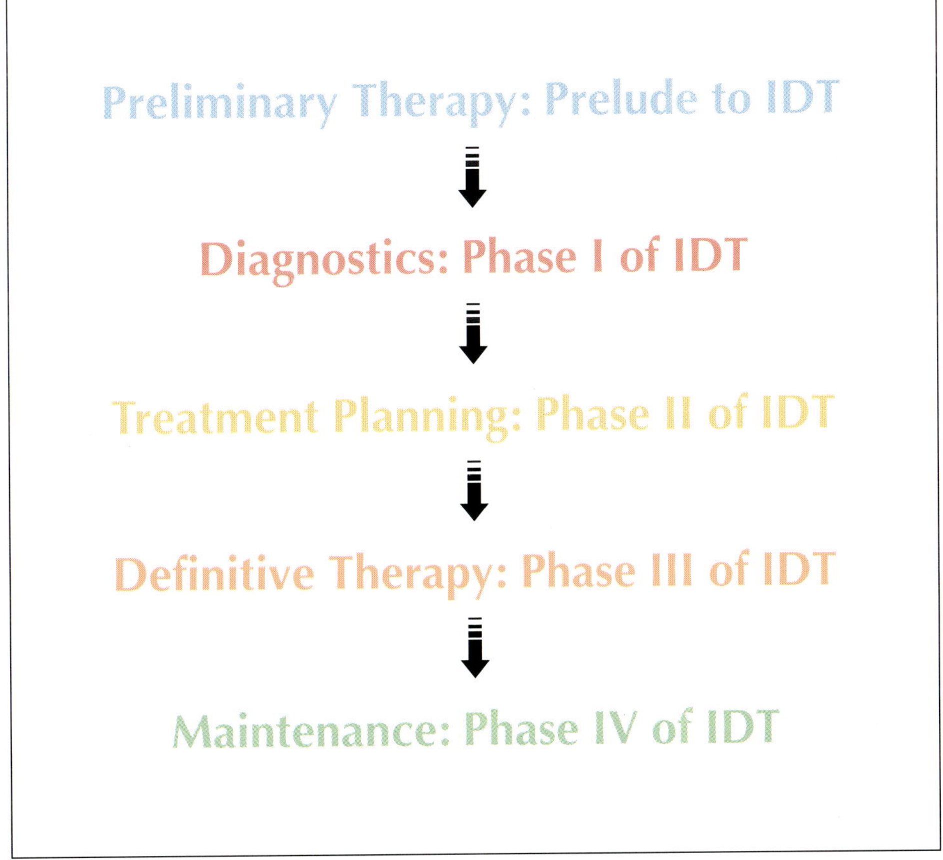

Fig 2-6 Interdisciplinary dentofacial therapy flowchart, showing the five stages of IDT.

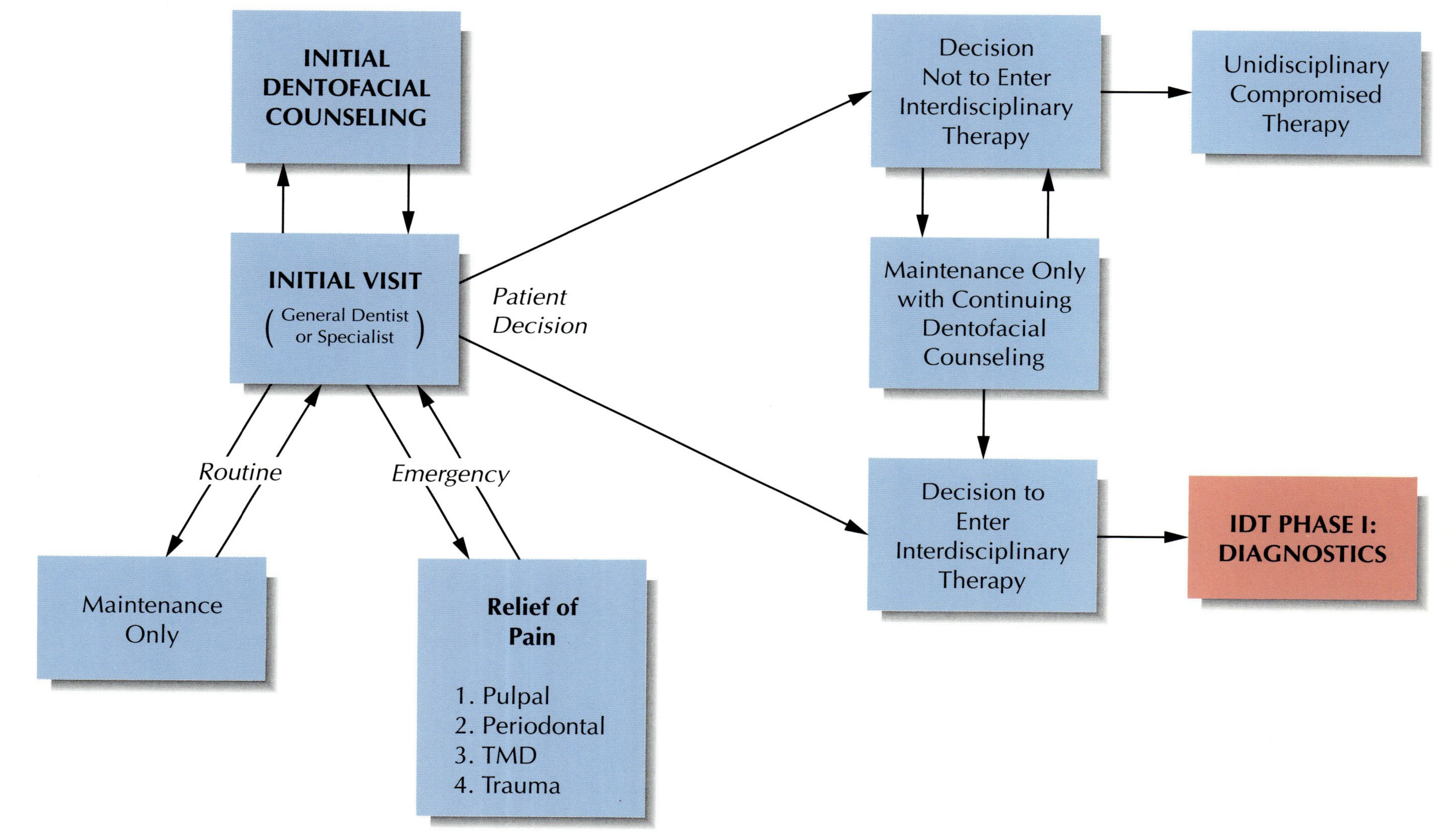

PRELIMINARY THERAPY: IDT PRELUDE

3

Preliminary Therapy

Prelude to IDT

Preliminary therapy entails the procedures necessary to get the patient into the interdisciplinary process. This therapy may be completed in the first appointment, or it may extend over several years until the patient accepts the idea of comprehensive dentofacial care.

Initial Visit

This visit may be the patient's first visit or it may be a visit for regularly scheduled dental maintenance. What distinguishes the initial visit is that it is the appointment at which the dental provider discovers the dentofacial problem and presents the option of comprehensive interdisciplinary therapy to the patient. This is the most important visit in the entire course of treatment, because this pivotal appointment may decide whether the patient will enter the interdisciplinary diagnostic process.

This patient visit will usually take place in the office of a general dentist for either emergency care or routine dental maintenance. It may be in the office of a specialist that the patient is seeing for an isolated problem. Occasionally, the patient will hear of comprehensive dentofacial treatment from other sources and seek the consultation of a general dentist or a specialist on their own. It makes no difference who the dental provider is at this initial visit, as long as he or she understands the magnitude and the mechanics of the appointment.

Relief of Pain

The primary concern of this appointment must be *the relief of pain*, if indicated. This should be done as conservatively and expeditiously as possible. Clinicians must train themselves to look at comprehensive patient care and put emergency treatment into its

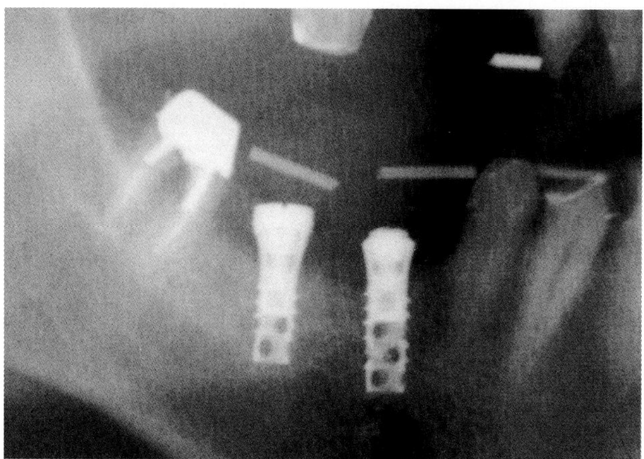

Fig 3-1 Whenever possible, hopeless teeth should not be extracted until a definitive treatment plan has been made, because these teeth may have several secondary uses in dentofacial therapy. In this example, a third molar that has been used as a terminal abutment for a long-span fixed partial denture is failing periodontally. At first impression, a clinician may feel that this tooth needs to be extracted as soon as possible. However, this failing tooth can play a key role in maintaining intra- and interarch stability during transitional implant therapy. It was maintained to support a provisional fixed partial denture during osseointegration of the implants placed in the missing first and second molar areas. If this tooth had been prematurely extracted, the patient would have had difficulty in mastication, and the opposing dentition may have supraerupted due to the inability to maintain occlusion provisionally during the osseotintegration phase of implant therapy.. The hopeless tooth will be extracted when the osseointegrated implants are surgically uncovered.
Restorative Dentist: Frank Higginbottom, DDS

proper perspective. At this point, the future importance or final position of the individual teeth is not yet known, because comprehensive diagnostic and treatment-planning procedures have not been performed. Therefore, the clinician should only initiate palliative procedures, including proper pharmacological management,[1] without performing definitive treatment that may compromise future interdisciplinary therapy. In this manner, proper treatment sequencing can lead to success, whereas performing definitive procedures out of sequence can lead to provider embarrassment, interdisciplinary friction, compromised results, and even failure.

If at all possible, teeth should not be extracted at this stage. This is because interdisciplinary therapy may be able to salvage them; and even if it cannot, hopeless or seemingly useless teeth may have secondary uses in dentofacial therapy. In some cases, these teeth may be temporarily retained to be used during orthodontic therapy for space maintenance, anchorage to facilitate difficult tooth movement, or esthetics in the initial stages of tooth movement (Fig 2-5d). Hopeless or otherwise unusable teeth can be used as temporary abutments for transitional restorations as part of implant therapy (Fig 3-1). Hopeless teeth may also be very important to maintain for orthognathic surgery (jaw repositioning), in which they may be helpful in establishing and maintaining vertical, anterior-posterior, and transverse movements of the jaw structures. At the very least, hopeless teeth can be used until the definitive therapy phase of IDT is initiated to maintain tooth positions and help prevent further collapse of the dental arches. In all these examples, the hopeless teeth will be extracted later in definitive therapy after their usefulness has been exhausted.

The emergency relief of pain can be broken down into four major categories depending on the problem. The four categories are *(1)* pulpal, *(2)* periodontal, *(3)* temporomandibular disorders and *(4)* trauma.

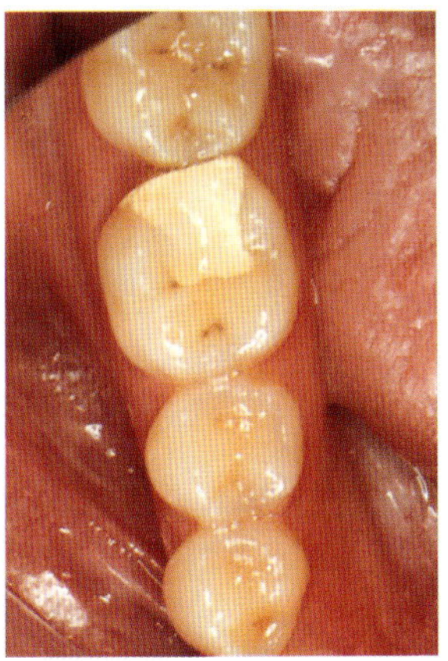

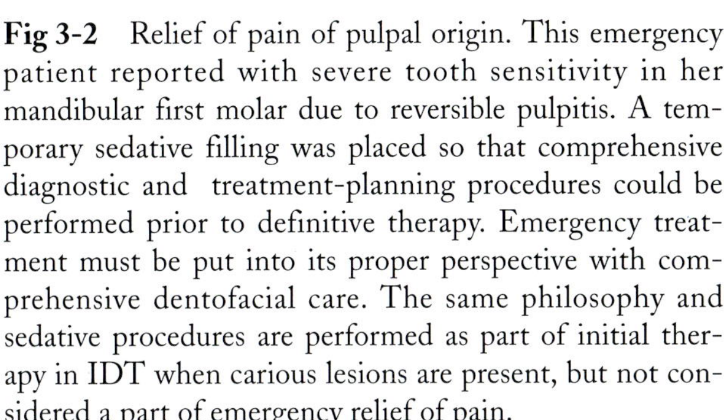

Fig 3-2 Relief of pain of pulpal origin. This emergency patient reported with severe tooth sensitivity in her mandibular first molar due to reversible pulpitis. A temporary sedative filling was placed so that comprehensive diagnostic and treatment-planning procedures could be performed prior to definitive therapy. Emergency treatment must be put into its proper perspective with comprehensive dentofacial care. The same philosophy and sedative procedures are performed as part of initial therapy in IDT when carious lesions are present, but not considered a part of emergency relief of pain.

Restorative Dentist: C.W. Dill, DDS

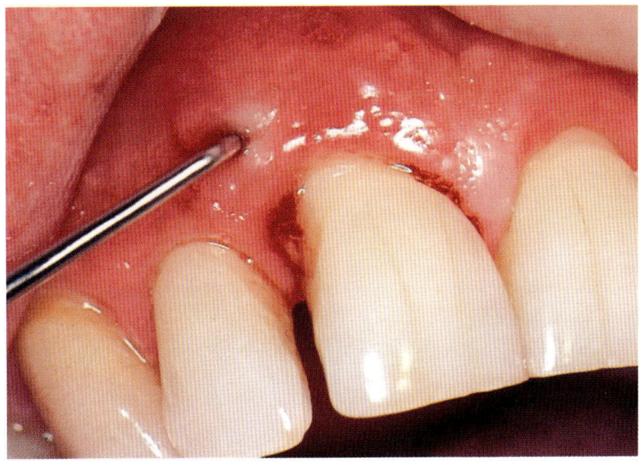

Fig 3-3 Relief of pain of periodontal origin. This patient presented with a periodontal abscess. Like the example in Fig 3-2, only palliative procedures were performed until a comprehensive evaluation and treatment plan could be made.

Periodontist: Charles A. White, DDS, MSD

Pulpal

When the patient presents with reversible pulpitis associated with a carious lesion, the caries should be excavated and a temporary sedative filling placed (Fig 3-2). If a patient has irreversible pulpitis and endodontic procedures are indicated, emergency treatment such as a pulpotomy, pulpectomy, incision and drainage, chemotherapy,[2] or trephination[3] may need to be performed. Permanent restorative or endodontic fillings should not be placed until the prognosis, relevance, and final position of the affected teeth have been determined through the interdisciplinary diagnostic and treatment-planning process.

Periodontal

The emergency pain may be of periodontal origin (Fig 3-3). Again, only palliative periodontal procedures should be performed.[4] As discussed previously, teeth should not be extracted until deemed necessary at a later stage in dentofacial therapy. Oral hygiene education, however, should begin as early in treatment as possible. Periodontal therapy will be discussed in detail later in this chapter.

Temporomandibular Disorders

Pain is frequently associated with one or more *temporomandibular disorders* (TMDs). This group of problems are usually more complex than the others, and may be symptoms of the overall dentofacial problems. When patients present with a complaint of temporomandibular pain, the clinician should allow adequate time for a thorough temporomandibular evaluation and differential diagnosis.[5] TMD pain should also be treated conservatively at the initial visit with various combinations of patient education, home care instructions, behavior modification, thermotherapy, medication, and/or occlusal splint therapy depending on the nature of the pain.[6,7] Occlusal splint therapy may later also function as a diagnostic tool in the treatment-planning process. More comprehensive TMD therapy may be performed as necessary in initial therapy of the diagnostics phase (discussed in greater detail in that section) after a general dentofacial evaluation has been completed.

Trauma

The problems associated with *trauma* can range from a chipped tooth to large continuity defects from severe dentofacial lacerations, fractures, and loss of soft tissues and/or dentosseous structures. Minor dentofacial trauma can usually be handled by properly evaluating the injuries and then applying the appropriate emergency therapy,[8,9] using the same conservative philosophy discussed previously. Major traumatic dental and facial deformities may require extensive planning and treatment by several dental and medical disciplines. Once the initial traumatic deformities have been stabilized, definitive therapy may be needed to reconstruct and rehabilitate the dentofacial structures.

Maxillofacial traumatology is an ever-growing area of specialization and needs its own prioritized assessment and treatment protocol.[10] Trauma must also, however, be treated to maximize and not compromise future dentofacial therapy. It is increasingly difficult to maintain this philosophy as the traumatic injuries increase to the life-threatening level. Obviously, life-threatening airway and bleeding injuries should be addressed expeditiously.[11] Once these problems are controlled, a thorough examination and treatment plan should be performed prior to initiating final emergency treatment. Complications and undesirable compromises in interdisciplinary therapy are frequently caused by inappropriate or inadequate care provided during emergency treatment of maxillofacial trauma.[12] Therefore, it is vitally important that all consultations and treatment plans are considered when treating maxillofacial trauma, so that optimal dentofacial results can be attained in the future.

These four categories of relief of pain address most of the problems that a patient would present with in a dentofacial emergency. However, clinicians must always keep in mind that pain may be associated with sinus disease, neurologic disease, neoplasms, or other significant pathologic disorders, such as a myocardial infarction.[13]

Initial Dentofacial Counseling

Almost as important as the relief of pain during the initial appointment is the initial dentofacial counseling. Dental providers and their staffs need to develop special behavioral and counseling skills when it comes to setting the stage for interdisciplinary dentofacial therapy. The strength of the initial provider's recommendations will frequently determine whether a patient will pursue and accept further treatment.[14] Obviously, the dental professionals who interact with the patient have to be committed to optimal dentofacial health, or they will not be able to relay its importance to their patients.

It has been pointed out that the patient's perception of the value of treatment is usually indicative of their future treatment appreciation and cooperation.[15] If the patient has a high value for treatment, then chances are much better that he or she will accept comprehensive care, cooperate more fully, and thereby finish with more optimal results. The initial provider and his or her staff need to develop a high degree of sophistication to optimize the patient's value of and appreciation for comprehensive therapy. Few patients present with a high perceived value of therapy. Instead, a high treatment value must usually be nurtured in the patient by the team members during the initial stages of IDT.

A patient's perceived value of treatment can be enhanced by *(1)* throughly educating the patient about his or her dentofacial needs; *(2)* increasing the patient's dental IQ; and *(3)* developing patient trust and confidence in the dentofacial providers. These major categories overlap, and can be achieved simultaneously through the following:

a. A positive, caring attitude of the provider and staff
b. Thorough examinations and consultations
c. Consultations with different specialists
d. Proper use of visual aids during consultation (preferably patient's own diagnostic records)
e. Printed patient literature
f. Before and after photographs of similar cases
g. Patient educational videotapes

Occasionally, nothing will work to elevate a particular patient's value of treatment. Extensive therapy for this type of patient probably should not be undertaken, because coercion generally leads to poor cooperation and results.[15]

Another important aspect of enhancing the patient's value of treatment is whether the provider should promote esthetic improvements at this time. A study of adult orthodontic patients found high treatment motivation in those individuals who were referred for esthetic improvements, but low motivation in individuals referred for physiologic correction.[16] Other studies found that the main factor for patients electing to proceed with jaw surgery is their desire to improve facial appearance.[17] Similar factors were found to be primary motivators in adults seeking orthodontic[18] and restorative therapies. With this information in mind, it behooves interdisciplinary providers to consider and promote esthetics in addition to physiologic health, which is their primary concern.

Patients can find many reasons to postpone extensive therapy. The initial provider must be forceful and assertive with recommendations about treatment to alert patients to the existing problems. If patients are just casually informed of their problems, they usually will not place enough importance on them to pursue further treatment. The initial provider should also follow up on the patient's progress soon after the recommendations have been made.

Sometimes after a dentist has gained a patient's trust and confidence, the patient will be reluctant to leave that office to be treated by other interdisciplinary team members. Patient anxieties can usually be relieved by informing the patient that he or she will be treated by an interdisciplinary team, of which the referring dentist will be an intimate part, to make sure that the patient gets the best results possible. It is also important to inform the patient of the other specialists' credentials and expertise in a positive way, so the patient can start developing trust and confidence in the rest of the interdisciplinary team.

Patients are likely to ask many questions concerning the treatment and its cost. The initial provider should address these questions briefly, without specifics. If the patient is given incorrect information, it may eventually lead to confusion and loss of confidence. Also, if too many specifics about treatment are given too early, the patient may become overwhelmed and apprehensive, especially if the patient's value of treatment has not yet been adequately developed. The specifics are always best handled by the expert in that particular area at a treatment plan consultation. Patients should be encouraged to go through the diagnostic and treatment-planning process so they can be fully educated about their specific dentofacial needs. Only then can the patient make an intelligent decision concerning dentofacial therapy and its relative importance to their unique circumstances.

If possible, treatment costs should not be discussed early in the IDT process, because the patient's perceived value of treatment usually is not yet high enough to accept justification of the cost, which can overwhelm the patient. A patient's concern about the cost of therapy can usually be relieved by explaining that, although it may be expensive, the financial burden may be lightened by spreading it out over several years. Also, it is obviously easier for the patient to begin the diagnostics and treatment-planning phases if the members of the interdisciplinary team agree to keep their diagnostic and consultation fees to a minimum. Once a patient is in the interdisciplinary flow and fully educated, that patient's perceived value of treatment will be enhanced, and the treatment acceptance rate will dramatically improve.

Patient Decision

The patient must now decide whether to enter into interdisciplinary therapy. Hopefully, the initial dentofacial counseling has elevated the patient's perceived value of treatment to a level where they will make the decision in favor of at least thinking about comprehensive treatment. At this point, a positive decision does not mean that the patient has accepted dentofacial therapy, but has merely agreed to undergo the diagnostics and treatment-planning phases. If a positive decision is made, the provider should then guide the patient into the diagnostics phase of IDT.

If the patient elects not to consider interdisciplinary therapy, an attempt should be made by the provider to subtly decline that as a definitive answer. Instead, he or she should continue to pursue the optimal goal of comprehensive therapy. This is done by performing only maintenance-type initial therapy, while continuing to provide dentofacial counseling to try to elevate the patient's perceived value of treatment to the point where he or she will enter the comprehensive process. This continued dentofacial counseling is most effective if the patient can be persuaded to visit with some of the other interdisciplinary providers to further elevate the patient's dental IQ and to reaffirm and strengthen the initial provider's counseling. Through this continuing process of education, care, and understanding, the patient will frequently decide to enter interdisciplinary therapy.

Occasionally, the patient will show some desire for comprehensive care but cannot go through it at that time. In these instances, the providers should attempt to perform therapy that will promote and maintain the oral environment until the patient can initiate interdisciplinary therapy. This will frequently require some creative planning so that providers do not perform any therapy that will compromise the future interdisciplinary therapy (Fig 3-4). If definitive fixed prosthodontic procedures must be performed at this stage, they should be done to idealize coronal anatomy in relation to the root structures (Fig 3-5).

Ultimately, the provider may have to decide that the patient will not elect to enter the interdisciplinary process. If this occurs, the provider may have to perform unidisciplinary compromised therapy. At this point, the provider can at least feel confident that through his or her efforts, the patient has made an educated decision.

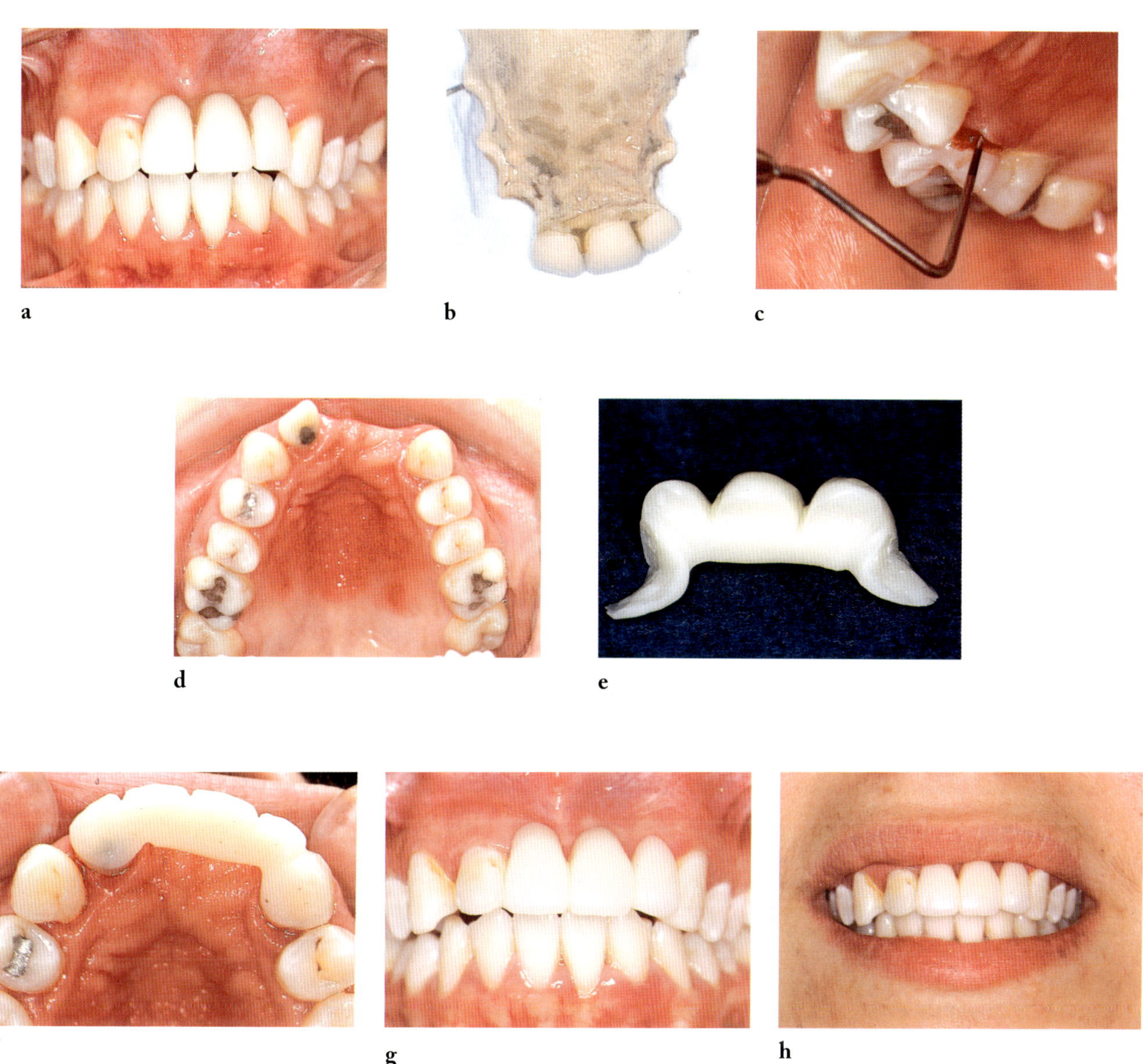

Fig 3-4 A 23-year-old female reported for dental therapy with periodontal, orthodontic, restorative, and financial problems. Instead of performing compromised unidisciplinary therapy, a creative treatment plan was formulated to allow optimal interdisciplinary care over an extended period of time that corresponded to the patient's financial means.

a Initial intraoral appearance. Teeth 11, 21, and 22 were avulsed in an accident at 8 years of age.

b Removable prosthesis worn continuously for 15 years.

c Severe periodontal problems were present only on palatal tissues. Patient was instructed to stop wearing prosthesis to allow successful periodontal therapy.

d Constructing a traditional fixed provisional restoration or another removable prosthesis might cause further irritation to the periodontal tissues. Instead, teeth 12 and 23 were prepared for a resin-retained fixed partial denture (FPD).

e A provisional composite-resin FPD was constructed directly in the mouth using a template made from a diagnostic waxup.

f to h The composite-resin FPD was bonded onto the prepared lingual surfaces of teeth 12 and 23. This provisional restoration will help esthetically maintain the dentition during initial periodontal therapy and until the patient can afford definitive orthodontic, periodontal, and restorative therapies. Once orthodontic therapy is initiated, the composite-resin FPD can be sectioned to allow proper positioning on the abutment teeth while the pontics are placed on the archwire to maintain esthetics. This type of creative problem solving can enable more patients to fit optimal interdisciplinary dentofacial therapy into their unique personal circumstances. The enhanced esthetics can also give the patient positive reinforcement about therapy and subsequently elevate their perceived value of treatment.

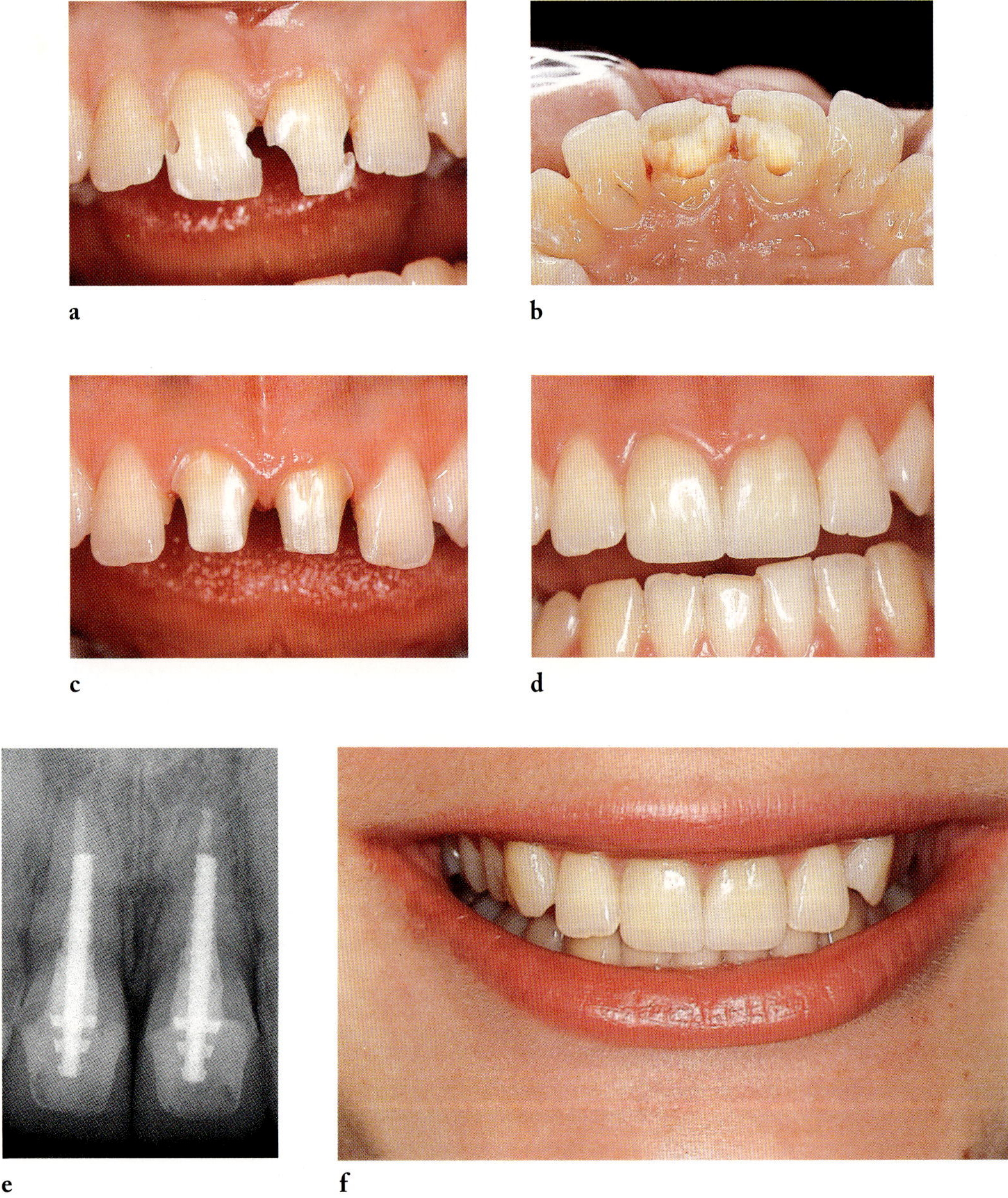

Fig 3-5 12-year-old female presented with severe restorative and orthodontic problems, but could only afford one therapy at that time. To further complicate these problems, the patient had a fragile self-image that made esthetics a primary concern. A treatment plan had to be formulated to esthetically restore the teeth without compromising future orthodontic therapy.

a, b Frontal and incisal views illustrating the severe breakdown of teeth 11 and 21.

c An endodontic post and a composite-resin buildup were bonded in place to reinforce the remaining tooth structure in preparation for definitive restorations.

d Resin-bonded all-ceramic crowns were used to restore the teeth and to provide optimal long-term dental and periodontal esthetics. Original coronal contours were duplicated so that proper root positioning could be accomplished in future orthodontic therapy.

e, f Final radiographic and clinical appearance of restorative result. If unidisciplinary compromised restorations would have been placed to restore the teeth and improve the coronal relationships, periodontal problems could have ensued as a result of establishing an improper restoration emergence profile. Unidisciplinary compromised restorations would also have to be replaced if orthodontic therapy was performed in the future, or their improper coronal morphology would prevent proper root positioning for future orthodontic therapy. This interdisciplinary treatment plan maintained esthetics while providing optimal dental and periodontal results without compromising future dentofacial therapy.

References

1. Gobetti JP. Controlling dental pain. J Am Dent Assoc 1992; 123:47–52.
2. Cohen S, Goerig AC. Endodontic emergencies. In: Cohen S, Burns RC (eds). Pathways of the Pulp, ed 5. St Louis: Mosby, 1991:25–47.
3. Harrison JW. Incision and drainage, and cortical trephination. In: Gutman JL, Harrison JW. Surgical Endodontics. Boston: Blackwell Scientific Publications, 1990: 387–396.
4. Wilson TG. Examination, diagnosis, classification, and disease activity for patients with periodontal diseases. In: Wilson TG. Dental Maintenance for Patients with Periodontal Diseases. Chicago: Quintessence, 1989: 17–37.
5. Cooper BC, Cooper DL. Multidisciplinary approach to the differential diagnosis of facial, head and neck pain. J Prosthet Dent 1991;66:72–78.
6. Dawson PE. Evaluation, Diagnosis, and Treatment of Occlusal Problems, ed 2. St Louis: Mosby, 1989.
7. Okeson JP. Management of Temporomandibular Disorders and Occlusion, ed 3. St Louis: Mosby, 1993.
8. Andreasen JO, Andreasen FM. Essentials of traumatic injuries to the teeth. Copenhagen: Munksgaard, 1990.
9. Fountain SB, Camp JH. Traumatic injuries. In: Cohen S, Burns RC (eds). Pathways to the Pulp, ed 5. St Louis: Mosby, 1991: 454.
10. Helfrick, JF. Early assessment and treatment planning of the maxillofacial trauma patient. In: Fonseca RJ, Walker RV (eds). Oral and Maxillofacial Trauma, vol 2. Philadelphia: Saunders, 1991.
11. Rajchel JL, Scully JR. Emergency airway management in the traumatized patient. In: Fonseca JR, Walker RV (eds). Oral and Maxillofacial Trauma, vol 1. Philadelphia: Saunders, 1991: 114–136.
12. Alpert B. Complications in the treatment of facial trauma. Oral Maxillofac Surg Clin N Am 1990;2:171–187.
13. Textbook of Advanced Cardiac Life Support. Dallas: American Heart Association, 1987.
14. Tayer BH, Burek MM. A survey of adults' attitudes toward orthodontic therapy. Am J Orthod 1981;79:305.
15. Vanarsdall RL, Musich DR. Adult orthodontics: diagnosis and treatment. In: Graber TM, Swain BF (eds). Orthodontics: Current Principles and Techniques. St Louis: Mosby, 1985: 791–856.
16. Barrer HG. The adult orthodontic patient. Am J Orthod 1977;72:617.
17. Jacobsen A. Psychological aspects of dentofacial esthetics and orthognathic surgery. Angle Orthod 1984;54:18–35.
18. McKiernan EXF, McKiernan F, Jones ML. Psychological profiles and motives of adults seeking orthodontic treatment. Int J Adult Orthod Orthognath Surg 1992; 7:187–198.

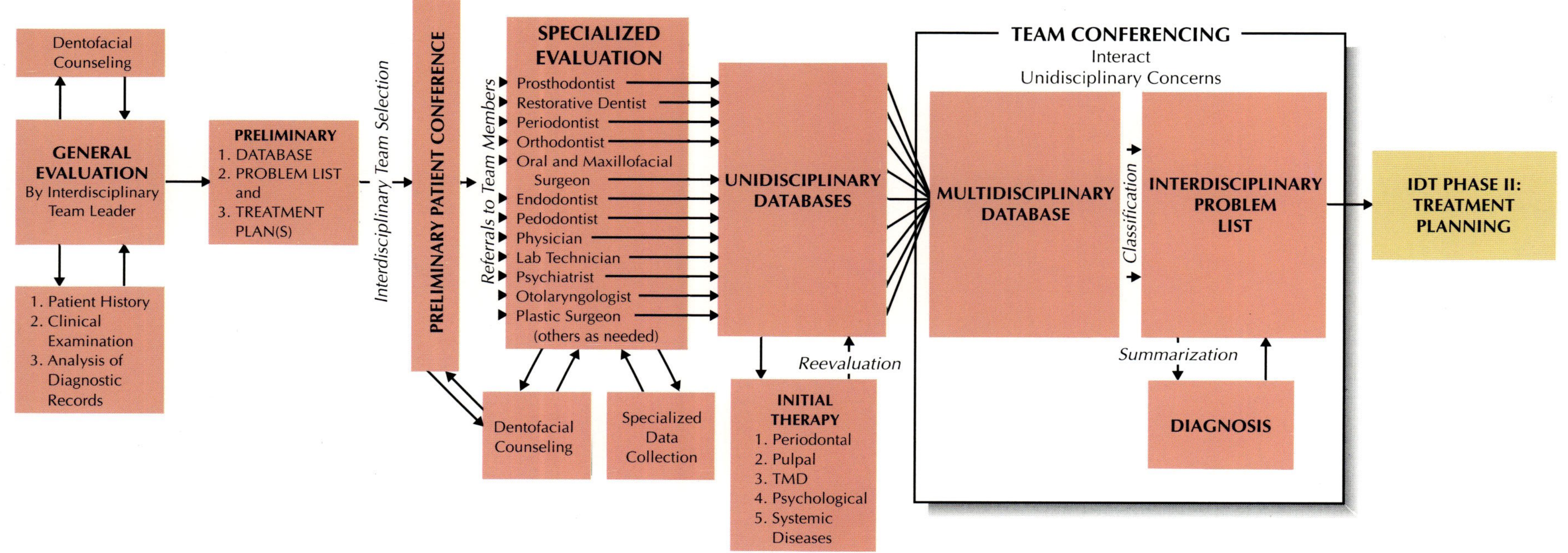

DIAGNOSTICS: IDT PHASE I

4

Diagnostics

Phase I of IDT

Once the preliminary treatment goals of relief of pain and initial dentofacial counseling have been accomplished, the patient is ready to proceed into the interdisciplinary dentofacial process. Optimal interdisciplinary dentofacial therapy consists of four distinct phases, the first of which is the diagnostics phase. The goals of this phase are to organize the interdisciplinary team, collect the database, and synthesize the problem list and diagnosis. The thoroughness of the diagnostic phase can prevent major complications and confusion in the definitive therapy phase.

General Dentofacial Evaluation

The first step in the diagnostics phase is the collection of the preliminary database by a thorough *general dentofacial evaluation* by the interdisciplinary team leader.

The interdisciplinary team leader can be the provider at the initial visit or a specialist to whom the initial provider referred the patient. The leader should understand the mechanics of interdisciplinary therapy and have an excellent comprehensive knowledge of different disciplines. Ideally, all members should be able to function as a team leader on an experienced interdisciplinary team. It is the leader's duty, in the diagnostics phase, to organize the rest of the team and coordinate their data collection. Later, in the treatment-planning and definitive-therapy phases of treatment, the leader will serve to maintain cohesion and interaction among the different team members to insure an organized progression of treatment planning and therapy, and ultimately lead the patient to optimal results. The team leader is an important position around which the interdisciplinary therapy will revolve.

The team leader will thoroughly evaluate the patient to amass pertinent information (both subjective and objective) related to the patient's physical, psychological, and dentofacial status. This information will make up the preliminary database and will be accumulated through *(1)* patient history *(2)* clinical examination, and *(3)* analysis of diagnostic records. Proffit, with the help of Ackerman, Epker, and Fields, has thoroughly described the database collection process, its development into a problem list, and the subsequent formulation of orthodontic and orthognathic treatment plans.[1–5] Portions of the data-collection and treatment-planning phases of this book were adapted and broadened from their work. Due to the broad perspective of data collection and treatment planning in interdisciplinary dentofacial therapy, they will only be briefly summarized in this text.

Patient History

The first portion of the preliminary database is collected through the *patient history*. In dentofacial therapy, the patient history is usually accumulated through questionnaires, patient interviews, and previous providers. The patient questionnaires should cover pertinent personal, social, and both past and present medical and dental information. It is often beneficial to the interdisciplinary team and the patient if the questionnaires of the various team members are combined and standardized so that all members use the same forms. This helps assure a consistent and comprehensive patient history from an interdisciplinary perspective. In addition, common interdisciplinary forms enable the team leader to send copies of the completed questionnaire to all the team members so that the patient doesn't have to fill out new ones at every specialized evaluation. This can lessen the burden of the diagnostic phase on the patient, and significantly enhance the patient's confidence in the team concept. Standardized forms and other aspects of coordinating an interdisciplinary team will be discussed in more detail in Chapter 8.

During the patient interview, the team leader should go over the completed questionnaire with the patient to help ensure accuracy and completeness of pertinent information.[6] Invaluable information can also be obtained through correspondence with previous providers. While all the information gathered in the history process is important, the patient's chief concern, motivation, and expectations for treatment[3] must be kept in mind throughout therapy. If these areas are not addressed and satisfied, the therapy may be a failure in the eyes of the patient, no matter how technically successful the interdisciplinary results are.

Clinical Examination

The second part of the database collection is the clinical examination of the patient. This examination needs to include a limited physical evaluation,[7] and thorough dentofacial, temporomandibular, occlusal, dental, and periodontal evaluations. The team leader may perform an abbreviated evaluation in one or more of these areas if a specialized evaluation by another team member is planned for that area. A detailed systematic process should be used for the patient history and clinical examination[8–11] (Fig 4-1) to make sure no important aspects are overlooked.

Analysis of Diagnostic Records

The database is completed through the *analysis of diagnostic records*. Not all of the possible dentofacial diagnostic records will be necessary for all patients, especially during the general evaluation, where the main focus is to get an overall picture of the patient's dentofacial problems. Later, in the specialized evaluations, more specific records can be made, but for now standard general evaluation diagnostic records will suffice (Fig 4-1). The leader must process these necessary diagnostic records and thoroughly analyze them to complete the preliminary database.

Dentofacial Counseling

It is critical to the success of interdisciplinary therapy that the team leader and future team members continuously build upon the *dentofacial counseling* started at the initial visit. Most people requiring comprehensive therapy have already had many years of negative conditioning toward comprehensive dental treatment. Negative conditioning can come from sources such as poor dental experiences and advice in the past, or from friends' and family members'

Chief Concern, Motivation for Treatment and Expectations

Medical and Dental Histories (must include temporomandibular dysfunction symptoms)

Limited Physical Evaluation

- Examine exposed body parts and physical characteristics
- Pulse
- Blood pressure
- Airway competency

Facial Evaluation (frontal and lateral views)

- Symmetry
- Proportionality
- Profile
- Lip support and competency

Smile Evaluation

- Symmetry
- Incisor and gingival exposure (lips slightly parted in repose and during smile)
- Symmetry and harmony of dentition and gingival tissues

Temporomandibular Evaluation

- Palpation of temporomandibular joints (TMJ) and masticatory muscles
- TMJ auscultation
- Mandibular range of motion and deviations
- TMJ loading
- Centric relation/maximum intercuspation discrepancy using an accurate and repeatable manipulation technique

Oral Evaluation

- Mucogingival evaluation
- Edentulous area evaluation (potential implant and prosthetic sites)
- Periodontal pocket and inflammation evaluation
- Dental evaluation (caries detection, status of existing restorations, wear, mobility, discoloration, etc)

Panoramic Radiograph

- Screening film for TMJ and pulpal pathology
- Analyze for pathologic lesions, impacted or supernumerary teeth, and angulations of teeth

Right Angle Periapical and Vertical Bitewing Radiographs

- Interproximal caries
- Interproximal bone levels, vertical defects, furcation involvement, etc
- Overhangs, overcontoured margins, subgingival calculus, etc
- Periapical lesions

Extraoral and Intraoral Photographs or Transparencies (Slides)

- Further evaluation and documentation of facial, smile, periodontal, and dental aspects

Accurate Study Casts Mounted in a Semi Adjustable Articulator Utilizing a Facebow Transfer and an Accurate and Repeatable Centric Relation Record

- Interarch relationships (Angles Classification, vertical and horizontal anterior overlap, crossbites, planes of occlusion, tooth-size discrepancies, etc)
- Intra-arch tooth relationships (symmetry, arch length/tooth size discrepancies, alignment, angulations, etc)
- Functional relationships (centric interferences, anterior coupling, working, balancing, and protrusive interferences, wear facets, etc)

Fig 4-1 Suggested diagnostic procedures and records needed for an adequate general evaluation. These records will provide the information needed to complete the preliminary database. It is imperative that a standard sequence be followed during a general evaluation so that no important information will be overlooked. A diagnostic procedure or record may be abbreviated or omitted during the general evaluation if it is to be performed later during a specialized evaluation by an expert in that area.

opinions of dentofacial therapy. This negative conditioning can eventually lead to distrust of providers or an unrealistic perceived discomfort.[12]

This conditioning must be overcome through positive enhancement of the patient's perceived value of treatment, as discussed earlier. Each member on the team must first gain the trust and confidence of the patient, then educate the patient about his or her specific needs and the various procedures currently available to meet those needs. The providers must make every attempt possible to interest and involve the patient interested in therapy. This can be greatly assisted by making esthetics improvement as early in treatment as possible (Fig 4-2). For example, discolored composite-resin restorations can be replaced and rough incisal edges smoothed in the diagnostics phase, as long as this will not potentially compromise future therapy. Improvements as small as these can often get a previously disinterested patient excited about dental health. This excitement must be nurtured throughout the interdisciplinary process by *(1)* further esthetic improvements whenever possible (Fig 4-3), *(2)* positive reinforcement for patient cooperation (such as oral hygiene), and *(3)* frequent progress reports to the patient.

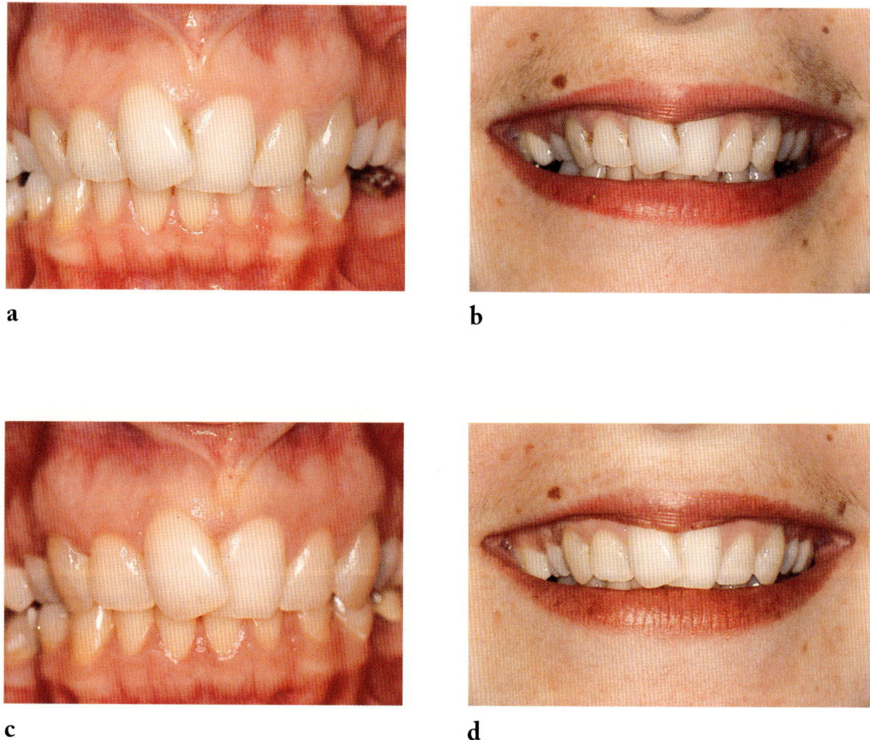

Fig 4-2 28-year-old female is in need of periodontal, orthodontic, orthognathic, surgical, and restorative aspects of interdisciplinary dentofacial therapy.

a, b Unsightly initial appearance of anterior dentition due to many defective and discolored composite-resin restorations.

c, d Improved appearance of anterior dentition following replacement of discolored restorations. This patient had lived with extensive dentofacial problems for a long time and had acquired a poor perceived value of therapy. The optimal interdisciplinary therapy that was eventually performed required a change in her attitude toward comprehensive care and a lot of patient dedication. Simple esthetic enhancements performed early in treatment can work wonders to motivate a patient about dentofacial health. Care must be taken at this stage in treatment to only perform early esthetic improvements that will not interfere with or compromise future interdisciplinary therapy.

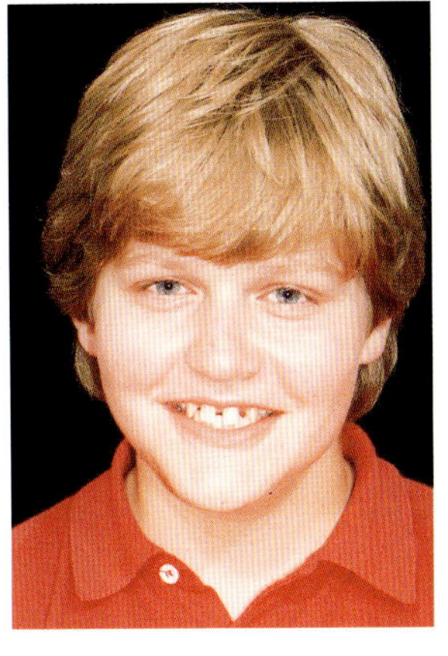

a

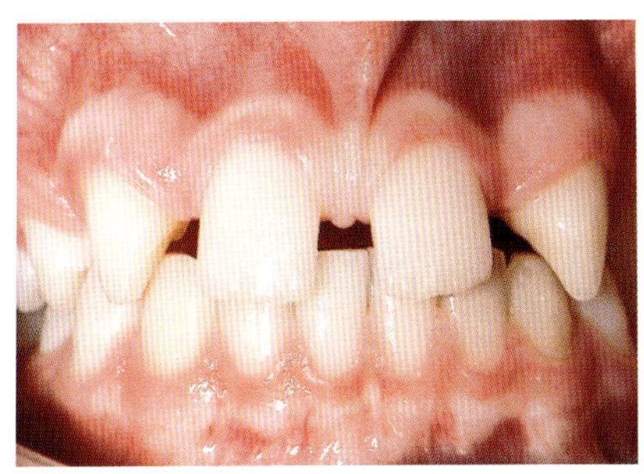

b

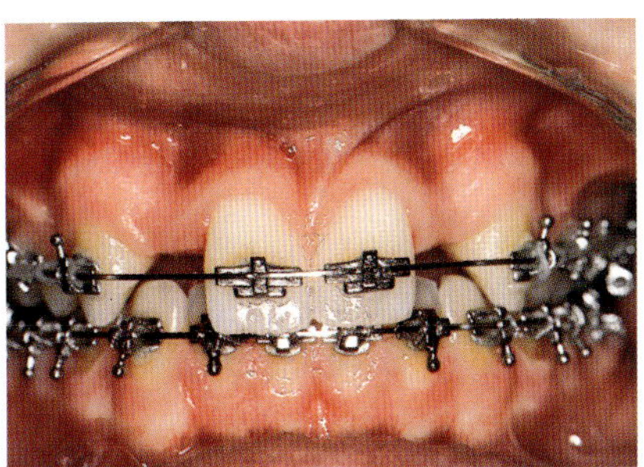

c

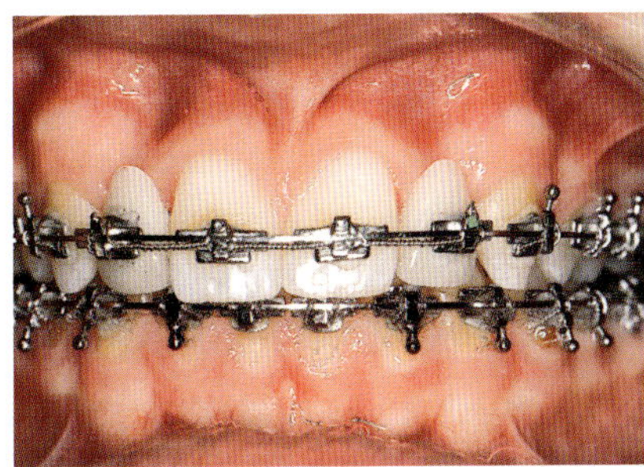

d

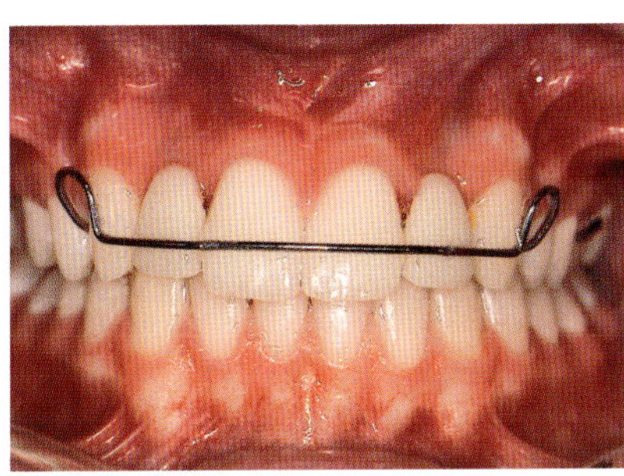

e

Fig 4-3

a 14-year-old male reported for orthodontic therapy with a low self-image and poor self-esteem.

b Initial appearance of dentition. Teeth 12 and 22 were congenitally missing.

c Orthodontic appliances were placed and spaces were opened to allow temporary replacement of the missing teeth.

d The restorative dentist selected appropriate denture teeth, which were optimally shaped and fitted with brackets so they could be fixed to the archwire. These preparatory restorative-type II procedures (discussed in Chapter 6) were performed to enhance esthetics and give the orthodontist the information necessary to position the dentition to accept optimal definitive restorative procedures.

e After orthodontic therapy was completed, the same denture teeth were added to a Hawley appliance to maintain esthetics and tooth positions until definitive periodontal and restorative therapies were completed. The appliance was also used by the restorative dentist as part of preparatory restorative-type III therapy (discussed in Chapter 6) . This aided the periodontist during ridge augmentation procedures by illustrating optimal cervical contours of the future prosthetic replacement teeth in the edentulous areas. [Note large labial defects in edentulous ridges *(d)* compared to same areas after one ridge augmentation procedure *(e)*.]

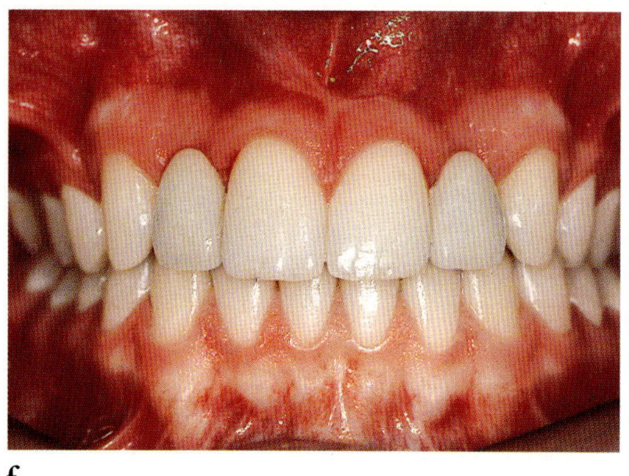
f

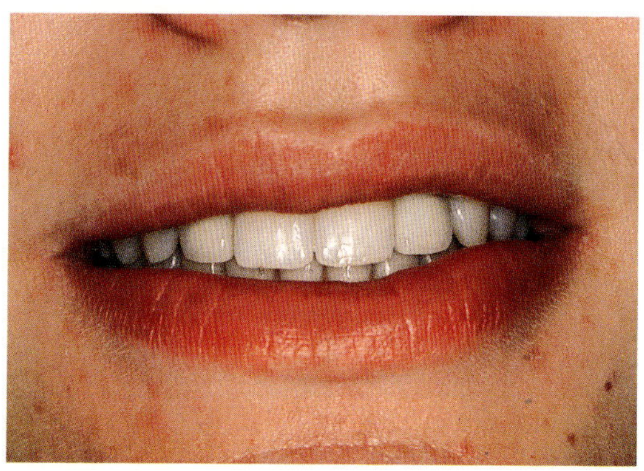
g

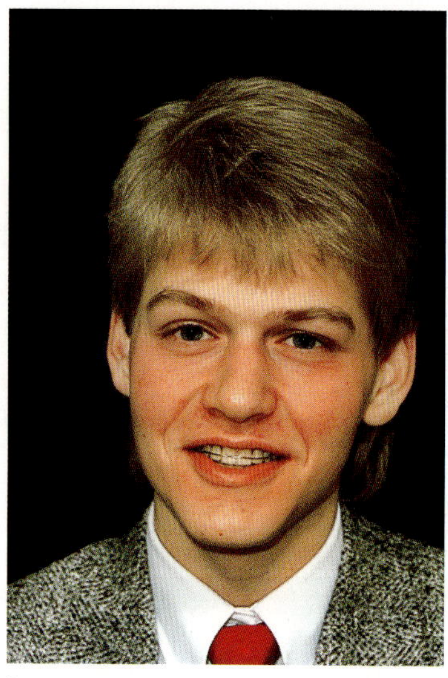
h

Fig 4-3 (continued)

f, g Final dental appearance after interdisciplinary therapy was completed. The missing teeth were conservatively restored with a resin-retained fixed partial denture to optimally maintain the health and esthetics of the abutment teeth.

h Final dentofacial appearance with Hawley retainer in place. Esthetic improvements were made as early and as frequently as possible during treatment to enhance and maintain the patient's motivation toward therapy. The patient's self-image and self-esteem were also greatly enhanced during therapy. Many positive psychological and physical changes were observed in the patient, (compare Figs 4-3a and 4-3h) including the intentional loss of 50 lb of excess weight.

Orthodontist: Robert L. Waugh, DMD, MS/*Periodontist:* Edward P. Allen, DDS, PhD
Restorative Dentist: Richard D. Roblee, DDS, MS/*Laboratory Technician:* Jeffrey Singler, CDT

Preliminary Database, Problem List, and Treatment Plan(s)

The team leader must organize the mass of information collected during the general evaluation into a useful *preliminary database* and derive the *dentofacial preliminary problem list* from the database. Not everything included on the problem list is necessarily a problem. Instead, the problem list should spell out pertinent factors associated with the patient that need to be taken into consideration when formulating the *treatment plans*. For example, a problem list may include the fact that the patient is an 18-year-old female. This patient's age and gender are not a problem; however, they are important to know because her dentofacial problems may be addressed differently than those of a 65-year-old male.

Once the preliminary problem list has been made, the leader should combine it with his or her experiences, creativity, and comprehensive knowledge of the different disciplines to formulate one or more preliminary treatment plan(s). The preliminary treatment plan(s) should include the potential definitive therapy options that may be available to the patient, as well as a detailed outline of the specialized evaluations, initial therapies, and other diagnostic procedures that must be completed before a definitive treatment plan can be made.

A thorough description of how interdisciplinary teams construct problem lists from databases and formulate treatment plans will be discussed later in this chapter and in Chapter 5. The same philosophy should be used here, except here the process is done solely by the team leader. This will serve as preliminary work which the team of experts can build upon or change during their specialized evaluations.

The process of synthesizing the database into a discrete list of problems and formulating preliminary treatment plans will suggest what expertise among the different disciplines will be needed to plan treatment optimally and treat the patient's unique dentofacial problems.

Interdisciplinary Team Selection

The leader now has all the information needed for *interdisciplinary team selection*. This selection process can have either a positive or a negative impact on the overall treatment. Each provider on the team must have an optimal level of skill in his or her area of expertise to be a positive factor. The interdisciplinary team (and the overall results) can only be as good as the weakest member's skills. Dental providers should not only have expertise and skill, they must have the patience and desire to satisfy the rigorous treatment demands of comprehensive interdisciplinary therapy.

It is possible that one team member will be able to adequately handle two areas of expertise, but this should be done very cautiously. For example, comprehensive therapy is often completed with apparent success, except that the periodontal tissues were not properly prepared or monitored. This can lead to devastating problems, because, in the presence of inflammation, a well-intended therapeutic procedure (such as orthodontic tooth movement) can act as a co-destructive factor and lead to rampant bone loss.[13–15] It is in the best interest of the patient and, in our litigious society, it is also in the best interest of the team to have an expert responsible for each aspect of therapy.

Occasionally, a seemingly insignificant problem will arise either before or during definitive therapy and an expert in a discipline other than the one needed will attempt to treat the new problem, either for monetary reasons or to save the patient a trip to another office. For example, during the course of caries control, the restorative dentist may discover a premolar with irreversible pulpitis. Instead of referring the problem to an endodontist, the restorative dentist may elect to perform the root canal therapy, even though it is not his or her area of expertise. Fate often has it that this will be the tooth that has recurrent problems (Fig 4-4). The problems could be due to ledging, a missed canal, or a poor fill, and the patient has to be referred to an endodontist, who

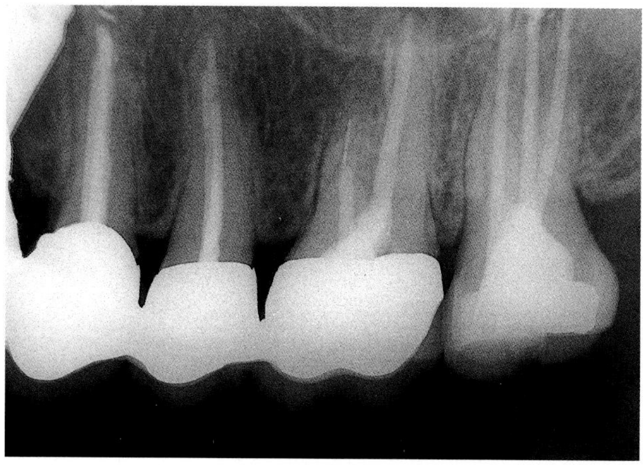

a

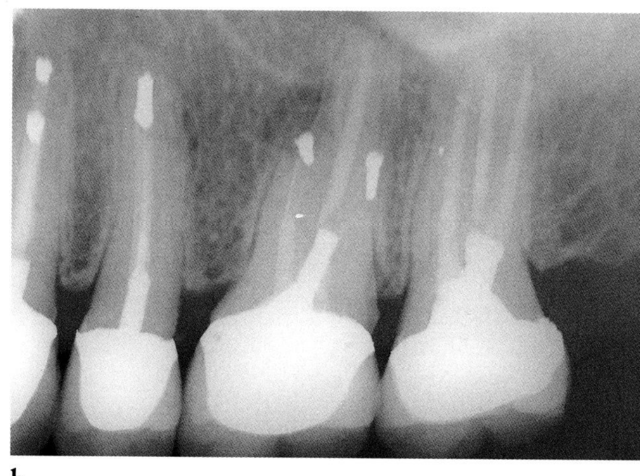

b

Fig 4-4

a Initial radiograph illustrating failing root canal therapies on teeth 24, 25, 26, and 27 that were performed by a provider other than an endodontic expert.

b Radiograph after endodontic retreatment. Teeth 24, 25, and 26 required root-end surgery, while tooth 27 was treated nonsurgically. The problems associated with the failed endodontic therapy led to loss of patient confidence in the initial provider, and subsequently the patient would not allow that provider to perform the planned full-mouth dental reconstruction. To help ensure optimal results with the fewest therapy-associated problems, each dentofacial problem should be dealt with by the team member who is the expert in that specific area.

Endodontist (surgical and nonsurgical retreatment only): James M. Tinnin, DDS, MSD
Restorative Dentist (retreatment only): Frank Higginbottom, DDS

will attempt to salvage the tooth. The treatment plan may be destroyed if the tooth is lost, and even if the tooth is saved, the sequence of events could cause the patient to discontinue treatment because of lost confidence and trust in the team. In the end, instead of gaining a root canal fee, the restorative dentist could lose an entire reconstruction. The risk/benefit ratio of having an expert treat each specific problem usually greatly weighs in favor of both the patient and the interdisciplinary team.

Preliminary Patient Conference

The team leader should see the patient for a *preliminary patient conference* after the preliminary treatment plan(s) have been completed. The purpose of this appointment is to explain to the patient his or her preliminary dentofacial problems and preliminary treatment options. The same philosophies are to be used here as were outlined in initial dentofacial counseling. The potential treatment options should be presented in a general strategy overview, without too much detail about each aspect of possible treatment. This generalized description is important, because the specific treatment plans can (and probably will) change after the specialized evaluations and initial therapies remaining in the diagnostic phase and the entire treatment-planning phase are completed. Also, the individual experts should ideally present the detailed description of their own specific therapies to prevent the patient from receiving misinformation.

The goal of the preliminary patient conference should be to further educate patients about their dentofacial needs and to further evaluate their perceived value of treatment. As a result, patients should better understand their roles in the remaining portions of the diagnostic and treatment-planning phases of IDT; this will facilitate the interdisciplinary process and help assure the patient's continuation in it. In addition, this appointment gives the patient an opportunity to ask questions and/or give feedback about the proposed therapy so that the team leader can further educate the patient and adjust the preliminary treatment plan(s) if appropriate.

The preliminary conference should end with the team leader making the appropriate referrals to the rest of the team. If possible, the leader's office should help the patient schedule the specialized evaluations with the other team members. This will help make sure the patient does not put off making the appointments. Knowing the schedule will also help the team leader track the patient and ensure that each team member gets the general evaluation records, the preliminary problem list, and the preliminary treatment plan(s) before their specialized evaluation. This will minimize confusion and duplication of diagnostic records and procedures by the individual providers, and will limit team members' frustration.

Specialized Evaluations

The patient will now undergo highly focused examinations in the *specialized evaluations.* These evaluations usually take place in the offices of the different team members, who will concentrate on specialized data collection. At the same time, the team must also continue the dentofacial counseling to further enhance the patient's perceived value of treatment.

Both the prosthodontist and the restorative dentist are shown in the flowchart for these examinations. It must be pointed out that even though it may be ideal for a prosthodontist to be on the interdisciplinary team, it is not always possible or necessary to do so. Whenever "restorative team member" is mentioned in this text, it refers to either a prosthodontist or a restorative dentist who is responsible for the restorative aspects of IDT. The restorative dentist must also be considered a "specialist" on an IDT team. To optimally fulfill this role, restorative dentists must expand on the expertise acquired in their formal dental education with extensive continuing education, literature review, and clinical experience. This is true for all other team members as well.

As mentioned earlier, the team leader should organize the specialized evaluations so that each specialist has access to previously made diagnostic records. Thus, each specialist can focus on collecting specialized data in his or her own area of expertise; expanding and building upon previous diagnostic procedures and records. For example, the orthodontic team member will use his or her expertise to expand the information gathered at general evaluations and make specialized records, such as a lateral cephalometric radiograph and analysis. Other specialized records, such as tomograms or magnetic resonance imaging of the temporomandibular joints that are considered adjunctive diagnostic procedures (treatment-planning phase), should be made now if needed to begin initial therapy. Biopsies of neoplasms should also be made as part of the specialized evaluations, so that further records and referrals can be made if indicated. Specialized evaluations usually require that the different team members clinically evaluate the patient, but some aspects can be analyzed by evaluating only the diagnostic records. For example, the laboratory technician can analyze the diagnostic records, without seeing the patient, and provide invaluable diagnostic information about possible prosthetic design to restore mutilated dentition.

During these evaluations, a team member will frequently discover another problem requiring the expertise of a discipline not included on the original team. This problem finding is a positive aspect of these highly specialized evaluations, which attempt to elicit all pertinent information associated with a patient's dentofacial needs. Additional team members, with the appropriate expertise and skills, should be selected as needed and included on the interdisciplinary team.

Unidisciplinary Databases

The end product of the specialized evaluations are *unidisciplinary databases.* Each of these databases should be strongly directed toward that particular team member's area of special interest. The biggest advantage to this style of data collection is that each aspect is evaluated individually. This helps prevent an obvious problem from overshadowing a less-obvious but equally-important problem. These less-obvious

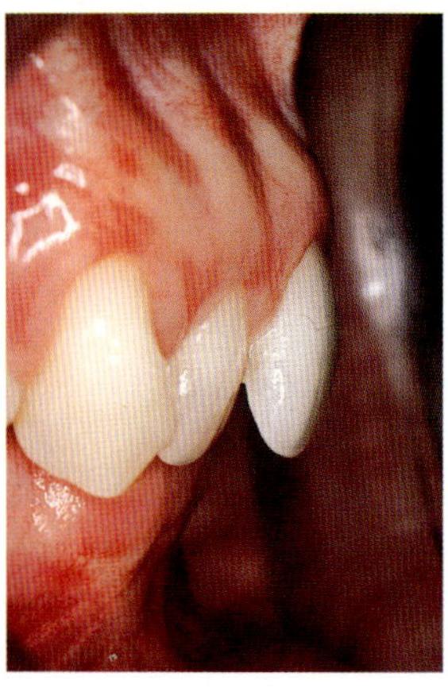

a

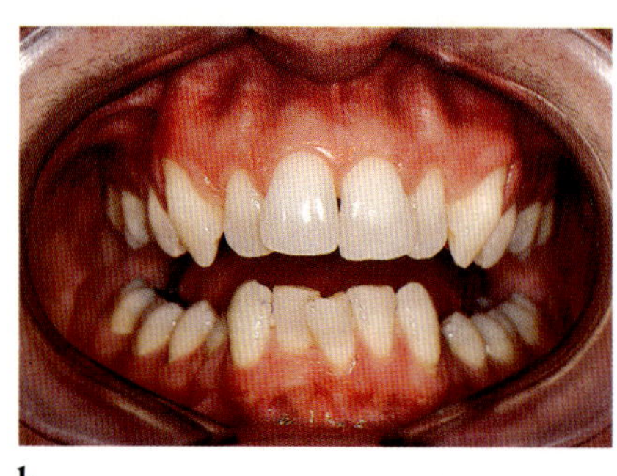

b

Fig 4-5

a, b Preoperative intraoral views of patient with Class II dental and skeletal discrepancies, in obvious need of orthodontic and orthognathic therapies. Using interdisciplinary specialized evaluations to have the various aspects of the dentofacial problems evaluated by expert in each area helps ensure that less-obvious problems (such as the insufficient attached gingiva in the anterior mandibular region, which may not be able to withstand the stresses of orthodontic and orthognathic therapies) are not overlooked.

problems can be easily overlooked in a general evaluation. For example, it is easy to see the obvious skeletal and dental problems in a patient with a severe Class II malocclusion, but it is also easy to overlook the possible existence of an insufficient amount of attached gingiva in the mandibular anterior region to withstand the stress of orthodontic and orthognathic surgical procedures (Fig 4-5). If this less-obvious problem is not found and the treatment plan adjusted accordingly, the patient's dental and skeletal Class II problem may be corrected, but with subsequent gingival stripping and eventual bone loss in the mandibular anterior region.

Initial Therapy

During the collection of the unidisciplinary databases, the appropriate team members should begin *initial therapy* to arrest active pathosis. The major categories of initial therapy are *(1)* periodontal, *(2)* pulpal, *(3)* temporomandibular disorders (TMD), *(4)* psychological, and *(5)* systemic disorders. Ideally, only minimal treatment is performed at this stage in the diagnostic process, because nothing should be done that may contradict or undermine the definitive treatment plan yet to be formulated. Initial therapy is therapeutic in nature, but it can also supply critical diagnostic information, such as the prognosis of pathologically involved teeth, periodontal tissues, or temporomandibular joints. This information is required before a definitive treatment plan can be made. Initial therapy for severe periodontal and TMD problems can last 12 months or more,[16] so initial therapy should be initiated early in IDT to minimize the length of the treatment-planning process.

Periodontal

The restoration of periodontal health is a prerequisite to all other dental therapies. Dental procedures performed in the presence of periodontal disease are often destined to fail, due to the loss of supporting structure. This is especially true in interdisciplinary therapy, in which procedures such as orthodontic tooth movement can act as co-destructive factors in the presence of periodontal inflammation and rapidly accelerate bone loss.[13-15] Orthodontic tooth movement and other definitive therapies can be accomplished without further attachment loss in periodontally compromised patients as long as the periodontium is healthy.[17] The goal of initial periodontal therapy is to nonsurgically control the clinical signs and symptoms of inflammation and reduce pocket-probing depths to allow periodontal stability and prepare for possible bony or soft tissue enhancement during the definitive therapy phase of IDT.

This is accomplished through meticulous personal plaque control by the patient and removal of tooth-bound accretions by the clinician, usually using closed-scaling and root-planing procedures.[18,19] A critical part of this treatment is educating the patient about the harmful effects of oral bacteria and teaching proper techniques for removal of bacterial plaque.[20,21] Contributing factors, like amalgam overhangs or poor crown margins, may have to be removed and temporized to facilitate soft tissue healing.[22] Conservative occlusal therapy with selective grinding or occlusal splints may be indicated when trauma from occlusion may be a contributing factor in periodontal destruction.[23-25] Periodontally hopeless teeth should not be extracted until it has been decided that they will be of no strategic value during the definitive therapy phase of IDT. Hopeless teeth should be extracted, however, when their retention jeopardizes the prognosis of the adjacent teeth.[26]

Periodontal surgery is usually contraindicated at this time, because initial periodontal therapy is necessary to provide valuable diagnostic information for developing an optimal definitive treatment plan for definitive periodontal therapy and the other definitive therapies. This information can include: *(1)* host susceptibility to periodontal disease(s), *(2)* the initial prognosis of periodontally involved teeth, and *(3)* the level of patient compliance. Also, periodontal surgery should not be performed on teeth until their strategic value (in addition to their initial prognosis) has been determined through the IDT diagnostic and treatment-planning procedures.

The success of the initial periodontal therapy should be evaluated at least 30 days after it is completed. In more advanced cases of periodontal disease, initial periodontal therapy alone may not successfully control periodontal problems. If signs of active disease[27-29] and/or pocket probing depths of 5 to 6 mm or greater remain after such initial therapy, more extensive definitive periodontal therapy may need to be performed in the definitive therapy phase of IDT. Which definitive periodontal therapies are needed will be decided as part of the treatment-planning phase of IDT. Some periodontal problems may require definitive periodontal surgical procedures to resolve them prior to orthodontics; these procedures will be performed as part of preparatory periodontal therapy.

Pulpal

Initial pulpal therapy is usually accomplished through the same endodontic and/or restorative procedures discussed earlier for relief of pain at the initial visit. Deep carious lesions that may be a threat to the pulp should be excavated and restored with a temporary sedative filling material (Fig 3-2). Endodontic procedures should be initiated[30,31] for asymptomatic and symptomatic necrotic pulps, and for retreatment of failing endodontically treated teeth[32] to control pathology and assess the initial prognosis of the affected teeth. Once again, final definitive restorative or endodontic procedures should ideally not be performed until after the definitive treatment plan has been formulated to prevent needless or incorrect definitive therapy from being performed. For example, after the definitive treatment plan is formulated, a tooth may be extracted for orthodontic reasons. If a definitive root-canal filling and/or a restoration had been recently performed on that tooth, it would be most embarrassing for the interdisciplinary team and could lead to a loss of patient confidence. However, it is important that all active pulpal pathology be resolved so that an initial prognosis can be made on the affected teeth.

Temporomandibular Disorders

Temporomandibular disorders (TMD) is a collective term embracing a number of clinical problems that involve the masticatory musculature and/or the temporomandibular joints (TMJ) and includes associated structures.[33,34] A universal etiology of TMD does not exist, but there are many known contributing factors. These factors may be related to trauma (macro and micro) and/or may be anatomic (including occlusion), pathophysiologic, and even psychosocial in origin. This complex multifactorial nature of TMD and orofacial pain frequently requires an interdisciplinary team for successful diagnosis, treatment, and maintenance.[35] Orofacial pain can be

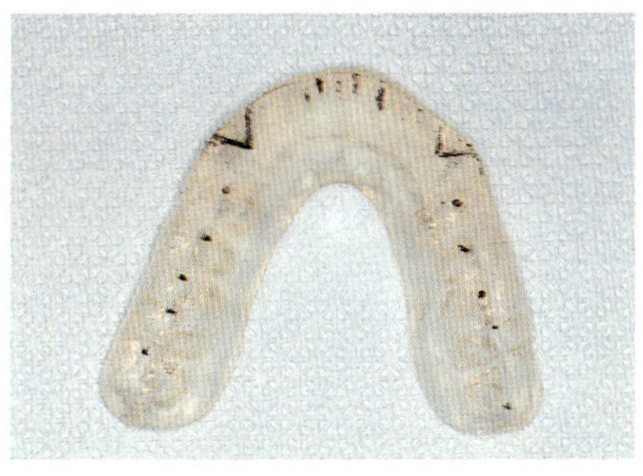

a

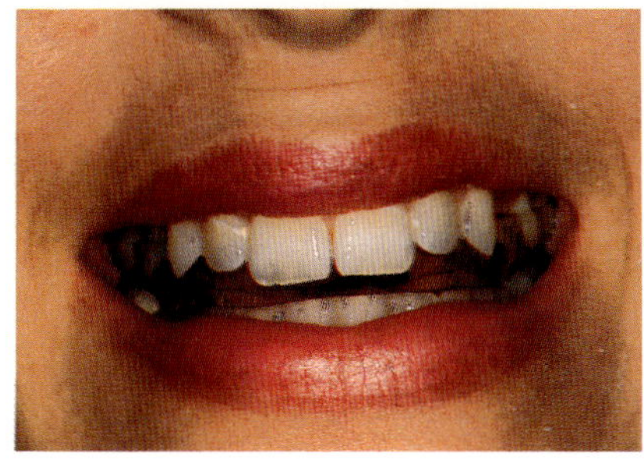

b

Fig 4-6 An occlusal splint or biteplane can be an invaluable therapeutic and diagnostic aid in the treatment of temporomandibular and occlusal disorders.

a Occlusal view of a properly adjusted centric-relation splint. There are even centric contacts throughout the posterior area, with lighter centric contacts in the anterior area. There is also anterior guidance for lateral and protrusive movements with posterior disocclusion.

b Smile of patient with esthetic occlusal splint in place. This splint was constructed so that the anterior teeth were not overlapped, and the acrylic resin was pressure-processed to make it as clear as possible. Extra care by the clinician to make the splint more esthetic will help ensure patient compliance. The patient may need to wear the splint from 2 to 9 months or more. *Orthodontist:* Richard D. Roblee, DDS, MS/*Laboratory Technician:* Cara Beaver

associated with pathology or disorders related to intracranial and extracranial structures (including TMD) and neurovascular, neuropathic, and psychogenic pain disorders.[36] The IDT team must thoroughly evaluate the patient's symptoms and determine if they are associated with any of these problems other than TMD. These other sources of orofacial pain can potentially be more serious in nature than TMD and the appropriate treatment and/or referrals should be initiated immediately.

There are many excellent references for the diagnosis and management of TMD and orofacial pain.[37] TMD symptoms should be resolved to an acceptable level and the occlusion stabilized in centric relation before the definitive treatment plan is finalized and the definitive therapy phase of IDT is initiated.[38,39] This may frequently be accomplished through conservative reversible treatment.[40,41] This conservative treatment varies according to the symptoms and history of each case, but it usually consists of various types of patient education and self-care, cognitive behavioral intervention, psychotherapy, pharmacotherapy, physical therapy, and/or orthopedic appliance therapy.[42] Orthopedic appliance therapy may be particularly useful in conservative TMD management when it is performed with an occlusal splint (biteplane) in centric relation, with proper anterior guidance in excursive movements (Fig 4-6).[43] This versatile appliance can also replace missing teeth by filling the edentulous area with denture teeth and/or a bulk of acrylic resin (Fig 4-7). The occlusal splint can be an invaluable therapeutic and diagnostic aid in interdisciplinary dentofacial therapy.

Through the proper use of an occlusal splint with certain TMDs, an "ideal" functional relationship may be established to assist the other conservative therapies in the resolution of TMD symptoms. Also, occlusal splint therapy should be continued until a stable interocclusal relationship has been attained. At that point, the occlusal splint therapy may be diagnostic in nature, demonstrating that the removal of occlusal discrepancies (in conjunction with other conservative therapy) has resolved the TMD symptoms. This can be verified by discontinuing appliance wear and seeing if the associated TMD symptoms return. Furthermore, with certain TMD and occlusal problems, occlusal splint therapy may help provide a stable condylar position, from which diagnostics, treatment planning, and therapy should be initiated. Occlusal splints are frequently used on TMD patients in the early stage of definitive therapies (such as orthodontics) to help maintain a stable condylar relationship until a proper dental occlusion is established. After definitive dentofacial therapy is completed, an occlusal splint may also be indicated for nighttime wear (night guard) (Figs 6-25w and

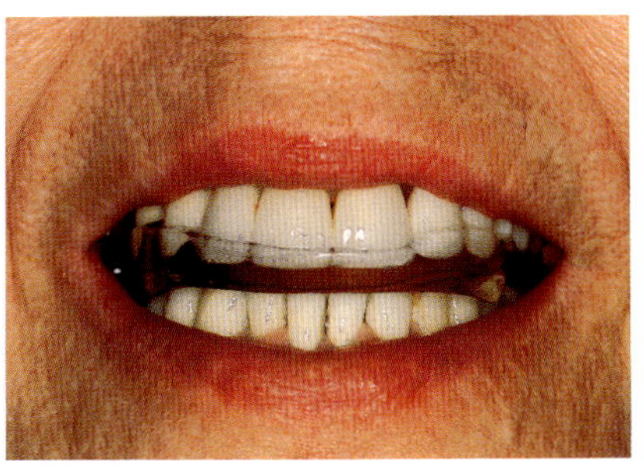
a

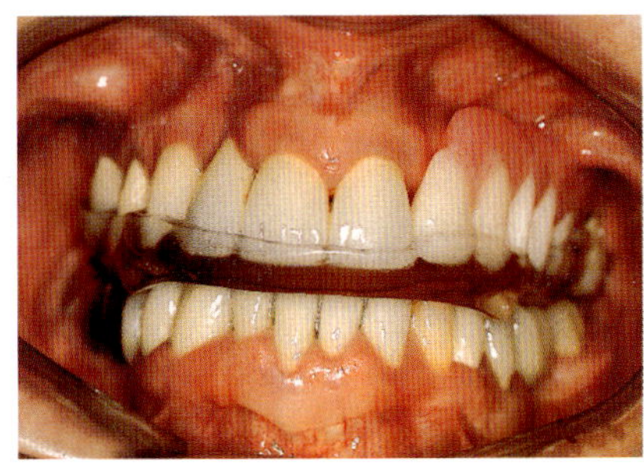
b

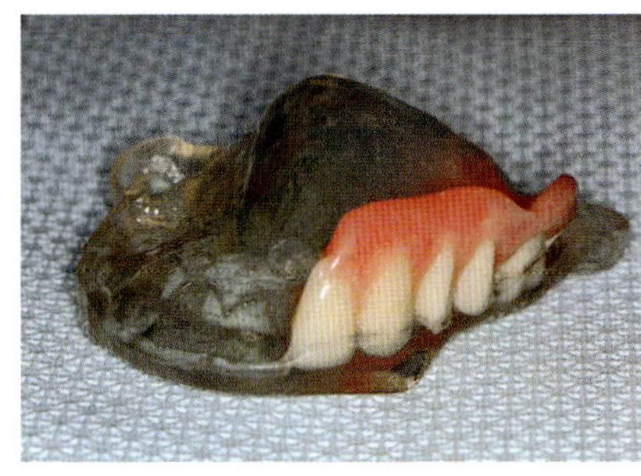
c

Fig 4-7 An occlusal splint can be a very versatile appliance.

a to c Smiling, intraoral, and extraoral views of an occlusal splint that replaced numerous missing teeth. Edentulous areas can be filled in by adding denture teeth and/or acrylic resin. This creative use of splint therapy can help reversibly establish a stable occlusal relationship when treating complicated occlusal discrepancies and mutilated dentition with missing teeth.
Restorative Dentist: C.W. Dill, DDS/*Laboratory Technician:* Richard D. Roblee, DDS, MS

6-25x) to maintain temporomandibular health and the dental result, especially when there is a nocturnal bruxing problem.

Conservative TMD therapy will usually last from 1 to 9 months, depending on the severity of the problems. Occasionally, conservative therapy will not successfully resolve the TMD symptoms. In these selected cases with confirmed degenerative TMD, invasive TMJ therapy may be needed, followed by conservative management until the TMD symptoms resolve and the occlusion stabilizes. Depending on the etiology and severity of the disorder, this invasive therapy may include a range of treatments, from simple joint injections to total joint reconstruction. Recent data suggests that some of these more difficult disorders can be resolved with more conservative surgical modalities, such as arthrocentesis[44] or arthroscopy.[45,46] If conservative therapy for a severe TMJ derangement has failed and specialized records or adjunctive diagnostic procedures have verified an internal derangement, more invasive surgical procedures may be indicated. TMJ arthrotomies, condylotomies, or grafting procedures, followed by conservative therpay, may be beneficial in controlling these TMD symptoms and stabilizing the TMJ.[47–49] Certain disorders in which the entire joint is degenerated or destroyed may even require a total joint reconstruction (Fig 6-26).[50] It must also be remembered that certain condylar pathology (ie, condylar hyperplasia, osteochondroma, idiopathic condylar resorption, etc) can cause a continuous shifting of the jaws and occlusal relationships (Fig 4-8).[51] This pathology will need to be eliminated and the occlusion stabilized before a predictable and stable dentofacial reconstruction can be accomplished. When the condylar pathology is related to systemic diseases such as rheumatoid or psoriatic arthritis, the disease process must also be properly managed as part of initial systemic disease therapy.

All the above procedures should usually be done as part of the initial therapy so that the dentofacial definitive treatment plan can be properly formulated from a proper and stable occlusal relationship. When TMD symptoms and the temporomandibular complex are not adequately stabilized, subsequent definitive treatment plans may be erroneously based on unstable or incorrect interocclusal relationships.[52] This can lead to tremendous complications and problems for an interdisciplinary team after definitive therapy has been initiated or completed. When this happens, the team must frequently go back to the diagnostic phase of IDT to properly address these problems. This change in treatment can be frustrating for both the team and the patient, and can lead to a loss of patient confidence in the team.

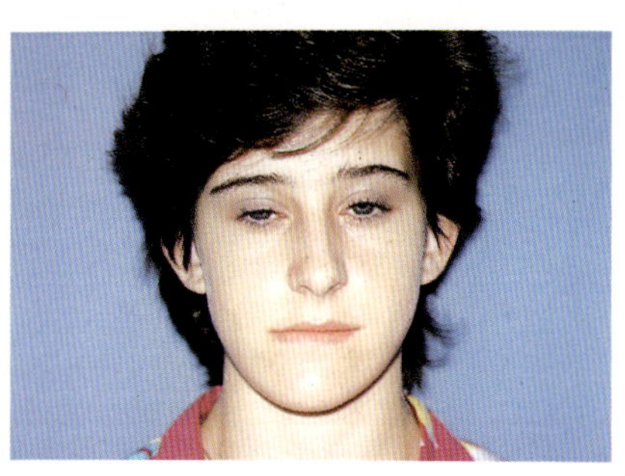

a

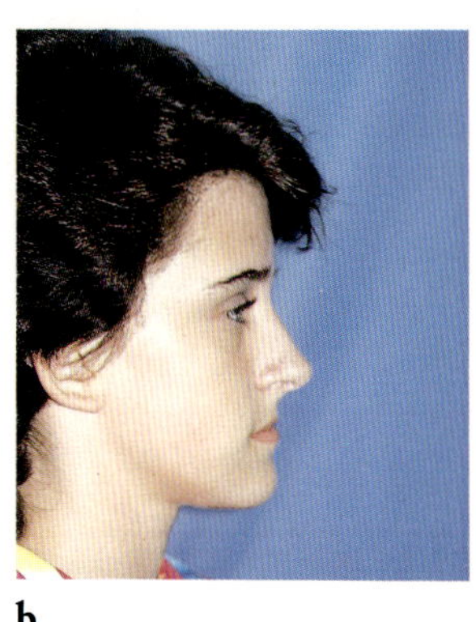

b

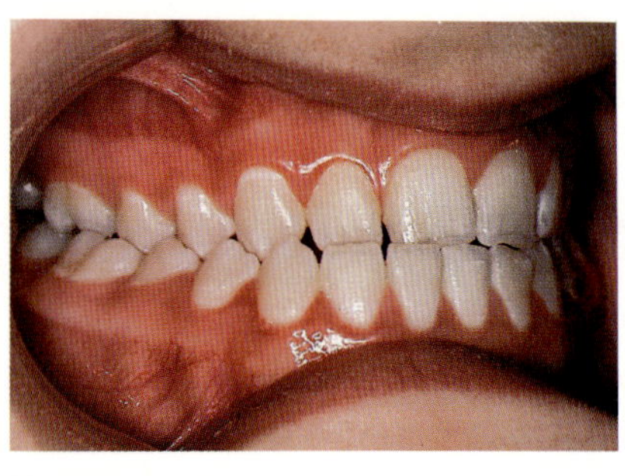

c

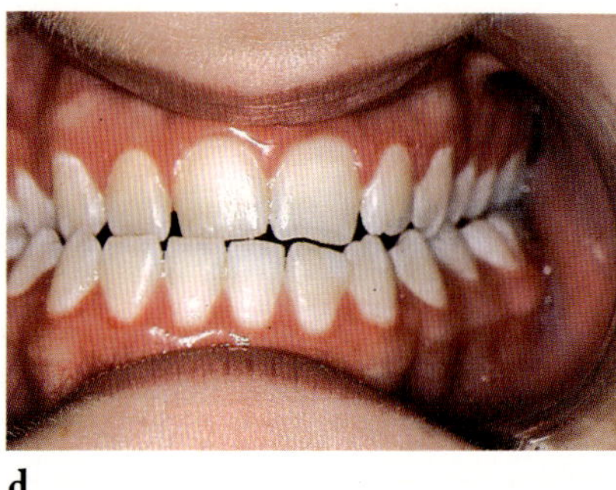

d

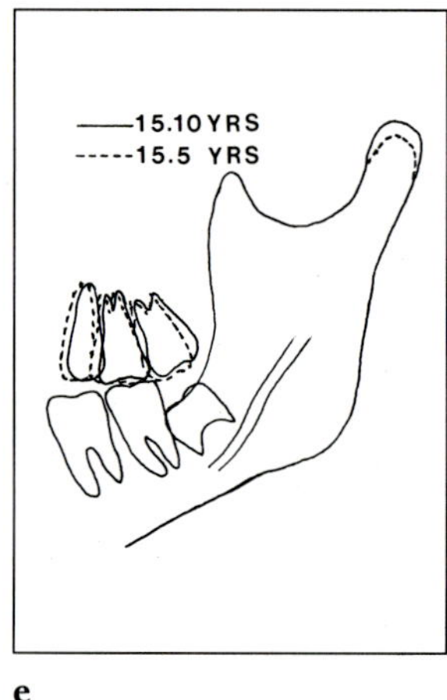

e

Fig 4-8

a to d Initial views of 15½-year-old female whose primary concerns are jaw malalignment, progressive worsening of facial asymmetry, headaches, and discomfort in and around her jaws. She has left condylar hyperplasia with mandibular deviated prognathism toward the right side. She also has anterior-posterior and transverse maxillary deficiencies with a right anterior crossbite and a bilateral posterior crossbite. The lower dental midline is shifted toward the right side and is progressively worsening. The anterior occlusal plane is canted, with the left side 1.5 mm lower than the right.

e Superimposition of 5-month serial cephalometric tomograms of the left TMJ, clearly demonstrating the excessive growth occurring as the result of left condylar hyperplasia.

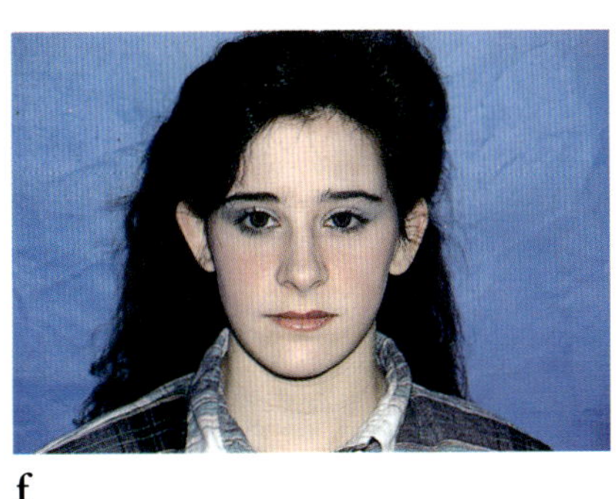
f

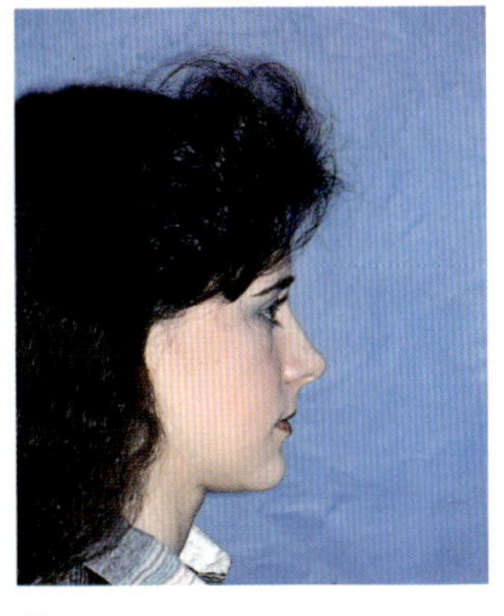
g

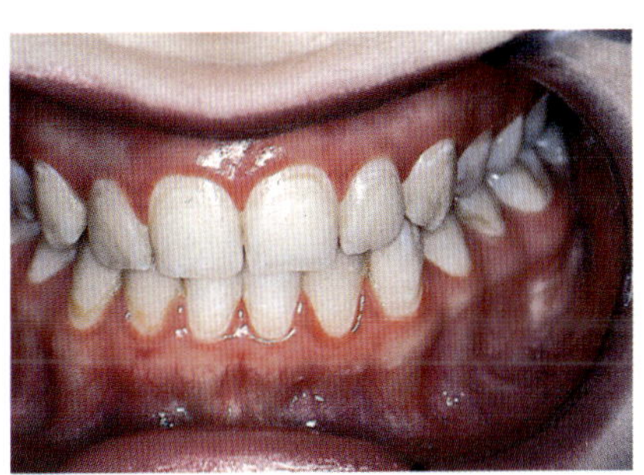
h

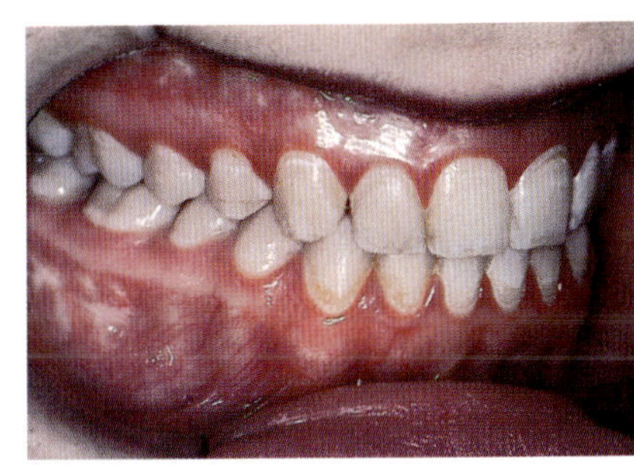
i

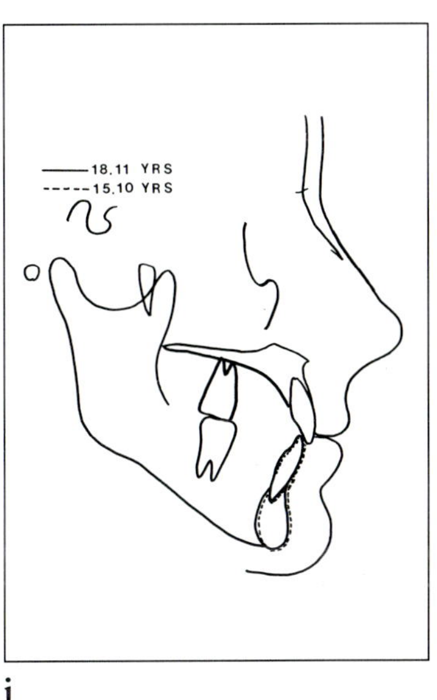

j

Fig 4-8 (continued)

f to i Posttreatment facial and intraoral views. A left mandibular high condylectomy was performed to remove the growth center of the hyperplastic condyle. Good functional and esthetic results were achieved though surgical orthodontic therapy, with a maxillary advancement and mandibular setback. The occlusion has remained stable following treatment, with a good Class I canine-molar relationship.

j Superimposition of the immediate postoperative and 3-year-postoperative cephalometric radiograph shows virtually no changes in position, except some settling of the mandible into occlusion.

Cases that exhibit progressive development of facial asymmetry are generally caused by *(1)* overgrowth of the condyle on one side, *(2)* resorption of the condyle on one side, *(3)* generalized asymmetric facial growth and development, *(4)* unilateral disruption of normal growth, *(5)* tumor, or *(6)* trauma (ie, fracture of the condyle). These pathological conditions can occur unilaterally, causing facial asymmetry, or bilaterally, causing a more symmetrical distortion of the mandible. This pathology needs to be eliminated before a stable reconstruction can be expected. Condylar hyperplasia usually becomes more evident and progressive around the pubertal growth spurt, but the abnormal growth can continue into the middle to late 20s. When the problems are directly related to the overgrowth of the condyle (condylar hyperplasia), removal of the growth center of the condyle (the top 3 to 4 mm of the condyle) will predictably stop mandibular growth. Many of these patients with condylar hyperplasia, condylar resorption, and other such conditions will frequently have an associated articular-disc displacement problem, which may also need to be addressed. These cases are sometimes treated at one surgical setting, but are more commonly performed in two surgical settings, first addressing the TMJ problem as part of initial therapy, then correcting the jaw malalignment concerns.

Oral and Maxillofacial Surgeon: Larry Wolford, DDS

Psychological

Psychological factors such as anxiety,[53] apprehension, frustration, hostility, anger, fear,[54] and depression[55] can often have a profound influence on the resolution of TMD symptoms. Many emotionally unbalanced patients may have psychological disturbances associated with dentofacial changes subsequent to orthognathic surgery.[56] Some patients have inappropriate motivations for and unrealistic expectations of esthetic dentofacial procedures. These and other areas of psychological therapy in dentistry[57] are continuously expanding. Failure to diagnose and address these psychological factors can greatly complicate dentofacial therapy and may even lead to its failure. Important psychological factors must be detected in the patient interview, then properly treated as part of the initial therapy.

Systemic Disease

There are a number of *systemic diseases* that can greatly influence dentofacial therapy and its success or failure. For example, diabetes or immunodeficiency diseases alter the body's ability to heal and to defend against infections. These same diseases may also predispose patients to periodontal disease.[58] Scleroderma or other connective tissue diseases may affect the quality of the soft tissues, making it very difficult to gain intraoral access to perform dentofacial therapy. Diseases such as rheumatoid arthritis (juvenile or adult onset) may cause destruction of the TMJ and lead to posterior shifting of the mandible and occlusal instability. Systemic disorders such as cardiovascular disease may weaken a patient's ability to withstand the physical stress of extensive interdisciplinary dentofacial therapy. To prevent complications, these and many other uncontrolled systemic diseases must be brought under control before dentofacial therapy is initiated; if they are not, the therapy should be modified accordingly. Interdisciplinary interaction with medical team members is necessary for the management of these disease processes.

Treated systemic diseases and other completed areas of initial therapy must be earmarked as special considerations. These special considerations must be closely monitored and addressed throughout the treatment-planning, definitive-therapy, and maintenance phases of IDT.

Reevaluation

After initial therapy is completed and the appropriate healing periods have elapsed, the patient should be reevaluated by the appropriate team members to assess the changes that have taken place during these various initial therapies. These changes should be added to the unidisciplinary databases and developed into the interdisciplinary problem list. The results of initial therapy can have a very profound effect on the definitive treatment plan(s), and so must not be overlooked.

The reevaluation is also an excellent opportunity for the providers to continue dentofacial counseling by furthering patient education and by providing positive reinforcement to the patient for the improvements made thus far. When properly handled, the patient's confidence in the providers and the patient's perceived value of treatment are usually greatly enhanced by this portion of treatment. If the interdisciplinary procedures have progressed properly to this point, the patient should be physically and psychologically prepared for the definitive patient consultation and subsequent definitive dentofacial therapy.

Multidisciplinary Database

At this point in the diagnostic phase, the initial therapy has been completed and the unidisciplinary databases have been compiled by the different team members. The highly specialized unidisciplinary databases are now combined to form the *multidisciplinary database.* An experienced team will usually have minimal interaction on the IDT case up to this point. Unlike the previous diagnostic procedures, success in the remaining phases of dentofacial therapy is dependent on the communication and interaction between all the different disciplines.

The most fundamental aspect of interdisciplinary therapy is communication between team members. This communication is the most effective means for overcoming the inherent shortsightedness of "specialty bias" in the different disciplines. It is at this point where the team concept becomes all-important to optimally diagnose and solve complex dentofacial problems.

Team Conferencing

The wide range and complexity of dentofacial problems necessitates a highly organized method of communication between the different team members so that all aspects can be equally voiced. This is performed through a method of team conferencing. *Team conferencing* must be highly structured or it will lead to lack of proper communication and ultimately to frustration and disappointing results. It is the responsibility of the team leader to maintain organization and quality in this communication.

Team conferences can take place through many different forms of communication. In situations where the different team members are separated by large distances, it is difficult to communicate face-to-face. In these circumstances, it is possible to communicate effectively by telephone and correspondence, especially since modern communication methods allow electronic transmission of large amounts of data and images quickly and easily.

Interdisciplinary team meetings are, however, by far the best means of team conferencing. An interdisciplinary study group can be formed that includes members from all the different disciplines. Interdisciplinary study group meetings can then be regularly scheduled to diagnose, formulate treatment plans, monitor the progress of therapy, and subsequently make modifications in treatment when needed in current interdisciplinary cases.

Regularly scheduled interdisciplinary meetings also set up an ideal format for the advancement of individual team members' knowledge and comprehension of dentofacial therapy. In addition to the discussion of current and posttreatment cases, members can present summaries of current advancements in their particular areas of expertise. This allows all members to stay abreast of the advancements being made in all the different disciplines. It is not necessary that an individual understand all the specifics of the other areas, but it is crucial that he or she be aware of the various treatment options the different disciplines have to offer and of their positive and negative effects on his or her area of expertise. This is an excellent way to enhance the concept of comprehensive dentofacial therapy and encourage improvement in the interdisciplinary treatment of complex dentofacial problems.

Interdisciplinary dentofacial therapy will be discussed in the remaining portion of this chapter and in Chapters 5, 6, and 7 from the perspective of a team that uses regular meetings. However, this same philosophy can be combined with the information in Chapter 8 to enable similar IDT results with a local or long-distance team.

Interdisciplinary Problem List

The interdisciplinary team must now interact to combine their unidisciplinary concerns (which make up the multidisciplinary database) and classify them into an *interdisciplinary problem list* (Fig 4-9). The database should be arranged by the team so that it gives a systematic description of the patient's problems that can be easily referred to during the treatment-planning process. The classification method also helps ensure that all important aspects have been evaluated and that nothing has been overlooked.

Some useful categories for classification are given in the following list.

1. chief concern/motivation/expectations
2. history (physical statistics, medical, dental)
3. facial/skeletal
4. temporomandibular
5. occlusion (static and functional)
6. periodontal
7. dental/implant

These categories are listed in the suggested order that they should be evaluated during a dentofacial general evaluation. As discussed earlier, not everything on the problem list is necessarily a problem, but everything on the problem list should be pertinent to the patient's diagnosis and treatment plan.

Diagnosis

The final process in the diagnostics phase of IDT is the summarization of the interdisciplinary problem list into a *diagnosis* (Fig 4-9). Related problems should be combined into a major problem area so that only highlights are described. The subsequent diagnosis provides a brief description of the particular case and a useful classification system for different cases, but does not provide all the necessary information for developing a treatment plan. The entire interdisciplinary problem list will be used to formulate the definitive treatment plan.

With a diagnosis attained, the diagnostics phase of IDT is complete. The information gained in this phase will be combined in the treatment-planning phase of IDT with the team's knowledge, creativity, and clinical experience to derive optimal solutions to the patient's dentofacial problems.

Fig 4-9 (opposite page) Examples of an interdisciplinary problem list and diagnosis based on the Case Summary in Fig 2-5. The IDT team should classify the unorganized information in the multidisciplinary database into an interdisciplinary problem list. This gives a detailed and easily referenced systematic description of the patient's dentofacial problems. The final process in the diagnostic phase of IDT is the summarization of the interdisciplinary problem list into a diagnosis. The diagnosis briefly describes the different cases and provides a useful system to classify them.

Interdisciplinary Problem List

Chief Concern(s)/Motivation/Expectation

- "My teeth are small and far apart."
- Self-motivated for treatment
- Expects a prettier smile

History

- 15-year-old white female
- Poor self-image due to unattractive smile
- Unremarkable medical, temporomandibular, and dental histories

Facial/Skeletal

- Concave profile with insufficient lip support and strong chin button
- Short upper lip
- Excessive incisor exposure with lips at rest
- Excessive gingival display during smile
- Class I skeletal relationship with bimaxillary dentoalveolar retrusion
- Maxillary and mandibular dentoalveolar extrusion of anterior segments

Temporomandibular

- Unremarkable

Occlusion

- Class I dental malrelationship
- Excessive anterior vertical overlap and insufficient anterior horizontal overlap
- Anterior crossbite 12, 32, and 53
- Unstable and traumatic interincisal relationship
- Initial centric contact is on left second molar and mandible shifts 1.5 mm anteriorly into maximum intercuspation position
- Traumatic functional occlusion with severe working and balancing interferences
- No anterior guidance

Periodontal

- Excessive free and attached gingival tissues throughout maxillary arch
- Minimal attached gingival tissues in mandibular anterior region

Dental/Implant

- Generalized microdontia with excess archlength and spacing in both arches
- Peg lateral incisors teeth 12 and 22
- Retroclined maxillary and mandibular incisors
- Retained maxillary primary canines with severe wear
- Defective restoration tooth 31
- Impacted maxillary canines and maxillary right second molar

Diagnosis

Class I skeletal and dental malrelationship with bimaxillary dentoalveolar retrusion, excessive gingival display, and microdontia

References

1. Proffit WR, Epker BN, Ackerman JL. Systematic description of dentofacial deformities: the data base. In: Bell WH, Proffit WR, White RP (eds): Surgical Correction of Dentofacial Deformities. Philadelphia: Saunders, 1980: 105–154.
2. Proffit WR, Fields HW. Orthodontic treatment planning: from problem list to final plan. In: Proffit WR. Contemporary Orthodontics, ed 2. St Louis: Mosby, 1992: 186–224.
3. Proffit WR, Ackerman JL. Orthodontic diagnosis: the development of a problem list. In: Proffit WR: Contemporary Orthodontics, ed 2. St Louis: Mosby, 1992: 139–185.
4. Proffit WR, Epker BN. Treatment planning for dentofacial deformities. In: Bell WH, Proffit WR, White RP (eds). Surgical Correction of Dentofacial Deformities. Philadelphia: Saunders, 1980: 155–199.
5. Proffit WR, Ackerman JL. Diagnosis and treatment planning in orthodontics. In: Graber TM, Swain BF (eds). Orthodontics—Current Principles and Techniques. St Louis: Mosby, 1985: 3–100.
6. Scully C, Boyle P. Reliability of a self-administered questionnaire for screening medical problems in dentistry. Community Dent Oral Epidemiol 1983;11:105–108.
7. Trieger N, Goldblatt L. The art of history taking. J Oral Surg 1978;36:118–124.
8. Roblee RD. The determination of the accuracy and reproducibility of six maxillomandibular relation techniques [master's thesis]. Dallas, Baylor College of Dentistry, 1989.
9. Allen EP. Use of mucogingival surgical procedures to enhance esthetics. Dent Clin North Am 1988;32:307–333.
10. Wilson TG. Examination, diagnosis, classification, and disease activity for patients with periodontal diseases. In: Wilson TG. Dental Maintenance for Patients with Periodontal Diseases. Chicago: Quintessence, 1989: 17–37.
11. Rudd KD, Morrow RM, Strunk RR. Accurate alginate impressions. J Pros Dent 1969;22:294–300.
12. Vanarsdall RL, Musich DR. Adult orthodontics: diagnosis and treatment. In: Graber TM, Swain BF (eds). Orthodontics: Current Principles and Techniques. St Louis: Mosby, 1985: 791–856.
13. Ericsson I, Thilander B. Orthodontic forces and recurrence of periodontal disease. Am J Orthod 1978;71:41–50.
14. Ericsson I, Thilander B, Lindhe J, Okamoto H. The effect of orthodontic tilting movements in the periodontal tissue of infected and non-infected dentitions in dogs. J Clin Periodontol 1977;4:278–293.
15. Ericsson I, Thilander B, Lindhe J. Periodontal conditions after orthodontic tooth movements in the dog. Angle Orthod 1978;48:210–218.
16. Kokich VC. Enhancing restorative, esthetic, and periodontal results with orthodontic treatment. In: Schluger S, Youdelis R, Page RC, Johnson RH (eds). Periodontal Diseases, ed 2. Philadelphia: Lea and Febiger, 1990: 433–460.
17. Boyd RL, Leggott PJ, Quinn RS, Eakle WS, Chambers D. Periodontal implications of orthodontic treatment in adults with reduced or normal periodontal tissues versus those of adolescents. Am J Orthod Dentofacial Orthop 1989; 96:191–199.
18. Rosling BG, McGuire MK. Mild chronic adult periodontitis. In: Wilson TG, Korman KS, Newman MG (eds). Advances in Periodontics. Chicago: Quintessence, 1992: 124–142.
19. Caffesse RG, Sweeney PL, Smith BA. Scaling and root planing with and without periodontal flap surgery. J Clin Periodontol 1986;13:205–210.
20. Wilson TG. Disruption or reduction of bacterial populations in the oral cavity. In: Wilson TG. Dental Maintenance for Patients with Periodontal Diseases. Chicago: Quintessence, 1989: 51–57.
21. Steffensen B, Sottosanti JS. Chronic gingivitis. In: Wilson TG, Korman KS, Newman MG (eds). Advances in Periodontics. Chicago: Quintessence, 1992: 103–123.
22. Brunsvold MA, Lane JJ. The prevalence of overhanging dental restorations and their relationships to periodontal disease. J Clin Periodontol 1990;17:67–72.
23. Lindhe J, Svanberg G. Influence of trauma from occlusion on progression of experimental periodontitis in the beagle dog. J Clin Periodontol 1974;1:3–14.
24. Amsterdam M, Vanarsdall RL. Periodontal prosthesis-twenty-five years in retrospect. Alpha Omegan, December 1974.
25. Caffesse RG, Fleszar TJ: Occlusal trauma. In: Wilson TG, Korman KS, Newman MG (eds). Advances in Periodontics. Chicago: Quintessence, 1992: 205–225.
26. Yulzari JC. Strategic extractions in periodontal prosthesis. Int J Periodont Rest Dent 1982;2:50–65.
27. Chaves ES, Caffesse RG, Morrison EC, Stults DL. Diagnostic discrimination of bleeding on probing during maintenance periodontal therapy. Am J Dent 1990;3:167–170.
28. Wilson TG, Glover ME. Treatment sequencing. In: Wilson TG. Dental Maintenance for Patients with Periodontal Diseases. Chicago: Quintessence, 1989: 41–50.
29. Williams RC, Kaldahl WB, Kalkwarf KL. Periodontal disease activity. In: Wilson TG, Korman KS, Newman MG (eds). Advances in Periodontics. Chicago: Quintessence, 1992; 58–73.
30. Goerig AC, Neaverth EJ. Case selection and treatment planning. In: Cohen S, Burns RC (eds). Pathways of the Pulp, ed 5. St Louis: Mosby, 1991: 48–60.
31. Glickman GN, Schwartz SF. Preparation for treatment. In: Cohen S, Burns RC (eds). Pathways of the Pulp, ed 5. St Louis: Mosby, 1991; 61–93.
32. Stabholz A, Friedman S, Tamse A. Endodontic failures and retreatment. In: Cohen S, Burns RC (eds): Pathways of the Pulp, ed 5. St Louis: Mosby, 1991; 738–797.
33. McNeill C (ed). Current Controversies in Temporomandibular Disorders. Chicago: Quintessence, 1992.
34. American Academy of Orofacial Pain. Temporomandibular Disorders: Guidelines for Classification, Assessment, and Management. Chicago: Quintessence, 1993.
35. Litrak H, Malament KA. Prosthodontic management of temporomandibular disorders and orofacial pain. J Prosthet Dent 1993;69:77–84.

36. Bell, WE. Orofacial Pain: Classification, Diagnosis, Management, ed 4. Chicago: Year Book Medical Publishers, 1989.
37. Travell, JG, Simons, DG. Myofacial Pain and Dysfunction: The trigger point manual. Baltimore: Williams and Wilkins, 1983.
38. Roth RH. Functional occlusion for the orthodontist. I-IV, J Clin Orthod 1981;15(1–4) 1981.
39. Williamson EH. Orthodontic implications in diagnosis, prevention, and treatment of TMJ dysfunction. In: Graber TM, Swain BF (eds). Orthodontics: Current Principles and Techniques. St. Louis: Mosby, 1985: 229–258.
40. Randolph CS, Greene CS, et al. Conservative management of temporomandibular disorders: A posttreatment comparison between patients from a university clinic and from private practice. Am J Orthod Dentofacial Orthop 1990;98:77–82.
41. Syrop SB. Nonsurgical management of temporomandibular disorders. In: Principles of Oral and Maxillofacial Surgery, vol 3. Philadelphia: Lippincott, 1992: 1905–1931.
42. Holmgren K, Sheikholeslam A, Riise C. Effect of a full-arch maxillary splint on parafunctional activity during sleep in patients with nocturnal bruxism and signs and symptoms of craniomandibular disorders. J Prosthet Dent 1993; 69:293–297.
43. Okun JH. Temporomandibular disorders. Am J Orthod Dentofacial Orthop 1992;102:475–476.
44. Nitzan DW, Dolwick MF, Martinez GA. Temporomandibular joint arthrocentesis: A simplified treatment for severe, limited mouth opening. J Oral Maxillofac Surg 1991;49:1163–1167.
45. Temporomandibular joint arthroscopy: A 6 year multicenter retrospective study of 4,831 joints. J Oral Maxillofac Surg 1992;50:926–930.
46. White RD. Retrospective analysis of 100 consecutive surgical arthroscopies of the temporomandibular joint. J Oral Maxillofac Surg 1989;47:1014–1021.
47. Keith, DA. Surgical management of degenerative joint disease. In: Principles of Oral and Maxillofacial Surgery, vol 3. Philadelphia: Lippincott, 1992: 1969–1987.
48. Hill SC. Surgical management of internal derangements of the temporomandibular joint. In: Bell WH (ed). Modern practice in orthognathic and reconstructive surgery. Philadelphia: Saunders, 1992: 702–715.
49. Piper MA. Microscopic disk preservation surgery of the temporomandibular joint. Oral Maxillofac Surg Clin N Am 1989;1:279–303.
50. McBride KL. Total joint reconstruction. In: Bell WH (ed). Modern Practice in Orthognathic and Reconstruction Surgery. Philadelphia: Saunders, 1992: 736–829.
51. Araz B, Nitzan DW, Brin I. Condylar hyperplasia: remodeling of facial structures following condylectomy: Two case reports. Int J Adult Orthod Orthognath Surg 1991;6:47–55.
52. Dryer EH. Importance of a stable maxillomandibular relation. J Prosthet Dent 1973;30:241–242.
53. Solberg WK, et al. Temporomandibular joint pain and dysfunction: a clinical study of emotional and occlusal components. J Prosthet Dent 1972;28:412.
54. Molin C, Edman G Schalling D. Psychological studies of patients with mandibular pain dysfunction syndrome (MDS). II: Tolerance for experimentally induced pain. Swed Dent J 1973;66:15–23.
55. Marbach JJ, Lund P. Depression, anhedonia and anxiety in temporomandibular joint and other facial pain syndromes. Pain 1981;11:73–84.
56. Peterson LJ, Topazian RG. Psychologic evaluation of candidates for dentofacial therapy. In: Bell WH, Proffit WR, White RP (eds). Surgical Correction of Dentofacial Deformities. Philadelphia: Saunders, 1980: 90–104.
57. McGlynn FD, Gale EN, Glaros AG, LeResche L, Massoth DL, Weiffenbach JM. Biobehavioural research in dentistry: some directions for the 1990's. Ann Behav Med 1990;12:133–140.
58. Ciancio SG. Detection and management of the high risk periodontal patient. Int Dent J 1991;41:300–304.

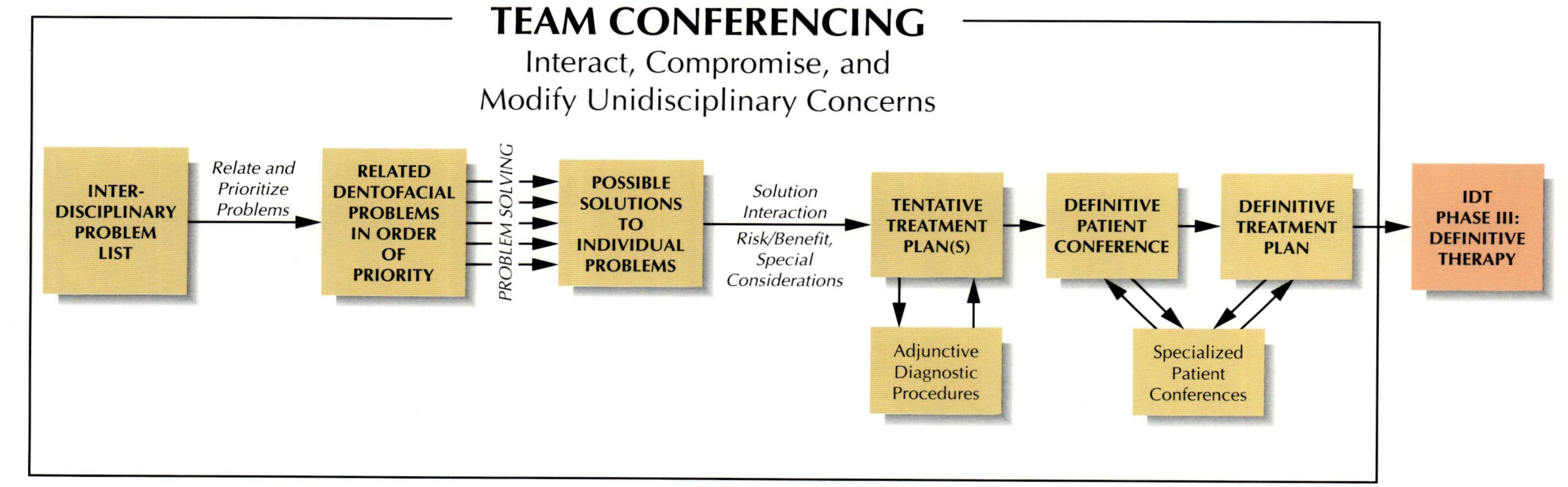

TREATMENT PLANNING: IDT PHASE II

5

Treatment Planning

Phase II of IDT

The treatment-planning process during the interdisciplinary team meetings or through interdisciplinary correspondence must follow a logical sequence to develop an interdisciplinary problem list into a definitive treatment plan. The main purpose of this sequence is to promote team conferencing through meetings and/or correspondence and enable individual team members to interact each member's unidisciplinary concerns. This interaction allows the members to debate the importance of the different dentofacial problems and therapies, compromise their unidisciplinary treatment goals into interdisciplinary treatment goals, and then modify their treatment strategy accordingly to arrive at an unbiased treatment plan that promotes optimal overall results. This interdisciplinary compromise is highly positive in nature. The individual concerns of the different members must be compromised according to their relative importance to the overall treatment.[1]

The format of treatment planning outlined in this chapter is a consistent and highly organized method of processing all the detailed information accumulated in the diagnostic phase. At first this format may seem long and cumbersome; however, interdisciplinary teams and individual providers should use it to develop their treatment-planning skills. With practice, this style can actually become second nature, and providers will be able to automatically go through the different steps in their minds. These learned treatment-planning skills can be a tremendous asset to providers, whether treating simple cases as individual providers, or using the knowledge and skills of an interdisciplinary team for more complex cases.

Interdisciplinary Problem List

The development of an interdisciplinary problem list was discussed in detail in Chapter 4. This list is a very useful and organized way to systematically describe a patient's dentofacial problems (Fig 5-1). Listing problems in this way helps ensure that all areas have been evaluated in the diagnostic phase.

The list also serves as a valuable reference throughout the treatment-planning and definitive-therapy phases of IDT (Fig 2-5). It is, however, an inefficient arrangement of problems from which to develop a treatment plan, because problems from different categories on the list are frequently related to each other in their overall dentofacial effect. For example, the excessive gingival exposure during smiling in Fig 2-5 is related to several problems listed in different categories: a short upper lip, dentoalveolar extrusion, and short clinical crowns with excessive gingival tissues. To efficiently address overall dentofacial problems while planning treatment, individual problems should be organized in relation to their overall effects. The interdisciplinary problem list also gives no information about the relative importance of each individual problem, thus further limiting its effectiveness in treatment planning. For these reasons, the team should relate and prioritize problems before formulating treatment plans.

Relate and Prioritize Problems

The first step in the treatment-planning phase of IDT is to relate problems on the interdisciplinary problem list. This is done by organizing the list into categories of the major effects of the combined problems with all related problems listed in these categories to define and modify the patient's unique dentofacial circumstances (Fig 5-2). When an underlying problem is related to two or more overall effects, it should be listed in each of the associated categories. If a problem is not related to any other problems (for example, an isolated carious lesion), it should be listed by itself. Patient history, statistics, and other information on the interdisciplinary problem list that are not actual problems (such as "15-year-old female" in Fig 2-5) do not need to be included on the list of related problems, because the team can easily refer to the interdisciplinary problem list if that information is needed while treatment planning. Relating problems by their overall effects will greatly facilitate the problem-solving process.

The next step is to prioritize the problems in order of importance. First, the groups of overall effects should be prioritized; then, the individual related problems that define and modify the overall effects should be prioritized within each group (Fig 5-2). The prioritization of the problems is important because it is frequently not possible to address all the problems associated with complex dentofacial treatment. Prioritization helps assure that the most important problems will be properly addressed.[1]

In the prioritization process, the individual team members debate the importance of each problem in reference to their own area of expertise. However, it is crucial that the patient's chief concern also be used for setting the priorities.[1] There is often a great deal of discrepancy between what the providers and the patient think are important. This prioritization process aids in best addressing everyone's concerns.

Problem Solving

The final list of related dentofacial problems in order of priority having been constructed, the team should list all possible solutions to individual problems (Fig 5-2).[1] This problem-solving exercise is invaluable for optimally planning treatment in a complex dentofacial case because it requires all team members to look at each problem individually. No problems should be overlooked, even the ones of lowest priority. One or more tentative treatment plans will be formulated as a result of the process. These treatment plans are called tentative because they are suggested as trials and will undergo much scrutiny before formulation of a definitive treatment plan. General therapeutic suggestions should be made during this problem-solving process, because the specifics of needed therapy will be ironed out after the tentative treatment plans become more focused.

The problem-solving exercise often allows the team to turn apparent disadvantages in the dentofacial case into advantages that will help solve other more complex problems (Fig 5-3). Treatment planning through problem solving is usually an enjoyable process, because the solutions and their interactions are often subjective in nature, and creativity and clinical experience are frequently as useful as pure dental knowledge. With all the different disciplines being represented, problem solving can be an educational experience in itself, and each individual member's knowledge of dentofacial problems and their solutions is sure to be enhanced.

Related Problems in Order of Priority

Excess archlength with spacing and subsequent dental instability

- Microdontia
- Peg lateral incisors 12 and 22

Excessive gingival display during smile

- Excessive incisor exposure with lips in repose
- Short upper lip
- Maxillary dentoalveolar extrusion of anterior segment
- Short clinical crowns with excessive free and attached gingiva in maxillary anterior segment

Traumatic functional occlusion with severe working and balancing interferences

- No anterior guidance
  - Impacted maxillary canines
  - Retained maxillary primary canines with severe wear
- Initial centric contact is on left second molars and mandible shifts 1.5 mm anteriorly into maximum intercuspation position
- Unstable and traumatic interincisal relationship
  - Retroclined maxillary and mandibular incisors
  - Excessive anterior vertical overlap
  - Insufficient anterior horizontal overlap
  - Maxillary and mandibular dentoalveolar extrusion
  - Anterior crossbite teeth 12, 32, and 53

Concave profile

- Insufficient lip support
  - Maxillary and mandibular dentoalveolar retrusion
  - Retroclined maxillary and mandibular incisors

Impacted maxillary right second molar

Minimal attached gingival tissues in mandibular anterior region

Defective restoration tooth 31

Fig 5-1 Example of skeletal problems in order of priority based on the Case Summary in Fig 2-5 (refere to the Problem List). To simplify the treatment-planning process, the individual problems on the interdisciplinary problem list are related to their overall effects. Then these overall effects and individual problems are prioritized to assure that the higher ranking problems will be properly addressed. The result is a list of related problems in order of priority that provides an efficient arrangement for optimal treatment-planning procedures.

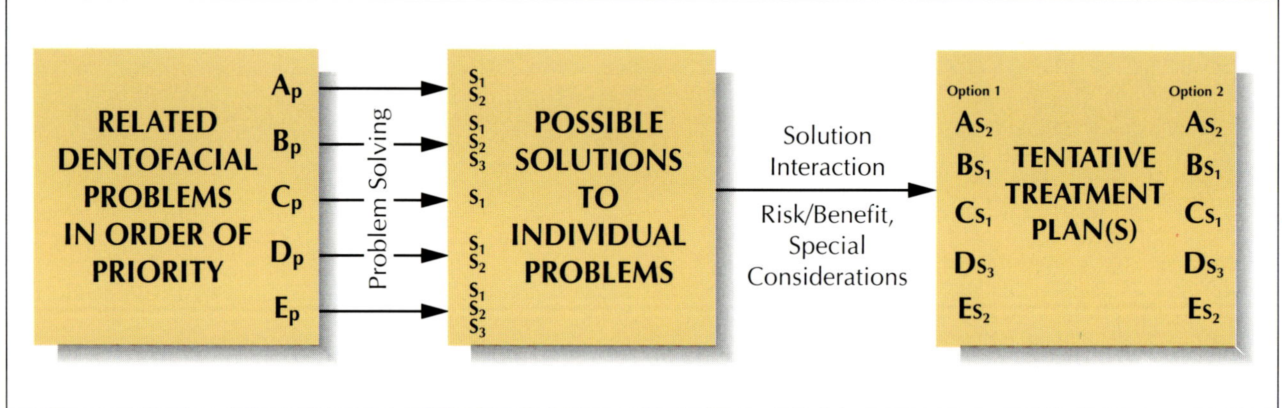

Fig 5-2 An interdisciplinary team must have a sophisticated method to address complex dentofacial problems so that they can consistently formulate the best treatment plan for each patient. The problem-solving approach to treatment planning is represented in the chart. The interdisciplinary problem list is an organized way to systematically describe patient's dentofacial problems and history; and it serves as a valuable and efficient reference throughout IDT. It is not, however, the most effective arrangement for treatment planning. To overcome this shortcoming, the problem list should be rearranged into a list of related dentofacial problems in order of priority, so that the team or individual members can undergo a more effective problem-solving exercise.

During problem solving, the team members will take each individual problem, in the new order, and list all possible solutions to that problem. At this point in the treatment-planning session, it is not important how the individual solutions to the various solutions interact with one another. After the list of all the possible solutions to individual problems has been completed, however, solution interaction should begin. This will evaluate the effects the individual problem solutions have on each other and on the overall problems. The solutions should be selected that will solve the greatest percentage of the highest-priority problems and give the best overall treatment result. These solutions must then undergo further scrutiny with risk/benefit and special-consideration analyses. The result of these analyses will be one or more tentative treatment plans. These plans are tentative because they are suggested as a trial. Tentative treatment plans should not be highly detailed until necessary adjunctive diagnostic procedures have been performed and the patient has made a final decision during the definitive patient conference. The resulting tentative treatment plan will then be expanded in its scope and detail, and developed into the definitive treatment plan.

This problem-solving approach to treatment planning is highly effective at developing the best overall treatment plan for each individual patient, whether it is performed by an individual provider or an IDT team. The team interaction during the problem-solving process is also one of the most useful tools for educating the individual team members about each other's therapy and the overall interdisciplinary process. With time, it will not be as necessary for the interdisciplinary team to go through this complex and time-consuming problem-solving process. As this approach to treatment planning becomes more second nature, the individual providers will begin to subconsciously evaluate and plan treatment for cases in this fashion.

Case Summary

Patient: J.D. is a 58-year-old female who reported for a second opinion concerning her dentofacial needs. She was told by another dental provider that her needs could only be fulfilled through full-mouth extractions and complete dentures. She reported that her dentofacial appearance had been rapidly declining over the last few years, especially since a unidisciplinary full-mouth reconstruction was performed a few years ago.

Chief Concern: "My smile is not as pretty as it used to be."

Abbreviated Problem List

- Class II skeletal relationship with high mandibular plane angle and increased lower face height
- Vertical maxillary excess ("gummy smile")
- Insufficient maxillary lip support
- Previously performed unidisciplinary full-mouth reconstruction
- Asymmetrical gingival contours
- Redundant soft tissue covering alveolar ridge in maxillary anterior edentulous area
- Severe maxillary and mandibular periodontal problems

Treatment Plan

Interdisciplinary Dentofacial Therapy

- Definitive Periodontal Therapy
    - Maxillary and mandibular soft tissue and osseous periodontal therapy
    - Extract teeth 17, 18, 25, and 27
    - Bone fill procedures on tooth 24
- Preparatory Restorative-Type III Therapy
    - Locate ideal dental relationships to allow optimal ridge recontouring procedures and healing
    - Decrease vertical dimension and enhance maxillary lip support
- Periodontal Plastic Surgery
    - Recontour redundant soft tissue ridge as dictated by the provisional restoration to allow eventual placement of optimal definitive restorations
- Definitive Restorative Therapy
    - Full-mouth reconstruction

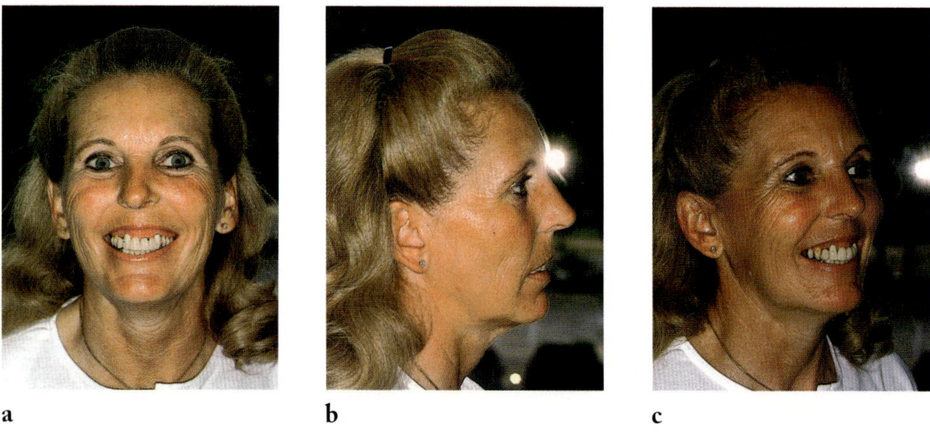

a b c

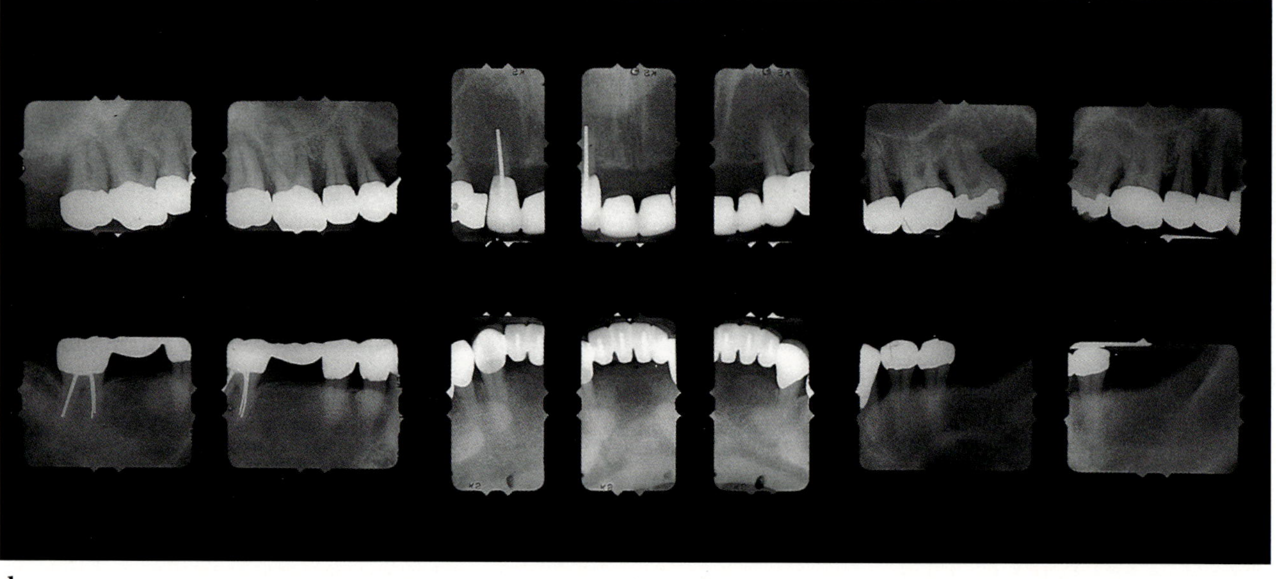

d

Fig 5-3

a to c Initial facial views illustrating vertical maxillary excess, increased lower face height, and asymmetrical gingival contours.

d Initial full-mouth radiographic survey illustrating the severe periodontal problems throughout the dentition and the redundant soft tissue in maxillary anterior edentulous area.

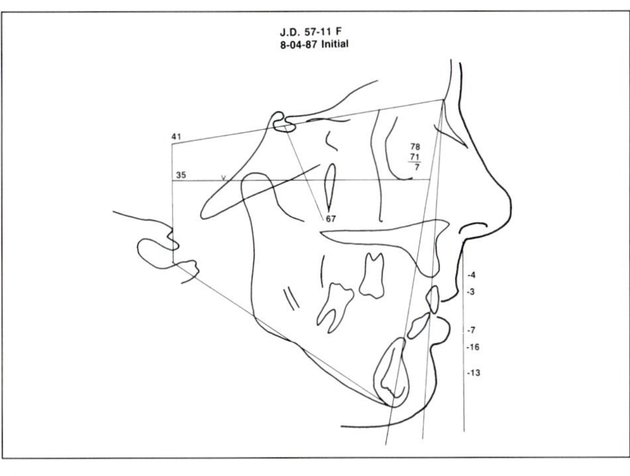

e

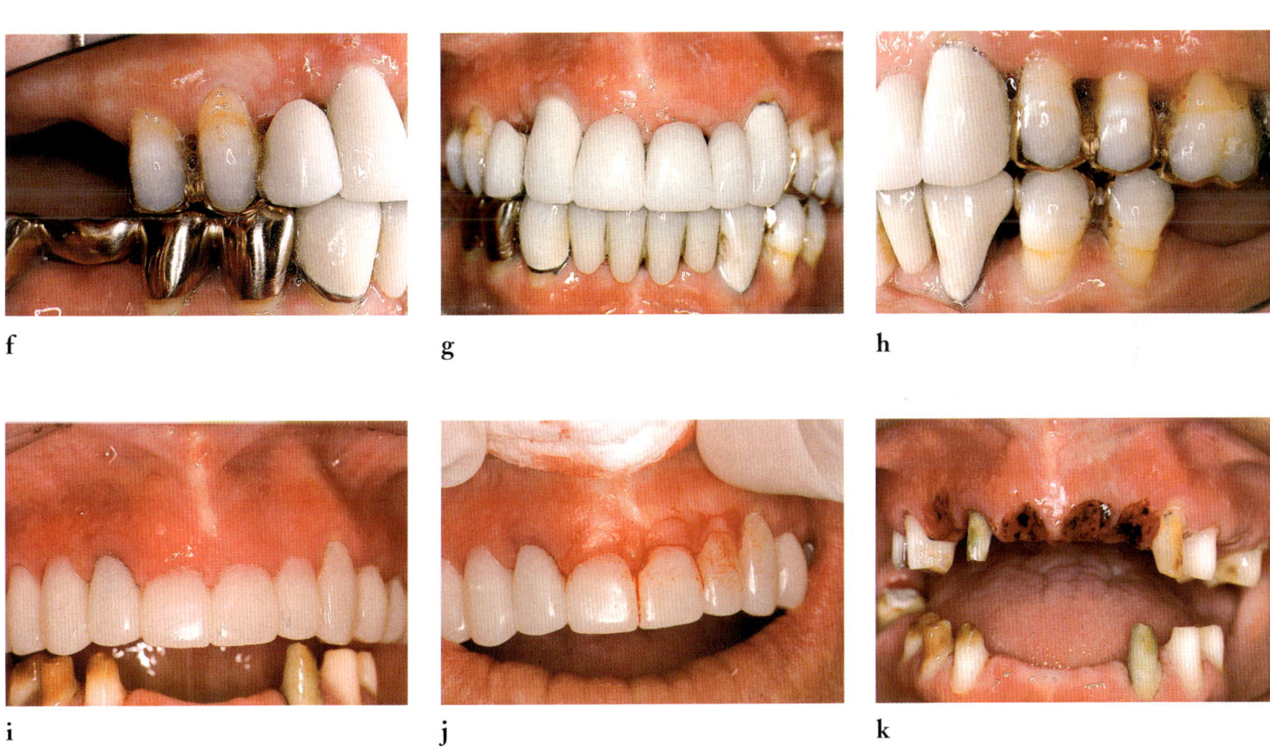

f g h

i j k

Fig 5-3 (continued)

e Initial cephalometric analysis.

f to h Intraoral appearance after the pathology control aspects of definitive periodontal therapy were completed.

i Provisional restorations were constructed to represent ideal maxillary incisal relationships (preparatory restorative-type III therapy) and to decrease lower face height approximately 4.5 mm.

j Optimal gingival relationships of the maxillary anterior pontics were marked on the alveolar ridge.

k Redundant soft tissue on the maxillary anterior alveolar ridge was recontoured with periodontal plastic procedures to allow placement of optimal-length pontics.

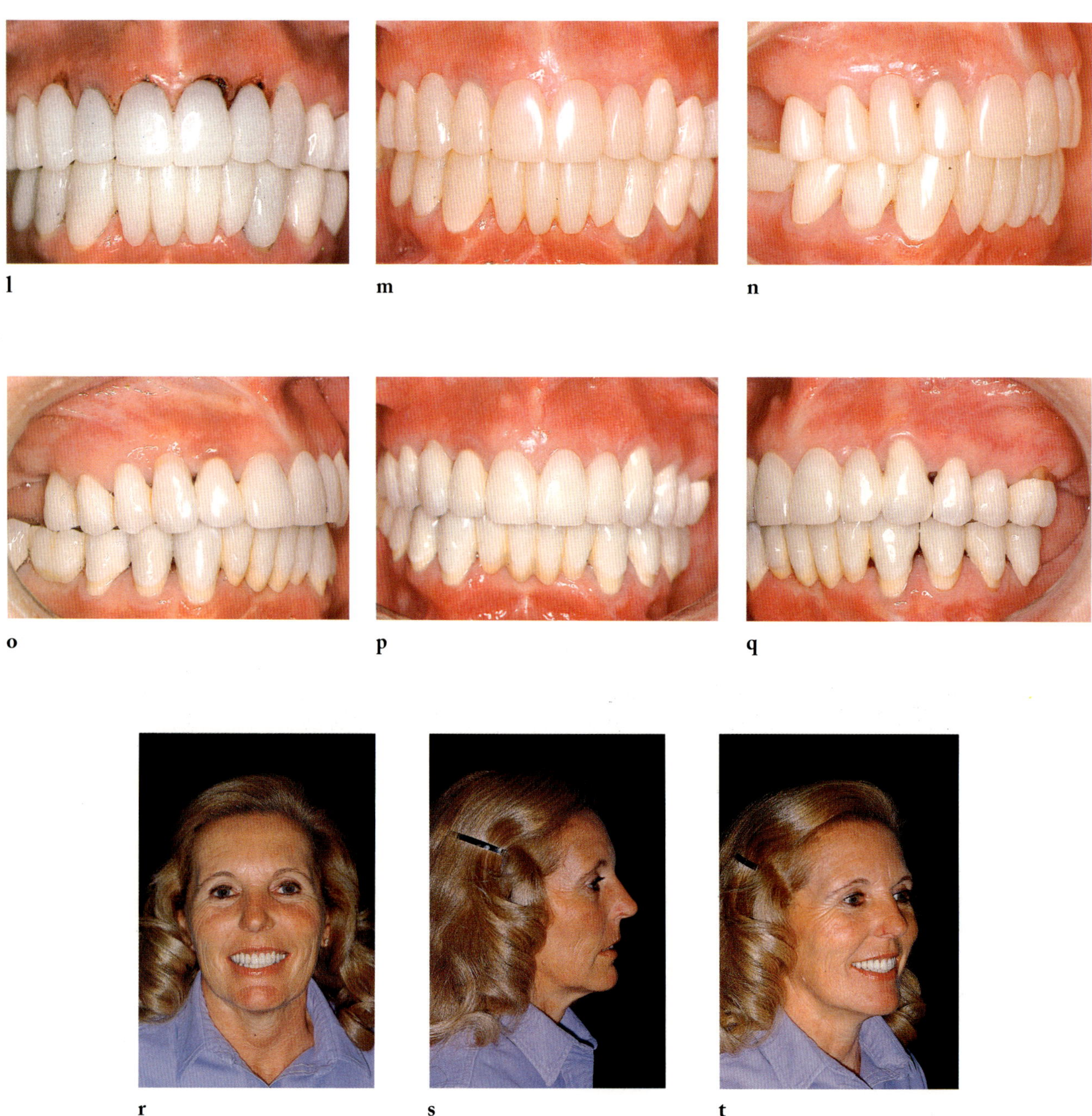

Fig 5-3 (continued)

l The provisional restorations shown in *i* were modified to extend into the newly recontoured soft tissue.

m, n Intraoral appearance 3 months after ridge-recontouring procedures and placement of the provisional restoration.

o to q Final intraoral appearance after definitive restorations were placed. Gingival contours and symmetry have been greatly enhanced and the pontics replacing teeth 11, 12, 21, and 23 appear to be coming directly out of the soft tissue.

r to t Final facial appearance illustrating significant reduction in the appearance of vertical maxillary excess. Lower face height has also been decreased and lip support has been enhanced. Note more youthful and relaxed appearance of patient.

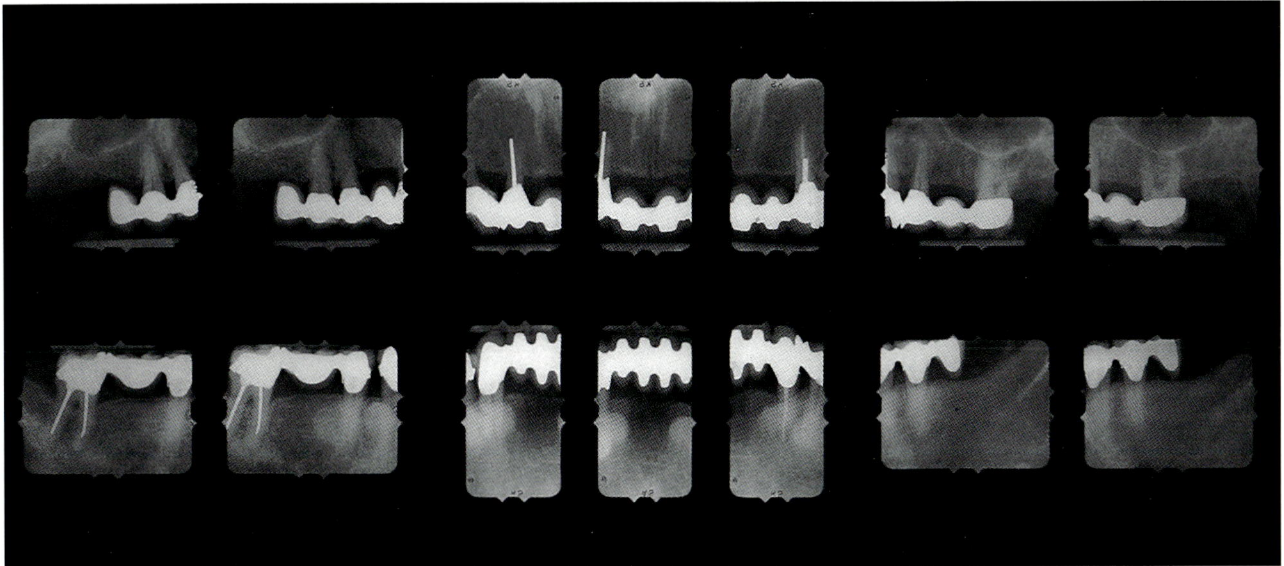

u

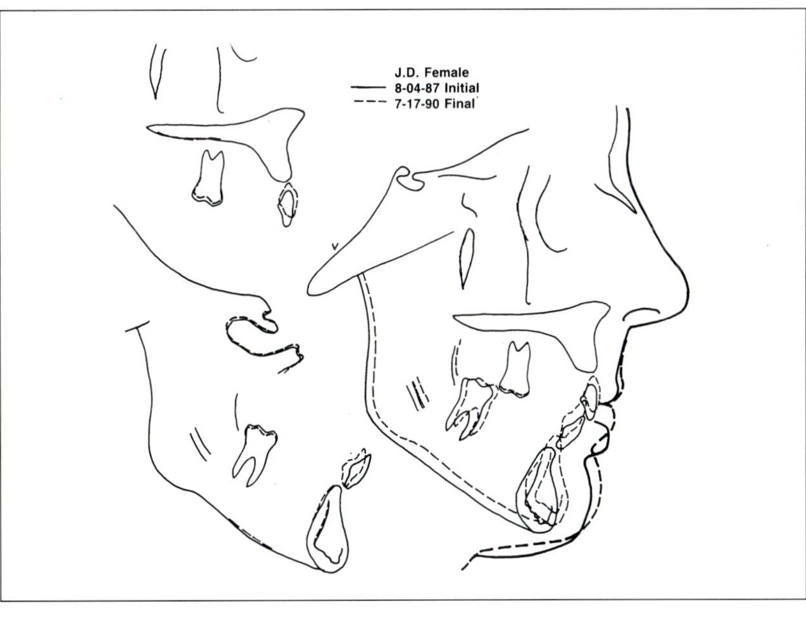

v

Fig 5-3 (continued)

u One year posttreatment full-mouth radiographic survey.

v Superimposition of initial and final cephalometric analyses. Note the effects of decreasing lower face height.

Periodontist (Periodontal Therapy): Robert Lee Johnson, DDS
Periodontist (Periodontal Plastic Surgery): Edward P. Allen, DDS, PhD
Restorative Dentist: Richard D. Roblee, DDS, MS/*Laboratory Technician:* Jeffrey Singler, CDT

Discussion

As in Fig 2-5, this case illustrates how an interdisciplinary team can conservatively correct complex dentofacial problems. Initially, it was thought that this patient needed a surgical maxillary impaction and advancement to provide optimal correction of her problems, but creative problem solving allowed the interdisciplinary team to solve this patient's problem without an orthognathic surgical procedure. This case is also a good example of how interdisciplinary diagnostics and problems solving can turn problems into advantages to help solve other problems. The redundant soft tissue in the anterior maxilla was first seen as a problem, but it was eventually used to solve optimally the other problems of asymmetrical gingival contours, "gummy smile," and excessive lower face height. It is felt that many of these problems were created iatrogenically during her previous unidisciplinary reconstruction. The previous restorative dentist had apparently viewed the redundant tissue as a problem, and subsequently opened the vertical dimension to place the maxillary anterior pontics in what he thought was the only relationship which would give them normal size. Through preparatory restorative procedures, the interdisciplinary restorative dentist was able to use his expertise in dental function and esthetics to give the periodontist the necessary information needed to optimally prepare the maxillary anterior soft tissue ridge to eventually accept an ideal dental reconstruction. The provisional restorations also served as an adjunctive diagnostic tool, testing the restorative changes in esthetic, periodontal, functional, and vertical relationships before definitive restorative therapy was performed. This case illustrates the importance of a thorough dentofacial evaluation when performing extensive surgical therapy or even when performing only restorative and/or periodontal therapy.

Solution Interaction

Each individual problem on the list of related problems in order of priority (Fig 5-2) should now have all of its possible solutions listed. At this point, the team must sift through all individual problem solutions and evaluate the effect they would have on each of the other problems.[2] The team must then be decided which solutions will solve the greatest percent of the highest-priority problems and give the best results. It is usually not possible to ideally solve all of a patient's dentofacial problems, but through the process described, the majority of the higher-priority problems will be appropriately addressed. To accomplish this, team members must continue to interact, compromise, and modify their unidisciplinary concerns. The team must also consider special considerations and the risk/benefit ratio while formulating treatment plans.[1,3]

Special Considerations

The special considerations are characteristics unique to a case that could have a major impact on the course of therapy, and which should be addressed at this point in treatment. (Fig 5-2) The patient's chief concern should have already been addressed in the prioritization of the problem list. However, the patient may have had other concerns that affect the treatment more than the final result; for example, a person who, due to their personal or professional needs must maintain high esthetics throughout treatment (Fig 5-4). A patient with these concerns obviously may require different treatment modalities (such as more esthetic ceramic or lingual, rather than metal, braces) to arrive at optimal results, compared to the patient without such concerns. These patients may require the interdisciplinary team to spend more time and creativity in the treatment-planning phase.

Other special concerns may be more of a physical than psychological nature. For example, the patient may have some type of systemic disorder (such as diabetes mellitus) that will have to be considered throughout treatment. In addition, the patient may be taking medication such as anticoagulants or steroids that must be considered in the treatment plan(s). The patient also may have specific periodontal, temporomandibular, or dental problems which may have to be monitored throughout therapy. The therapy must be adjusted so that it does not exacerbate these problems. If any of these concerns is overlooked, it may lead to compromise or failure of the overall therapy, and treatment could potentially cause more harm than good.

Risk/Benefit Ratio

The team needs to evaluate the risk/benefit ratio of the treatment options to provide an optimal treatment plan to the patient (Fig 5-2). Obviously, all treatment should provide the greatest benefit to the patient possible; however, this must be accomplished so that the amount of risk (and expense) to the patient does not outweigh the benefit. In fact, the team must weigh all the different factors and decide if some problems are even worth addressing at all. This must be assessed openly and honestly among the team members, and eventually with the patient. The risk/benefit analysis is particularly effective when performed in an interdisciplinary environment because the risks are evaluated from many different perspectives. One solution may often create more problems than it solves, including potential complications, discomfort, invasiveness, or interference with another aspect of therapy. If the risk to the patient is much greater than the potential benefit to the patient, it is obviously not a good solution. Conversely, if the risk is high but the potential benefit is considered to be even higher, then the solution may merit consideration. Expenses or problems for the patient, such as money, cooperation, discomfort, and treatment time,[1,3] must also be considered in this analysis.

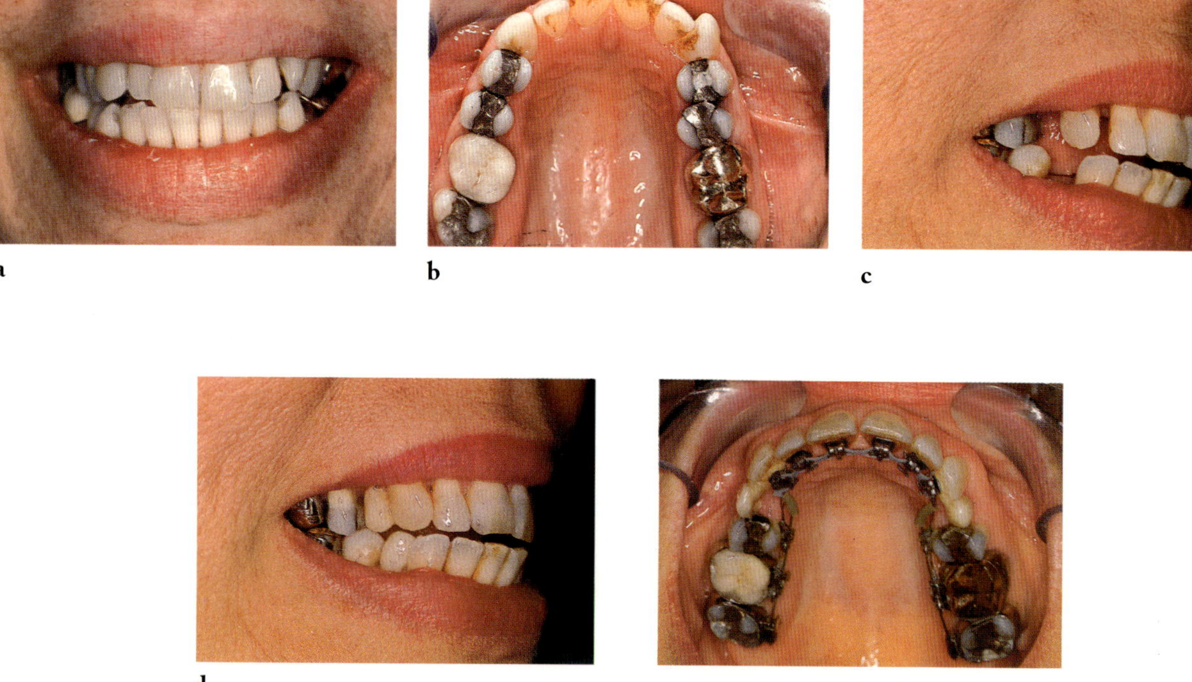

Fig 5-4

This patient presented with the special concern of maintaining high esthetics throughout therapy due to her professional needs. She could not tolerate the appearance of braces or extraction sites that would be present during traditional orthodontic extraction therapy.

a, b Initial smiling and maxillary occlusal views illustrating the severely crowded and rotated dentition.

c Lateral smiling view after lingual orthodontic appliances were placed and four first premolars extracted.

d Lateral smiling view after direct composite-resin pontics were bonded to the distal maxillary and mandibular canines to esthetically fill the extraction site.

e Occlusal view of pontics in place in conjunction with lingual orthodontics. The first premolar pontics will be gradually reduced on distal aspect to maintain esthetics while performing orthodontic space closure. Special concerns must be considered during treatment planning, as they can have a major impact on the course of therapy.

Adjunctive Diagnostic Procedures

At this point in the treatment-planning process, one or more adjunctive diagnostic procedures (Fig 5-5) may be necessary to work out the specifics suggested in the tentative treatment plans. Adjunctive diagnostic procedures may include any or all of the following procedures.

1. diagnostic waxup on dental casts to illustrate possible prosthetic changes (Fig 2-5k)[4];
2. orthodontic diagnostic setup of dental casts to illustrate orthodontic changes in the positions of teeth (Fig 6-24d);
3. surgical repositioning of dental casts to simulate orthognathic surgical procedures (Figs 5-5a.1 and 5-5a.2)[5–7];
4. tomograms (linear or multidirectional) or computed tomograms (CT scan) to evaluate the status of temporomandibular joints (Figs 5-5b and 5-5c)[8] and head and neck pathology (Figs 5-5d.1 and 5-5d.2), or to evaluate the regional anatomy on patients who may receive dental implants (Fig 5-5e.1 and 5-5e.2),[9–14] or prosthetic temporomandibular joint replacements
5. magnetic resonance imaging (MRI) for evaluating the integrity of condyle-disc relationships and for diagnosing the overall hard and soft tissue pathology of the temporomandibular joints (Figs 5-5f.1 and 5-5f.2),[15,16] and the head and neck region[17];
6. cephalometric predictions to illustrate orthodontic and surgical changes in the dental, skeletal, and soft tissue components (Fig 6-26g)[18];
7. computer imaging to simulate dentofacial esthetics following dental, skeletal, and soft tissue changes (Fig 5-6)[19];
8. other miscellaneous diagnostic procedures

These adjunctive procedures can provide invaluable information about the potential treatment options and their eventual results. For example, the diagnostic waxup can give the restorative dentist realistic information as to whether reconstruction is even a viable option; a diagnostic setup can give the orthodontist exact information on the direction and quantity of necessary tooth movement. In certain circumstances, one or more of these diagnostic procedures may have already been performed during the specialized evaluations in the diagnostic phase. Adjunctive diagnostic procedures also provide useful visual aids for the team during treatment-planning sessions and for the patient during dentofacial counseling and consultations. This is especially true with the advent of computer imaging that can easily simulate restorative, periodontal, orthodontic, and surgical changes for the patient (Fig 5-6).

Tentative Treatment Plan(s)

Several *tentative treatment plans* can usually be derived through the problem solving process (Fig 5-2). Again, these treatment plans are tentative, because they have been suggested as trials. These different plans usually have varying degrees of risks, expenses, and benefits for the patient. Frequently, the patient will have to make the final determination of the definitive treatment plan during the definitive patient conference according to what they perceive as being ideal for them (Fig 5-7).

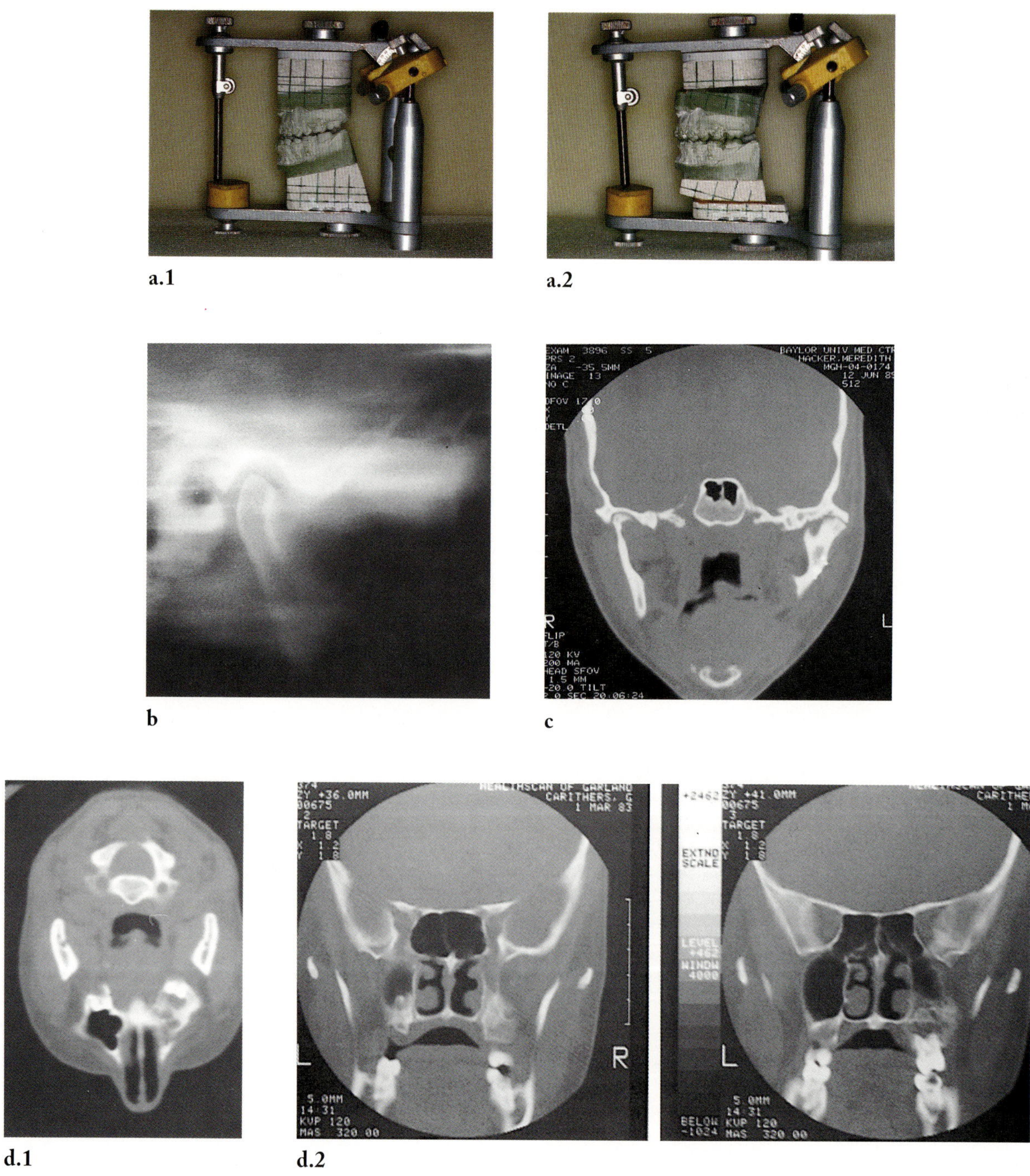

Fig 5-5 Adjunctive diagnostic procedures can provide invaluable information to the interdisciplinary team during the treatment-planning and definitive-therapy phases of treatment.

a.1 Mounted dental models and appropriate reference lines will allow orthognathic model surgery to predict hard tissue changes and to construct the surgical splint to be accurately performed, and to be correlated to the surgical treatment objective. (*Oral and Maxillofacial Surgeon:* Larry M. Wolford, DDS)

a.2 Model surgery was performed to simulate repositioning of the mandibular and maxillary components. These changes should correlate to the surgical treatment objective. (*Oral and Maxillofacial Surgeon:* Larry M. Wolford, DDS)

b Linear tomogram of the right TMJ demonstrates good morphology of the condyle and fossa with good joint space. A slight flattening of the antero-superior aspect of the condylar head is noted.

c Coronal (antero-posterior) CT scan through the TMJs shows relatively normal architecture of the right TMJ, although the condylar head is slightly small. The left TMJ has significant osteoarthritic changes with severe fibrous ankylosis.

d.1, d.2 CT scan of head and maxilla illustrating configuration of cementifying fibroma in the right posterior maxilla.(Courtesy of D. Lamar Byrd, DDS)

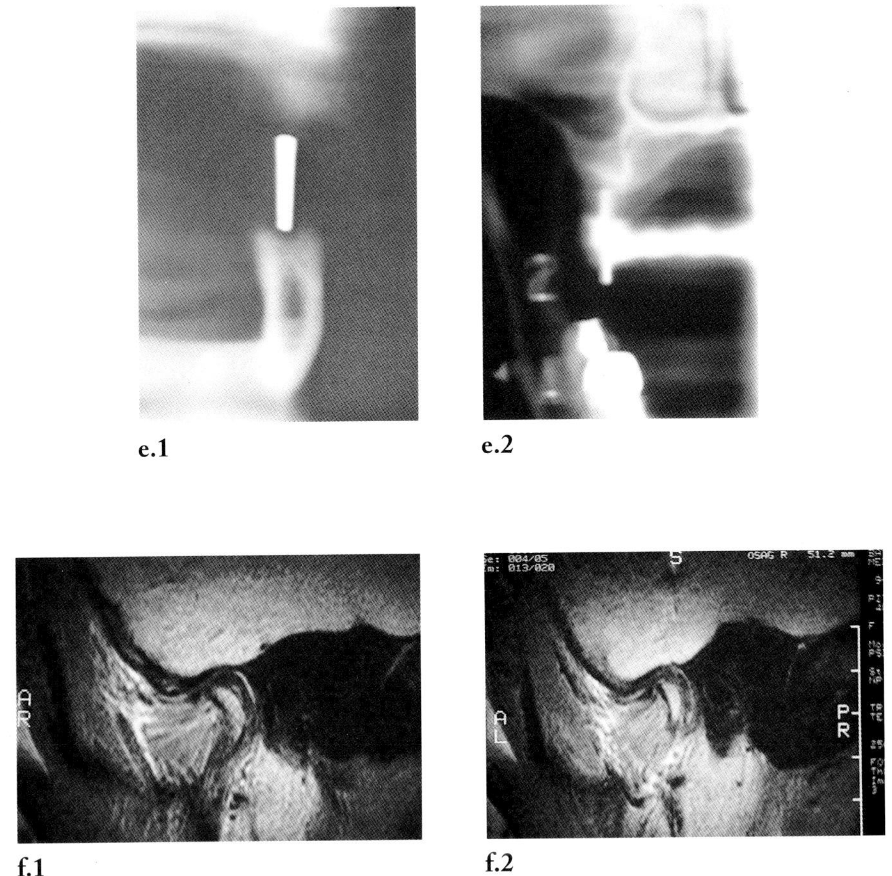

Fig 5-5 (continued)

e Linear tomograms can help determine configurations of regional anatomy and acceptability of proposed implant sites.

e.1 Mandibular first molar area with implant template in place. Note configuration of osseous tissues and mandibular canal.

e.2 Maxillary premolar area with implant templates in place. Note depth and width of bone and location of maxillary sinuses. (Courtesy of Richard W. Greenan.)

f Magnetic resonance image (MRI) of temporomandibular joints. MRIs are extremely useful for evaluating the integrity of the soft tissues of the TMJs.

f.1 A relatively normal MRI is seen with the articular disc in proper position. The posterior band is superior to the head of the condyle.

f.2 An anteriorly displaced disc is seen with the posterior band anterior to the head of the condyle and the anterior band on the anterior slope of the articular eminence. There are significant degenerative changes of the head of the condyle.

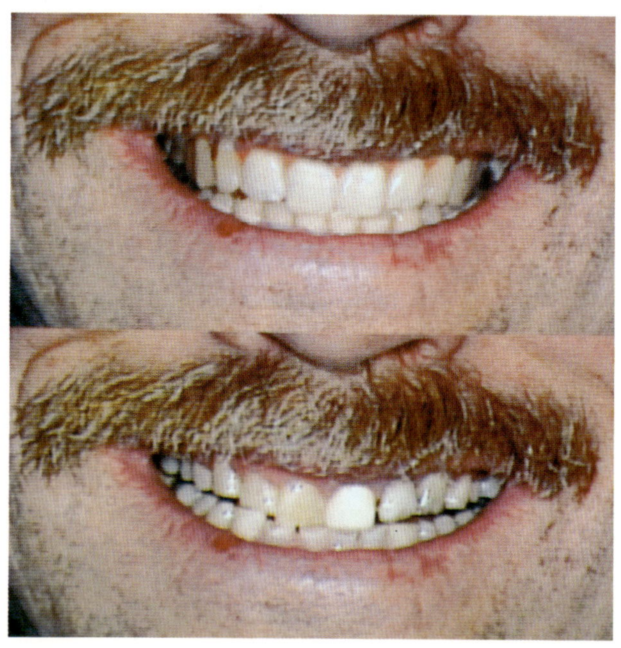

a

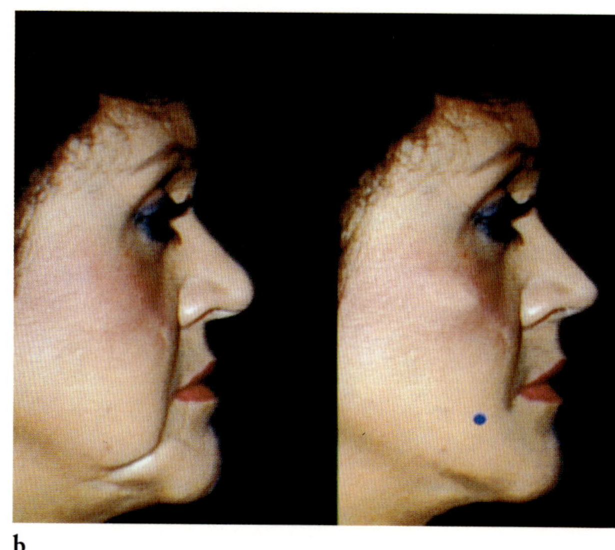

b

Fig 5-6

The adjunctive diagnostic procedure of computer imaging can be a powerful visual aid for educating patients of their dentofacial problems and potential treatment options during dentofacial counseling and patient consultations. Computer imaging can effectively simulate proposed periodontal, restorative, orthodontic and surgical changes for the patient and the interdisciplinary team. In both *a* and *b*, computer imaging was very successful in enhancing the patient's perceived value of treatment, and helped motivate both patients to accept comprehensive care.

a Split photograph of before and after imaging views of smile. Computer imaging was used to illustrate the esthetic results that could be obtained with periodontal plastic procedures (to properly align gingival contours and reduce "gummy smile") and a full-mouth dental reconstruction.

b Split photograph of before and after imaging of a patient who was in a severe auto accident twenty years ago and has subsequent dental, skeletal, and soft tissue deformities. Computer imaging was used to illustrate the resultant effects on the soft tissue profile of properly aligning the dentition and a maxillary advancement. Also imaged were the predicted changes predicted from the adjunctive facial cosmetic surgical procedures of a rhinoplasty, rhytidectomy (face lift), and a scar revision.

Case Summary

Patient: L.C. was a 28-year-old female who reported for dentofacial therapy primarily for esthetic reasons.

Chief Concern: "I don't like my smile."

Abbreviated Problem List

- Flat upper lip with deficient chin button
- Class II skeletal tendency with slightly retrognathic mandible
- Mildly canted plane of occlusion with left side superior to right side
- Full-step Class II dental relationship with excessive vertical and horizontal anterior overlap
- Mild to moderate maxillary archlength deficiency
- Defective restoration of tooth 7 with periodontal inflammation
- Moderate incisal wear on tooth 8 from traumatic occlusion

Treatment Plan

Interdisciplinary Dentofacial Therapy

- Presurgical non-extraction orthodontic therapy to align dentition
- Orthognathic surgery
  - Mandibular advancement
- Postsurgical orthodontic therapy to finalize occlusion
- Periodontal plastic surgery
  - Esthetic gingival recontouring on tooth 21 to lengthen crown and compensate for incisal wear
- Definitive restorative therapy
  - Esthetic dental recontouring in anterior maxilla to feminize and create better balance, symmetry, and horizontal alignment
  - Vital bleaching therapy on maxillary dentition
  - All-porcelain resin-bonded ceramic restoration on tooth 12

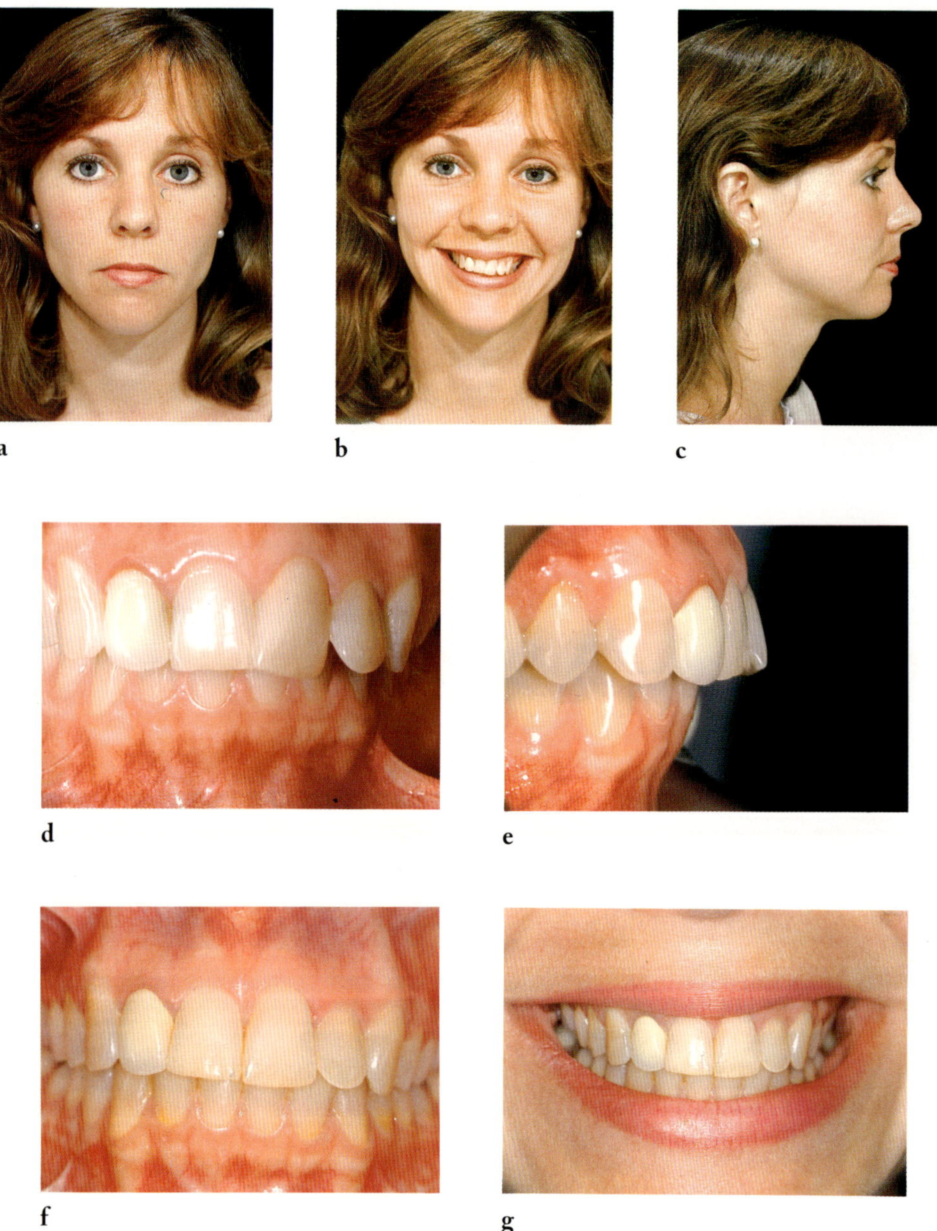

Fig 5-7 L.C. is a 28 year-old female who wanted to improve the esthetics of her smile and chin.

a to c Initial facial views illustrating good symmetry and proportionality, with a mild Class II skeletal relationship. The anterior occlusal plane appears slightly canted, with the right side being more superior to the left.

d, e Initial intraoral appearance with full-step Class II dental relationship and excessive vertical and horizontal anterior overlap. There is mild to moderate anterior crowding in the maxillary arch, with generalized discolored teeth and a defective crown on tooth 12.

f, g Dental views following full-mouth orthodontic therapy and a mandibular advancement. Dental appearance has improved but still has several shortcomings. Maxillary anterior dentition appears discolored, unbalanced, and poorly shaped, and the maxillary anterior plane of occlusion still appears to be slightly canted.

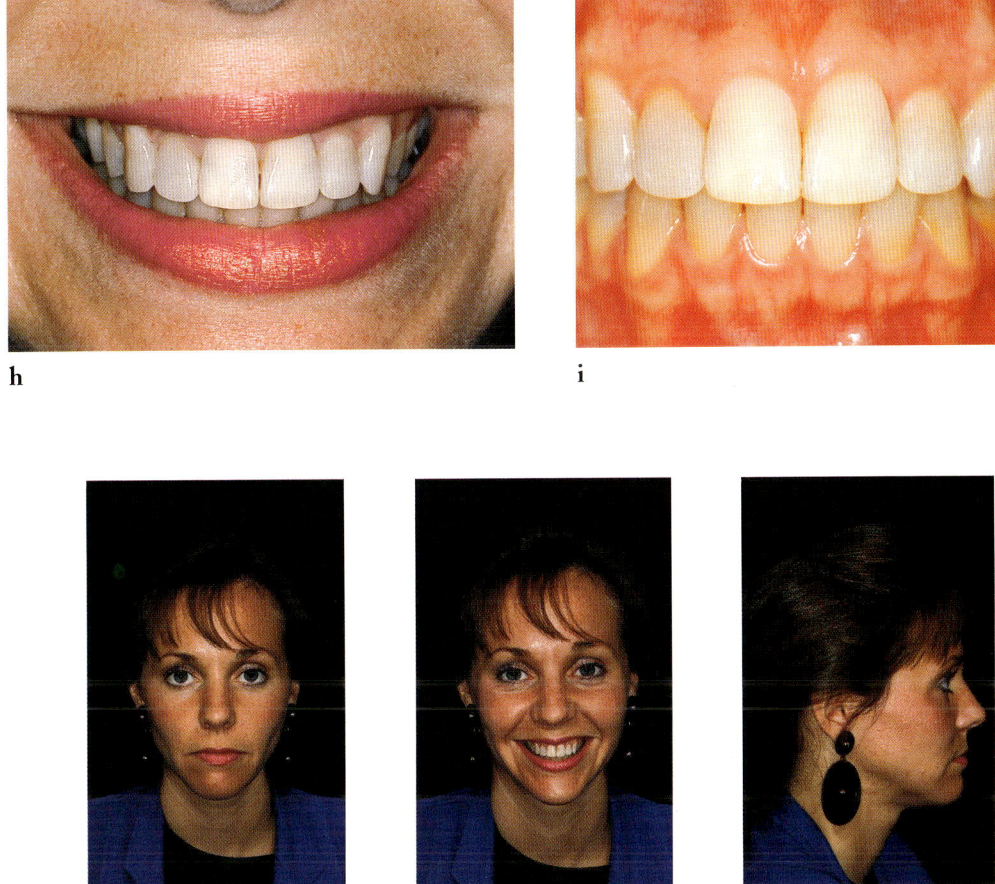

h i

j k l

Fig 5-7

h, i Final dental appearance following conservative periodontal and restorative therapy. Tooth 11 was lengthened by gingival recontouring procedures. The defective crown on tooth 12 was replaced with an all-porcelain resin-bonded restoration. The maxillary anterior dentition was esthetically recontoured to feminize contours and to create better symmetry and balance. Bleaching procedures were also performed on the maxillary dentition.

j to l Frontal facial views illustrating enhanced dentofacial esthetics.

Orthodontist: Alan C. Jensen, DDS, MSD/*Oral and Maxillofacial Surgeon:* Sterling R. Schow, DMD
Periodontist: Edward P. Allen, DDS, PhD/*Restorative Dentist:* Richard D. Roblee, DDS, MS
Laboratory Technician: Jeffrey Singler, CDT

Discussion

This case illustrates several important aspects about interdisciplinary therapy. It shows the importance of including the patient in the treatment-planning process. The patient had to make the final decision whether to have orthodontic extraction therapy or an orthognathic procedure to treat her Class II dental and skeletal relationships. The interdisciplinary team preliminarily agreed that orthognathic surgery was not needed to have a successful result. After the interdisciplinary team thoroughly educated the patient about her dentofacial problems, treatment options, and the associated risks and benefits of therapy, she chose to have the mandibular advancement procedure because of the high importance she placed on maximizing the dentofacial esthetic improvements. Another important point is this case illustrates that interdisciplinary treatment planning can attain optimal results through conservative therapy. This is illuminated by the results of the periodontal and restorative procedures. Dental problems such as the ones that remained after orthodontic and orthognathic surgical therapies were completed are typically overlooked or handled through extensive restorative procedures. This case shows that through the interdisciplinary approach, each team member can build upon the previous team member's therapy and turn mediocre results into outstanding results. This is illustrated by the esthetic improvements made by the restorative and periodontal team members after orthodontic and orthognathic procedures were completed. None of the team members could have attained this level of result without each one of the other team members' help. Interdisciplinary dentofacial therapy can build moderate improvements into outstanding improvements.

Definitive Patient Conference

The *definitive patient conference* to discuss the tentative treatment plans is a critical appointment. It will usually determine not only the definitive treatment plan but whether the patient will even enter the definitive therapy phase of IDT. The time spent at this conference advising the patient is often as important as the definitive therapy in achieving optimal dentofacial treatment results. This conference must highlight and summarize all dentofacial counseling to date.

A multispecialist consultation is the most effective for answering all questions and considering all the benefits and risks associated with therapy. It is also the most effective for developing the patient's trust in the providers and enhancing the patient's perceived value of therapy. Realistically, however, a multispecialist consultation is extremely difficult to organize, due to the constraints of the individual providers. For this reason, the patient conference is usually administered by the interdisciplinary team leader, and followed by specialized patient conferences with the other team members as needed. A one-on-one conference can be very effective when properly performed. The provider should be extremely careful not to discuss another member's treatment or fees in detail, as this could lead to misinformation, confusion, and an eventual loss of patient confidence. Financial matters are best handled by individual team members.

At the conference, the provider should present the detailed diagnostic findings to fully educate the patient as to his or her dentofacial needs, thus enhancing the perceived value of treatment. Use of actual diagnostic records as visual aids in the patient conference is extremely effective for communicating the problems to the patient, as well as for building the patient's confidence in the team by demonstrating the thoroughness of the diagnostic process.

Once the patient fully understands his or her dentofacial needs, the team leader needs to present the tentative treatment plans. Again, care must be taken not to give too many specifics in areas where the provider is not an expert. When more specifics about a patient's treatment or financial obligations with other providers are necessary, the patient should be referred for a specialized patient conference with the appropriate team member. All pertinent information about each of the treatment plans should be discussed with the patient. These include: *(1)* rationaled for rationale; *(2)* overall treatment plan summaries; *(3)* detailed discussion of risk/benefits to patient; *(4)* expense to patient (monetary fees associated with that provider, time involved, and cooperation needed); and *(5)* expected discomfort. Failure to adequately educate the patient can lead to confusion, disappointment, and noncompliance. This thorough consultation is an effective form of positive reconditioning in which founded or unfounded apprehension from previous negative conditioning can be overcome.

The end result of this thorough patient conference should be a patient who is highly educated about his or her dentofacial needs and the potential treatment plans, and who can now make an intelligent decision as to what is most important to him or her. The interdisciplinary team must always remember that what is important to them may not be important to the patient. The provider in the conference should listen and understand the concerns of the patient so that he or she can make a joint decision with the patient as to which treatment options will best address the greatest number of pertinent factors. After this has been decided, the treatment sequence that best conforms to the patient's schedule and financial constraints can be formulated.

Thus, the first thing that must be agreed upon at the definitive patient conference is the patient's final destination in dentofacial therapy, which decides the scope and level of the treatment. The exact route can then be mapped out to best reach that destination, taking into consideration the patient's specific needs.

For example, a common area of difficulty in IDT is that patients will often have to pay the bulk of expenses themselves, especially when orthodontic therapy or cosmetic procedures are involved. This presents a large obstacle, but this can usually be overcome by comprehensive dentofacial therapy that is spread out over a period of years. If carefully planned, the treatment time can usually be extended so that the rate of therapy conforms to the patient's financial means (Fig 6-30). The ability of the team to sequence treatment in relation to the patient's financial means can frequently determine whether the patient will be able to accept optimal dentofacial therapy.

Only through this thorough process of patient consultation can a mutual understanding between the providers and the patient be established concerning dentofacial needs, treatment possibilities, and various concerns. This will help insure not only acceptance of definitive treatment but also a smooth progression of therapy, with a higher rate of patient compliance and appreciation.

If the patient cannot accept optimal definitive therapy for some reason, then a secondary treatment plan will have to be formulated to best meet the patient's needs. If possible, this secondary plan should attempt to maintain the dentofacial status of the patient without compromising the possibility of future optimal dentofacial therapy (Fig 3-6). In this way, the patient can still have optimal treatment in the future without having to redo the therapy that was performed as a secondary measure.

After the definitive treatment plan has been formulated and decided upon, the patient should have specialized consultations as necessary with each of the major providers. This will allow the patient to more fully understand the details of each aspect of therapy, as well as the financial and physical obligations.

At this point, the team leader should summarize the interdisciplinary problem list and delineate the definitive treatment plan by making a detailed outline of the sequence of therapy and listing the providers responsible for each aspect. This summary and outline will serve as a map for the individual providers to follow during treatment. It is frequently helpful to provide the patient with a copy of this summary and outline to further enhance participation in therapy. Interdisciplinary summaries, outlines and other correspondence are discussed in detail in Chapter 8.

References

1. Proffit WR, Fields HW. Orthodontic treatment planning: from problem list to final plan. In: Proffit WR. Contemporary Orthodontics, ed 2. St Louis: Mosby, 1992: 186–224.
2. Proffit WR, Ackerman JL. Orthodontic diagnosis: the development of a problem list. In: Proffit WR: Contemporary Orthodontics, ed 2. St Louis: Mosby, 1992: 139–185.
3. Proffit WR, Epker BN. Treatment planning for dentofacial deformities. In: Bell WH, Proffit WR, White RP (eds). Surgical Correction of Dentofacial Deformities. Philadelphia: Saunders, 1980: 155–199.
4. Stuart CE. Full Mouth Waxing Technique. Chicago: Quintessence, 1983.
5. Hohl TA. Use of an adjustable (anatomic) articulator for cast prediction in segmental surgery. In: Bell WH, Proffit WR, White RP (eds). Surgical Correction of Dentofacial Deformities. Philadelphia: Saunders, 1980:169–177.
6. Hill SC. Cephalometric planning and model surgery. In: Bell WH (ed). Surgical Correction of Dentofacial Deformities—New Concepts. Philadelphia: Saunders, 1985: 210–226.
7. Amvar M, Harris M. Model surgery for orthognathic planning. Br J Oral Maxillofac Surg 1990; 28:383–397.
8. Christionsen EL, Thompson JR. Temporomandibular Joint Imaging. St. Louis: Mosby, 1990.
9. Schwarz MS, Rothman SLC, Rhodes ML, Chatetz N. Computed tomography: part 1. Preoperative assessment of the mandible for endosseous implant surgery. Int J Oral Maxillofac Implants 1987;2:137–141.
10. Schwarz MS, et al. Computed tomography: part II. Preoperative assessment of the maxilla for endosseous implant surgery. Int J Oral Maxillofac Implants 1987;2:143–148.
11. Eckerdal O, Kvint S. Pre-surgical planning for osseointegrated implants in the maxilla. Int J Oral Surg 1986;15:722–726.
12. Engelman MJ, Sorenson JA, Moy P. Optimum placement of osseointegrated implants. J Prosthet Dent 1988;59:467–473.
13. Petrikowski CG, Pharoah MJ, Schmitt A, Pre-surgical radiographic assessment for implants. J Prosthet Dent 1989; 61:59–64.
14. Kassebaum DK, Nummikoski PV, Triplett RG, Langlais RP. Cross-sectional radiography for implant site assessment. Oral Surg 1990;70:674–678.
15. Musgrave MT, Westesson PL, et al. Improved magnetic resonance imaging of the temporomandibular joint by oblique scanning planes. Oral Surg Oral Med Oral Pathol 1991; 71:525–528.
16. Wilk RM, Harms SE, Wolford LM. Magnetic resonance imaging of the temporomandibular joint using a surface coil. J Oral Maxillofac Surg 1986;44:935–943.
17. Westesson PL. Diagnostic imaging of oral malignancies. Oral and Maxillofac Surg Clin N Am 1993;5:207–228.
18. Wolford LM, Hilliard FW, Dugan DJ. Surgical Treatment Objective: A Systematic Approach to the Prediction Tracing. St Louis: Mosby, 1984.
19. Sarver DM, Johnston MW. Video imaging: techniques for superimposition of cephalometric radiography and profile images. Int J Adult Orthod Orthognath Surg 1990; 5: 241–248.

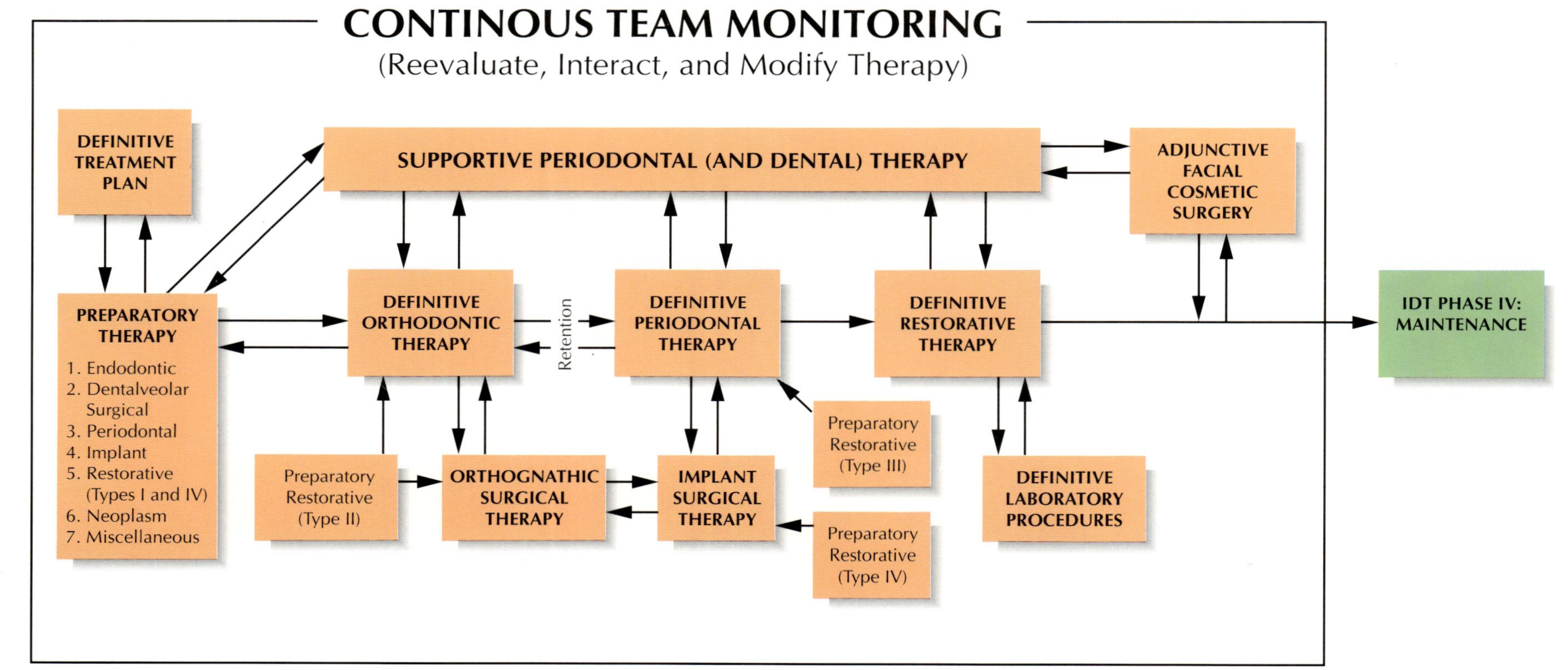

DEFINITIVE THERAPY: IDT PHASE III

6

Definitive Therapy

Phase III of IDT

With all of the diagnostic and treatment-planning procedures completed, definitive therapy can be initiated. The definitive-therapy phase is similar to the treatment-planning phase in that its success depends on how well the individual team members interact and cooperate. Communication between the different providers during this phase is as important as during any other phase of dentofacial therapy. Definitive therapy must be characterized by continuous team monitoring, which includes: *(1)* reevaluating the progress of treatment at every appointment, *(2)* interacting about pertinent findings with the other team members, and *(3)* modifying the original treatment plan to best accomplish the original goals of therapy using the information acquired in the monitoring process.

Continuous team monitoring allows adjustments to be made in the original treatment plan to compensate for unforeseen difficulties or for better-than-expected results during therapy. This enables definitive therapy to progress as smoothly and as efficiently as possible. The definitive treatment plan, no matter how well-conceived, cannot be expected to foresee all circumstances that may arise during the course of treatment.

Before any aspect of definitive therapy is completed, it is also extremely beneficial to include the next provider in the final stages of the current therapy. For example, the restorative dentist must be consulted during the finishing stages of orthodontic therapy to ensure that the dental alignment that will allow the best restorative result is produced. Not to consult the next provider would be against the philosophy of ideal interdisciplinary therapy, because the next provider can best interpret what he or she needs to optimally complete the therapy. Lack of communication in this phase can lead to frustration, compromise, and failure of subsequent treatment, whereas proper interaction allows greater efficiency during treatment, leading to optimal results in a shorter treatment time. Shorter treatment times are possible because without interaction, individual aspects of therapy can actually be overtreated. Interactive communication between providers allows for acceptable interdisciplinary compromises to be made in the different providers' therapies, allowing attainment of the optimal result as quickly as possible.

Supportive Periodontal (and Dental) Therapy (SPT)

Inadequate periodontal and dental maintenance can lead to severe problems or even failure during definitive therapy. Because of this, the entire interdisciplinary team must share responsibility for the health care of the dentition and its supporting tissues. Every member must monitor the periodontal and dental status during each visit to make sure that no problems go untreated. This periodontal and dental maintenance is now termed *supportive periodontal treatment* or SPT.[1,2] Despite the lack of the word "dental" in SPT, dental checks and therapy are an integral part of the treatment.

SPT is especially important during active orthodontic therapy, because the appliances can interfere with oral hygiene and cause mechanical irritation, and tooth movement adds to the potential for occlusal trauma. Inadequate oral hygiene, in combination with orthodontic mechanics, can lead to devastating effects on the supporting tissues and possible tooth loss.[3] Effective oral hygiene is indispensable if periodontal damage and caries are to be prevented during orthodontic therapy[4,5] and other definitive therapies. Rotary electric toothbrushes have been found to be more effective than manual toothbrushes for reducing plaque accumulations during orthodontic therapy.[6] Other procedures performed by the patient in addition to excellent oral hygiene, such as chlorhexidine mouth rinses, can significantly enhance periodontal inflammation control.[7] Fluoride can reduce white spot lesions (decalcification) frequently associated with orthodontic appliances.[8,9]

Plaque-control instructions should be repeated and positively reinforced as often as possible by every team member to improve and maintain an adequate tissue response[10] and prevent caries. Positive reinforcement can enhance the patient's overall involvement and perceived value of treatment. One of the interdisciplinary team goals should be to keep the gingival tissues free from clinical signs of inflammation during therapy. This means that there should be no bleeding upon probing[11] and no increases in pocket-probing depths (Fig 6-1).[12,13]

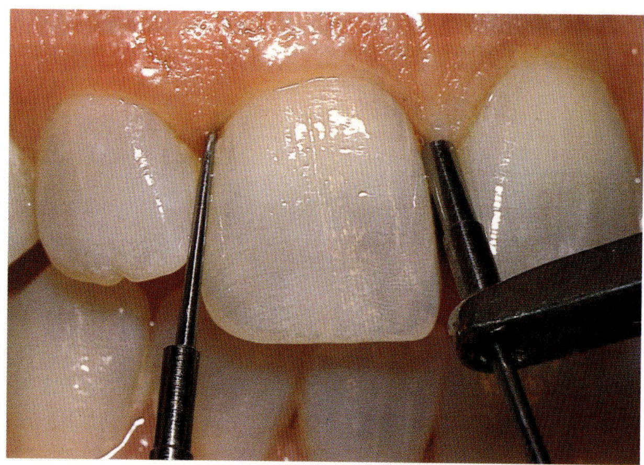

Fig 6-1 Increases in pocket-probing depths and bleeding upon probing are signs of active periodontal inflammation and should be accurately monitored. The use of pressure-sensitive probes allows the clinician to gain more reproducible information concerning pocket-probing depths. The device shown in this illustration is linked to a computer that provides the most accurate data currently possible.

Periodontist: Thomas G. Wilson, Jr, DDS

In addition to oral hygiene, periodontal, and dental evaluations at every appointment, it is important that the patients have regularly scheduled SPT appointments. A traditional 6- to 12-month maintenance interval is usually not adequate for adult patients undergoing interdisciplinary therapy, especially when they have preexisting periodontal problems. The correct time between visits should be based on disease activity, not on the calendar.[2] They may need to be seen as frequently as every 2 to 3 months to control inflammation.[1,14,15] This has been substantiated by Mousques and coworkers,[16] who found that the disruption of bacterial formations every 60 to 90 days helped keep periodontal tissues healthy.

The practitioner primarily responsible for SPT depends on the type and severity of the disease. In general terms, the more aggressive the periodontal disease, the more the periodontist should be responsible for SPT.[17] The patient receiving SPT exclusively from the periodontist should see the restorative dentist periodically to oversee maintenance of the dentition. This shared maintenance is best because it adds different dental and periodontal perspectives and keeps the periodontist and restorative dentist informed about the progression of treatment. All other team members must help ensure that patients follow through with these regular maintenance appointments.

At SPT appointments, a thorough scaling and root planing should be performed, especially where there are signs of active disease. Surgical removal of hyperplastic gingival tissues that are interfering with orthodontic therapy or causing difficulty in maintenance of proper oral hygiene may also be necessary[15] (Fig 2-5e). Wilson has described a typical SPT visit for a patient with inflammatory periodontal disease.[18] A patient undergoing interdisciplinary dentofacial therapy should be treated with the same thoroughness. In addition to monitoring and maintaining periodontal health, the dentition must be clinically and radiographically monitored on a regular basis for caries, decalcification, root resorption associated with orthodontics,[2,19] and endodontic problems. Also, the temporomandibular complex must be regularly evaluated for disorders. Maintenance therapy should be provided as needed for any problems that may be found, and should be performed in its proper relation to interdisciplinary dentofacial care. This maintenance therapy during definitive therapy, such as caries control while in full orthodontic appliances, usually requires more creativity by team members, but it can and must be accomplished in a timely fashion.[21]

Finally, it is important that all pertinent SPT findings are communicated to the other team members. This team conferencing will assist in the overall care and maintenance so that each team member's therapy can be customized to the patient's needs.

Preparatory Therapy

The first objective of the definitive therapy phase of IDT is to optimally prepare the dental, osseous, and soft tissue components for the various individual definitive therapies that are to be performed. This preparation must be done in a way that most facilitates and least compromises any future therapy. The goal of this preparatory therapy is to optimize the planned definitive therapies and enhance the overall long-term prognosis. Some definitive therapy may be performed in this stage, since the definitive treatment plan has been formulated and the strategic importance of each tooth has been determined. However, definitive therapy should only be performed at this stage if it can be done without compromising future therapy (outlined in the definitive treatment plan). The categories of preparatory therapy include: *(1)* endodontic, *(2)* dentoalveolar surgical, *(3)* periodontal, *(4)* implant, *(5)* restorative Type I and Type IV, *(6)* neoplasm, and *(7)* miscellaneous.

The exact order of the different types of preparatory therapy varies according to each patient's specific needs, and should be outlined by the interdisciplinary team during treatment planning. Some aspects of preparatory therapy may be postponed until definitive therapy if needed. For example, the preparatory dentoalveolar surgical therapy of extracting a hopeless tooth may not be performed until after definitive implant therapy is completed if the tooth has a secondary use as a transitional abutment in transitional implant therapy (Fig 6-38). Also, if further definitive therapy is not planned, then preparatory therapy would be considered definitive; for example, if third molars are extracted without any further therapy planned.

Endodontic Therapy

Endodontic therapy is a critical aspect of foundation dentistry, and its importance in IDT must not be underestimated. Preparatory endodontic therapy is the definitive phase of endodontic therapy. It involves the proper preparation of canals[22] requiring endodontic therapy (if not already performed during relief of pain or initial pulpal therapy), their definitive filling,[23] and subsequent post reinforcement[24] if indicated. Obturation of the canals should be accomplished with gutta percha filling material using a three-dimensional condensing technique. This is critical for maximizing the long-term success of endodontic therapy and for helping ensure the success of IDT, especially when orthodontic tooth movement is planned. Orthodontic tooth movement can occasionally cause some resorption in the apical portion of the root and expose the root-canal system.[20] If a three-dimensional technique with gutta percha has not been used, the canal may start to leak after root resorption occurs,which can eventually lead to failure of the endodontic therapy. In some cases, teeth undergoing endodontic therapy may require surgical root-end therapy to control periradicular inflammation and/or remove periradicular lesions not amenable to nonsurgical endodontic therapy.

If the coronal aspect of the tooth needs to be reinforced after the canal has been successfully treated, a post should be inserted if indicated,[24] so that the restorative dentist can place a crown buildup. Except in cases where surgical root-end therapy is indicated, endodontic pathology should have already been arrested as part of the initial pulpal therapy. The goal of preparatory endodontic therapy is to restore and maintain the endodontically treated canals in a nonpathological state.

Dentoalveolar Surgical Therapy

Preparatory dentoalveolar surgical therapy includes the following procedures:

a. necessary extraction of teeth;
b. root amputation or sectioning (bicuspidization);
c. surgical endodontic therapy (apicoectomies and other root-end procedures);
d. uncovering of impacted teeth.

These procedures are performed by various team members with the appropriate expertise. As previously stated, the extraction of teeth should not be performed until this time because their prognosis and possible secondary uses in dentofacial therapy have not been fully known until this point. Any teeth that have been given a hopeless prognosis and cannot be used secondarily to assist in dentofacial therapy should be removed at this stage. Useless teeth should also be extracted at this time, including the removal of impacted third molars,[25,26] other impacted teeth,[27] unopposed terminal teeth, malformed or fused teeth, and malaligned and interfering ankylosed teeth. Impacted teeth can have a devastating effect on an individual's dentition, jaws, and overall health. There are many indications (as well as contraindications) for the removal of impacted teeth.[27]

The timing of dental extraction in interdisciplinary therapy may be critical in preventing or minimizing complications in the various therapies. For example, third molars should be extracted with minimal bone loss at least 9 months prior to a sagittal split osteotomy to allow good bone healing prior to surgery. In some cases, however, third molars can be removed at the time of the orthognathic surgical procedures without compromising the surgery, thus eliminating a separate surgical procedure. Impacted and partially impacted teeth that are in an area that is to undergo radiation therapy should be removed at least 2 weeks before radiation is initiated to minimize problems associated with delayed healing and osteoradionecrosis. Teeth may also have to be removed to make room for proper orthodontic correction, in cases of severe dental crowding asymmetries, and/or to orthodontically decompensate the dentition in preparation for orthognathic surgical procedures. Teeth extracted for orthodontic reasons should be removed as late in therapy as possible, because extraction often leads to rapid alveolar bone loss and remodeling, which can compromise the orthodontic movement of adjacent teeth if performed early. No matter what the reason for the extractions, a conscious effort should be made to eliminate or lessen the creation of a defect within the residual ridge.[28]

Occasionally a multirooted tooth may require that roots be separated or removed subsequent to localized periodontal and/or carious involvement (Fig 6-2), failed endodontic therapy, vertical fracture in one root, or other reasons.[29] Using this approach for salvaging roots that can support fixed prosthodontics will often eliminate the need for a removable prosthesis or osseointegrated implants. Root resection is highly successful when performed properly[29] and maintained with optimal oral hygiene and precise restorative techniques.[30,31] Remaining roots can even be orthodontically moved into better relationship to facilitate proper periodontal maintenance and placement of optimal prostheses (Fig 6-2).

Surgical endodontic therapy,[29,32–34] including apicoectomies and other root-end procedures, may be needed to control inflammation caused by noxious stimuli that cannot be managed by nonsurgical endodontic therapy. This surgery should not be performed until the definitive treatment plan has been completed to make sure that surgery is not performed on a tooth that may be extracted for other reasons. In some cases, this surgery may also be necessary to remove neoplasms and cysts associated with teeth undergoing endodontic treatment. The objectives of surgical endodontic therapies are to remove the noxious stimuli, seal the apex of the root, and leave the surgical site in a state that will permit proper healing.

Impacted teeth that are going to be orthodontically brought into the arch can be uncovered at this time, or it may be more advantageous to wait until some initial stages of definitive orthodontic therapy has been performed to make room in the dental arch and to set up orthodontic anchorage. This uncovering may require soft and hard tissue removal to expose the clinical crown and allow access for placement of orthodontic appliances on the impacted tooth[35–38] (Fig 2-5c).

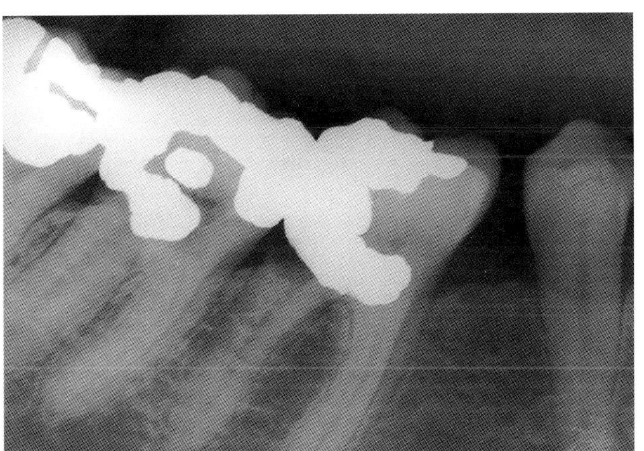

a

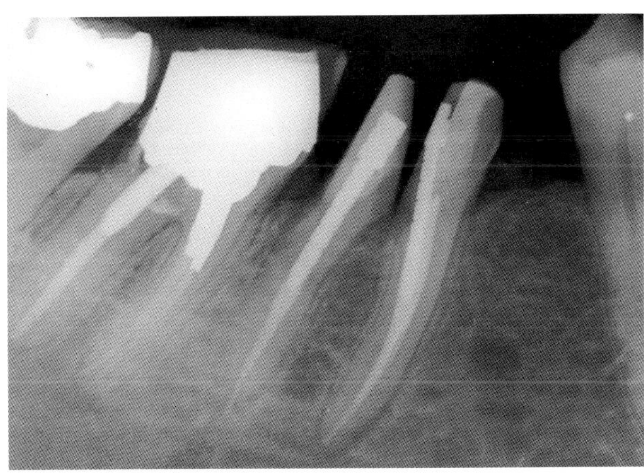

b

Fig 6-2

a Initial radiograph of a 63-year-old female with numerous dental problems. The second premolar was lost at an early age and all three molars had subsequently tipped forward, forming mesial pseudopockets. The first and second molars both had rampant recurrent decay that extended to the crestal bone and also involved the furcation on the first molar. Both of these molars were nonvital and had periapical abscesses.

b Radiograph taken after completion of preparatory therapy. This interdisciplinary stage of treatment included preparing the first and second molars with endodontic therapy, post-and-core reinforcement, and sectioning of the mesial and distal roots of the first molar. The teeth are now ready to be orthodontically uprighted and extruded. In addition, the sectioned roots will be orthodontically separated so that they can be restored with two individual crowns. Minor crown-lengthening procedures may still need to be performed after orthodontic therapy to level the crestal bone and allow proper restoration without violating the biologic width. This treatment plan promoted optimal resolution of the problems and allows the individual restoration of the involved teeth without utilizing fixed partial dentures.

Endodontist: James Tinnin, DDS/*Periodontist:* Gary Renegar, DDS/*Orthodontist:* Richard D. Roblee, DDS, MS
Restorative Dentist: Michael Carter, DDS

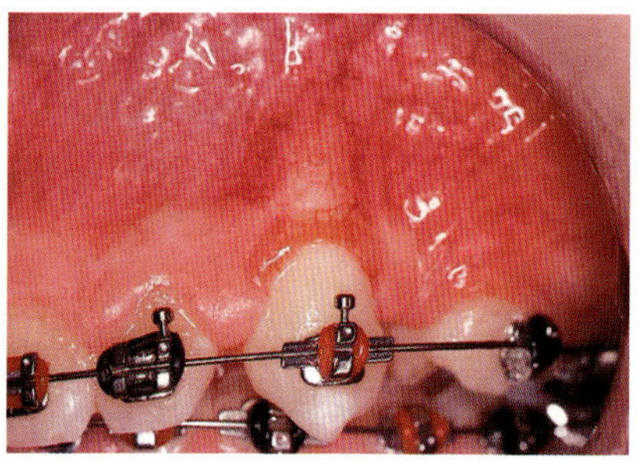
a

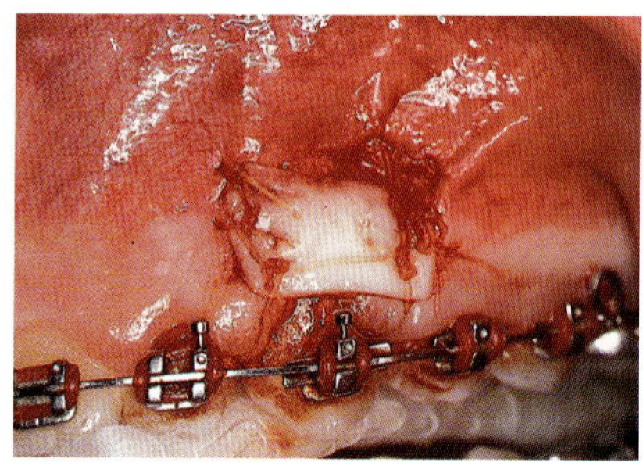
b

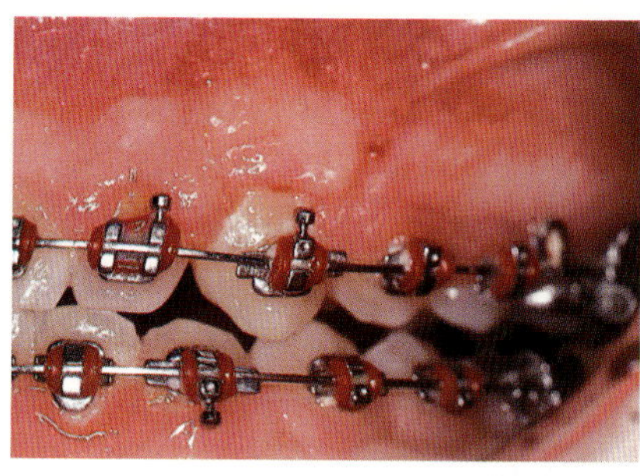
c

Fig 6-3 Gingival graft.

a Maxillary canine with a prominent root and absence of attached gingiva.

b Free gingival graft sutured with resorbable sutures.

c One month postoperative, the graft has provided adequate dimensions of gingiva where none existed, and there is a good color blend with the adjacent gingiva. For the most predicatble results, preorthodontic prophylactic surgical procedures such as this and that in Fig 6-4 should ideally be performed during preparatory periodontal therapy before orthodontic therapy is initiated. If orthodontics is not planned, these procedures should be done as part of definitive periodontal therapy. *Periodontist:* Edward P. Allen, DDS, PhD

Periodontal Therapy

Preparatory periodontal therapy usually involves mucogingival (and occasionally osseous) procedures that enable the remaining definitive dentofacial procedures to be performed more easily, more predictably, and more therapeutically, with minimal deleterious effects on the periodontal tissues. The preparatory periodontal procedures described below are performed separately from definitive periodontal therapy (described later in this chapter) only when preparing for definitive orthodontic therapy with or without preparatory implant or orthognathic surgical therapies. Otherwise, the procedures in preparatory periodontal therapy are performed as part of definitive periodontal therapy.

There are four main categories of preparatory periodontal therapy: *(1)* preorthodontic inflammation control and/or excessive probing-depth reduction that could not be managed with initial periodontal therapy; *(2)* preorthodontic stabilization of potential soft tissue problem areas; *(3)* facilitation of orthodontic therapy and *(4)* augmentation of preorthodontic implant recipient sites.

Preorthodontic Inflammation Control and/or Excessive Probing-Depth Reduction

Flap and osseous surgery for pocket reduction is usually contraindicated at this stage, because orthodontic tooth movement can often improve the osseous topography and minimize the need for later surgery.[39] Even periodontal surgeries that affect only the soft tissues should be postponed until after definitive orthodontic therapy if possible, because these surgeries can allow periodontal fibers to reorganize to the new tooth positions and help prevent orthodontic relapse.[40,41] Some periodontal problems may, however, require some definitive periodontal surgery before initiating orthodontics.[42]

Periodontal inflammation must be controlled prior to and maintained throughout definitive orthodontic therapy. This inflammation control is important because orthodontic tooth movement can act as a co-destructive factor in the presence of periodontal inflammation and can rapidly accelerate bone loss.[43–45] If signs of active periodontal disease[11–13] or pocket-probing depths of 5 to 6 mm or greater remain after initial periodontal therapy, scaling and root planing using a flap approach,[46] or even more extensive definitive periodontal therapy procedures (such as regenerative, resective, or soft tissue surgical procedures) may need to be performed[47–49] as part of preparatory periodontal therapy.

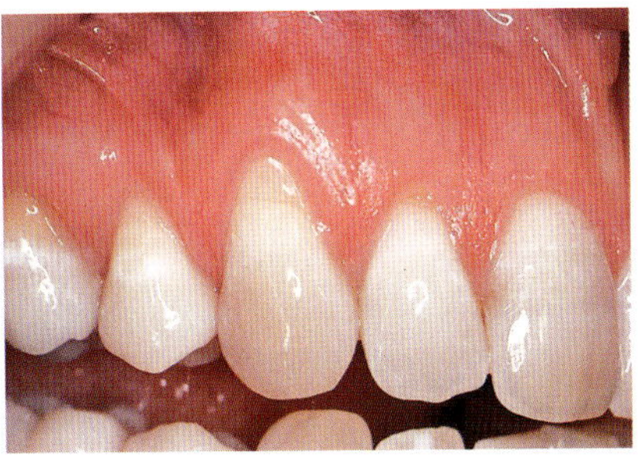
a

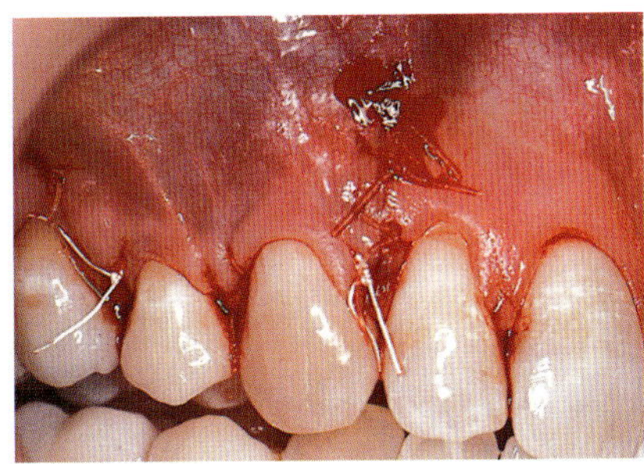
b

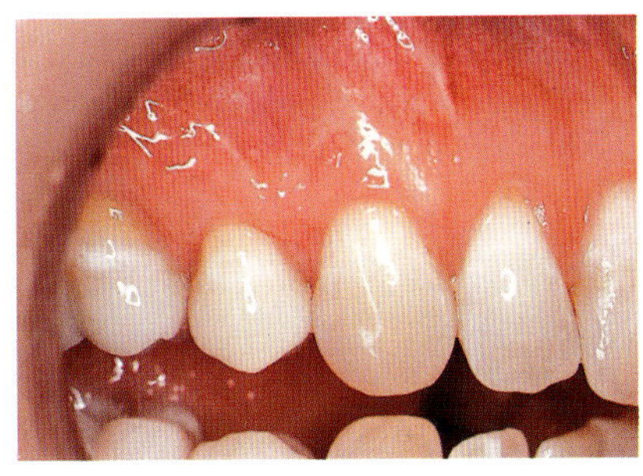
c

Fig 6-4 Coronally positioned flap.
a Gingival recession on the facial aspect of the canine and first premolar.
b A split-thickness flap has been coronally advanced to cover the exposed roots of the canine and first premolar.
c At 3 months postoperative, there is complete root coverage and excellent esthetics.
Periodontist: Edward P. Allen, DDS, PhD

Preorthodontic Stabilization of Potential Soft Tissue Problem Areas

Preparatory periodontal procedures for preorthodontic stabilization of potential soft tissue problem areas may include therapy for: *(a)* inadequate keratinized gingiva, *(b)* gingival recession, and *(c)* abnormal frenum attachment. These surgical procedures are usually performed only after periodontal inflammation and its etiologic factors have been brought under control. Inflammation control should have already been accomplished as part of initial periodontal therapy. In cases where inflammation or excessive probing depths were not resolved by initial periodontal therapy, these procedures can often be performed in conjunction with the definitive periodontal therapy procedures discussed in the previous paragraph.

The techniques for covering broad areas of root surfaces exposed after gingival recession have improved, but root coverage is still not always possible. Keratinized epithelium may be more resistant to the spread of inflammation into deeper structures than gingival mucosa.[50] Hence, the prognoses for successful gingival grafting procedures and prevention of gingival recession are better if preventive mucogingival procedures are done to reinforce the keratinized epithelium prior to definitive dentofacial therapy (such as orthodontic tooth movement or subgingival placement of crown margins), rather than performing corrective therapy after more damage is done. It has been suggested that the minimal zone required for periodontal health is 1 mm of free gingiva and 1 mm of attached gingiva.[51] Anything less may lead to a dramatic increase in the tendency for gingival tissues to recede as a result of orthodontic tooth movement.[52] To complicate this problem further, orthodontic appliances and dental restorations (especially provisional restorations) can cause mechanical as well as chemical (through increased plaque retention) irritation to the gingival tissues, subsequently exacerbate periodontal inflammation, and increase the chances of gingival recession and bone loss. Prophylactic surgical procedures that will supply an adequate band of keratinized tissue should be performed at this time if orthodontic therapy is planned (Fig 6-3). If orthodontic therapy is not indicated, these procedures should be done as part of definitive periodontal therapy.

The question of whether to perform gingival grafting procedures is much easier to decide when gingival recession is already present. In these cases, procedures often should be performed if there is more than 1 mm of recession with or without an adequate band of attached gingiva, especially if the recession appears to be progressing. There are many excellent techniques available to graft soft tissue over denuded root surfaces.[53–56] Root coverage can frequently be attained in the presence of inadequate attached gingiva by using a free soft tissue autograft

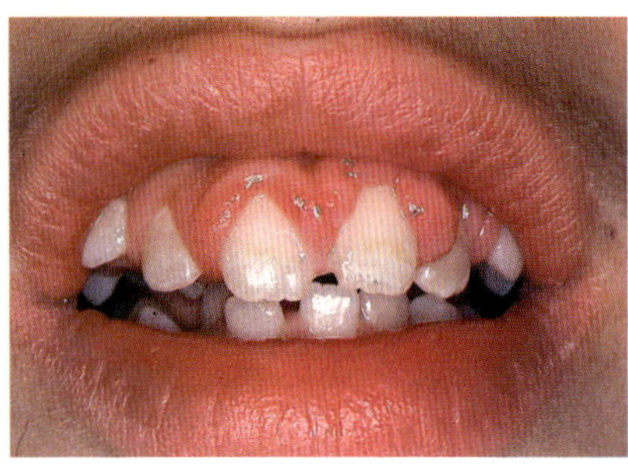

a

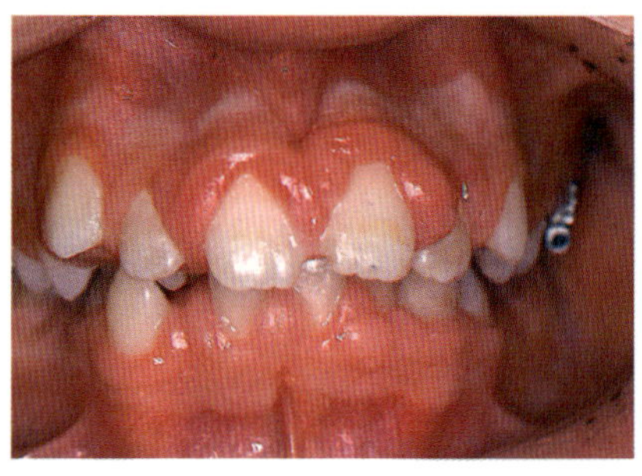

b

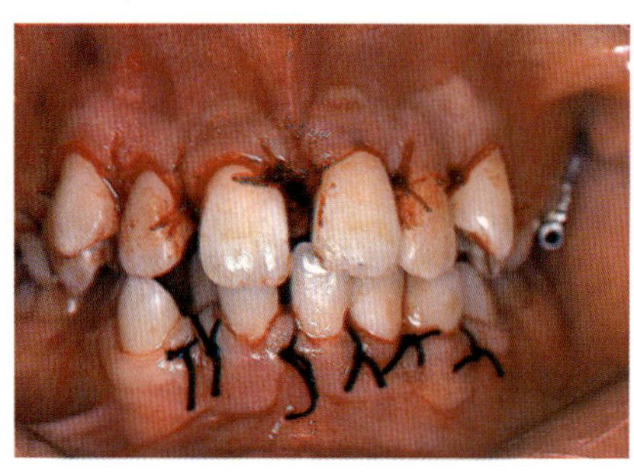

c

Fig 6-5 Preparatory periodontal therapy for facilitation of orthodontic therapy.

a, b Severe gingival enlargement prior to orthodontic treatment, which would interfere with the orthodontic appliances and affect tooth movement.

c Excessive gingiva excised by an internally beveled flap, exposing the normal crown length and restoring the normal gingival form.

Periodontist: Edward P. Allen, DDS, PhD

following citric acid application (Fig 6-3).[53] However, a coronally positioned flap[57,58] is the most effective and esthetic means of repairing gingival recession when marginal tissues are adequate and healthy (Fig 6-4). Another useful technique for covering root surfaces is to coronally reposition a previously placed autogenous gingival graft.[59]

A high marginal attachment of the frenum has been said to be an etiologic factor in gingival recession when it causes mobility of the marginal tissues and/or when there is an inadequate zone of attached gingiva or recession in relation to it.[60] This problem is most common in the mandibular anterior area and it can frequently be treated with a free gingival graft.[61] Also, a thick frenum is commonly associated with a maxillary midline diastema and may slow orthodontic tooth movement or be responsible for the reopening of spaces after orthodontic closure.[60] When attempting to close these maxillary midline diastemas, the current consensus is that nothing should be done for this type of frenum until after all six permanent anterior teeth have fully erupted and failed to close the diastema, and then only in conjunction with orthodontic therapy.[62] To help prevent relapse problems, a frenectomy procedure,[63] occasionally along with a gingival graft, should be performed as part of definitive periodontal therapy toward the end of active orthodontic therapy after the diastema has been closed.

Facilitation of Orthodontic Therapy

Procedures performed at this time to facilitate orthodontic therapy include: *(a)* treatment for insufficient clinical crown height where bone removal is not needed, and/or *(b)* thick tissues in edentulous areas. Clinical crown heights are often too short to allow proper placement of orthodontic appliances. This can be caused by an excessively wide band of keratinized gingiva covering a significant portion of the anatomical crown. In these cases, gingival recontouring should be performed by soft tissue excision[64] (Fig 6-5). In some cases, bone will need to be removed to provide adequate height.[65]

Areas of excessively thick tissues should be reduced in preparation for orthodontic therapy if tooth movement into the area is planned.[60] Thick gingiva impedes tooth movement, and as a result, gingiva accumulates interproximally between two orthodontically approximated teeth.[66,67] This can cause "bunching up" of the thick tissue and subsequently lead to slowing of tooth movement,[67] orthodontic relapse,[62] and the formation of pseudopockets. This thick tissue is frequently found distal to the terminal molars or in edentulous areas. In cases where the thick tissue is not excessive, removal (if necessary) should be postponed until toward the end of active orthodontic therapy as part of definitive periodontal therapy.[60,67]

Augmentation of Preorthodontic Implant Recipient Sites

If implants are to be placed prior to orthodontic therapy (preparatory implant therapy), then placement may have to be preceded at this time by soft or hard tissue augmentation of the recipient site (definitive periodontal therapy). This should be performed as soon as possible to shorten treatment time, because the augmentation and the implant require extensive individual healing periods. A minimum of 30 days healing for soft tissue augmentations and 6 to 18 months healing for hard tissue augmentations (depending on the nature and extent of the graft) are required before implants can be placed. In some cases, it is possible to do the augmentation and implant placement simultaneously to save time and minimize the number of surgeries.

These augmentation procedures are occasionally performed as part of preparatory periodontal therapy when implants are to be placed prior to or during orthodontic therapy for orthodontic or orthognathic anchorage and/or restorative purposes. However, these augmentation procedures are most often done in conjunction with definitive periodontal therapy.

Implant Therapy

Placement of root-form endosseous implants is frequently performed as part of preparatory therapy. Implants may be used for orthodontic anchorage (Fig 6-6),[68,69] stability for orthognathic surgery, and/or for future prosthetic abutments.[70] Implant placement may have to be postponed until later in therapy if placing them at this time would interfere with orthodontic therapy, or if orthodontic therapy is needed to make space for the implant. Dental implants should be placed as early in therapy as possible to allow proper healing and to shorten treatment time. Also, whenever possible, implants should be placed and/or uncovered in conjunction with other surgical procedures to reduce the number of surgeries.

Restorative Therapy

Preparatory restorative therapy uses restorative principles, knowledge and procedures to facilitate the planned definitive therapies in producing optimal dentofacial results. It can be relatively complex in nature, especially in patients requiring orthodontics, orthognathic surgery, dental implants, and/or periodontal therapy. For simplification, preparatory restorative therapy can be broken down into four distinct types (Fig 6-7). Not all of the different types of preparatory restorative therapy are required in all cases. The types necessary for the planned definitive therapies of each case and their sequencing should be outlined in the definitive treatment plan. The necessary types may be performed simultaneously or sequenced individually, or in any combination, throughout the definitive therapy phase of IDT, depending on the characteristics of each individual case.

Preparatory Restorative-Type I

At this point, caries control should already have been completed as part of initial therapy. *Preparatory restorative-type I therapy* should now be performed to prepare the teeth to withstand the stresses of the planned definitive therapies, and at the same time facilitate future therapy while minimizing any potential iatrogenic side effects to the dentition and their supporting structures. This type of preparatory therapy is particularly important when definitive orthodontic, implant, and/or periodontic therapies are planned, because these definitive therapies usually take an extended period of time to complete, and the integrity of the teeth must be maintained in a healthy and noninterfering state to help prevent unexpected complications (such as recurrent decay, tooth fracture, drifting of the teeth, etc). In addition, this type I therapy should facilitate periodontal maintenance, or even help reestablish periodontal health, during definitive therapy by removing restorative overhangs and establishing restorative contours that are conducive to periodontal health.

Preparatory restorative-type I therapy can also facilitate almost any of the therapies (in addition to orthodontic, periodontal, and implant) performed in the definitive therapy phase of IDT. For example, proper isolation during root-canal therapy may not be possible if the tooth is severely broken down.

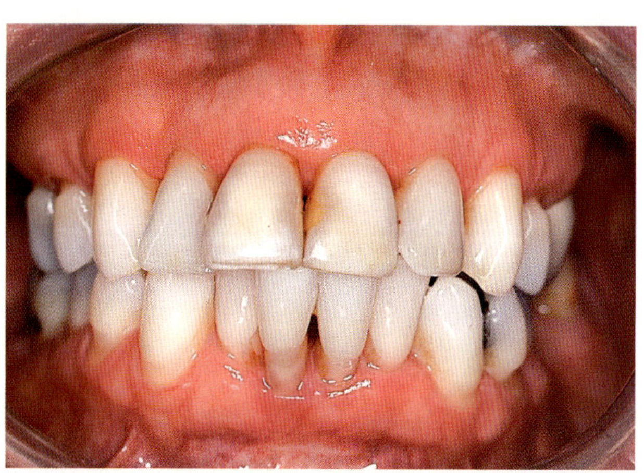

a

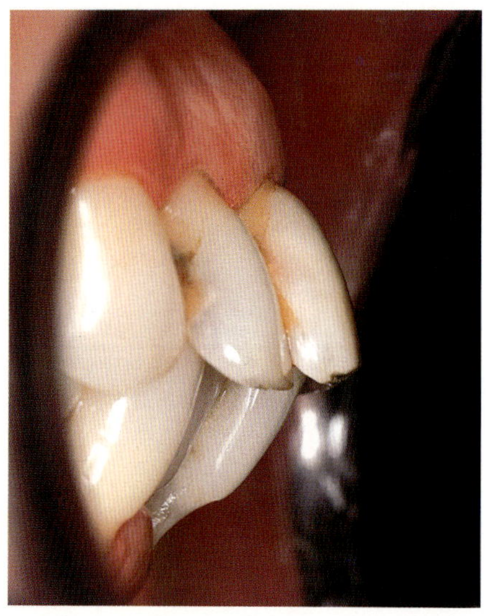

b

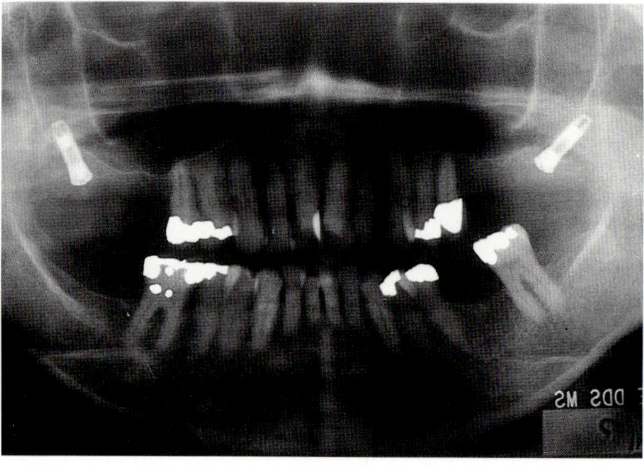

c

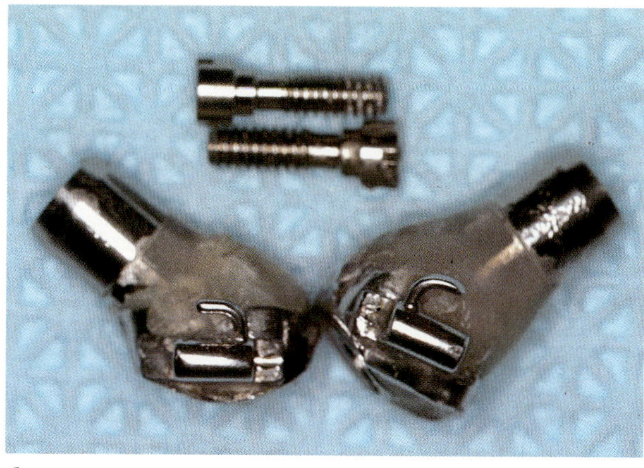

d

Fig 6-6 Orthodontic therapy utilizing endosseous implants for anchorage.

a, b Initial intraoral views showing mutilated dentition. This patient presented with significant bone loss from previous periodontal problems and periodontal therapy. Patient also lost all maxillary molars which, in addition to the bone loss, led to insufficient occlusal support and anterior drifting of dentition, creating a bimaxillary dentoalveolar protrusion.

c Initial panoramic radiographs illustrating significant bone loss and low maxillary sinus. Due to poor health of patient, she elected not to have extensive sinus procedures to allow proper implant placement in edentulous areas. Instead, endosseous root-form implants were placed bilaterally into maxillary tuberosseous areas for orthodontic anchorage.

d Implant attachments were constructed that allowed placement of orthodontic appliances bilaterally onto osseointegrated implants.

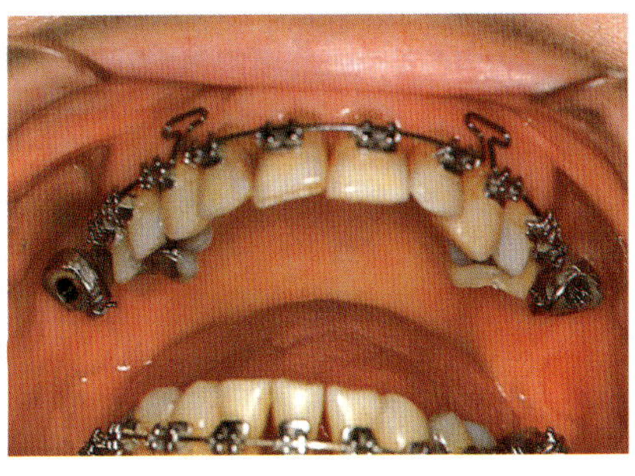
e

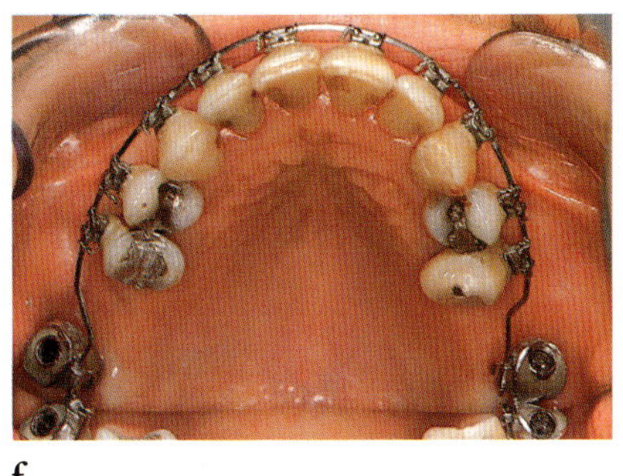
f

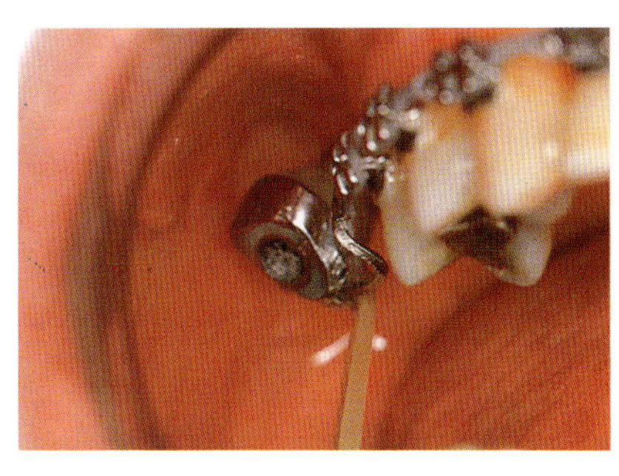
g

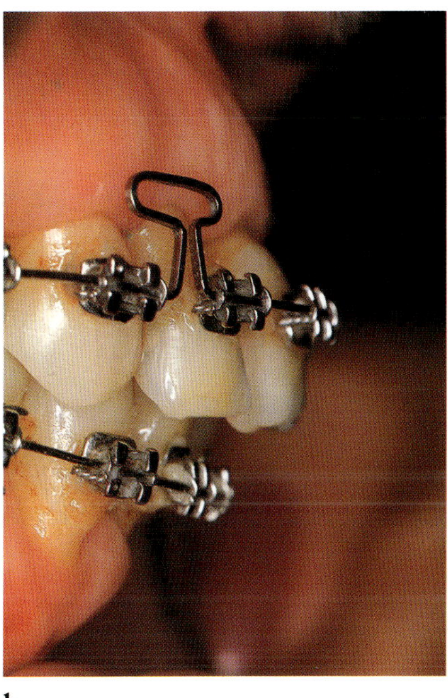
h

Fig 6-6 (continued)

e to g Intraoral progress views illustrating use of implants for orthodontic anchorage in the retraction of maxillary and mandibular dentition.

h Progress view of interincisal relationships with decreased maxillary and mandibular dentoalveolar protrusion. The dentition will continue to be retracted until an ideal interincisal relationship can be obtained, and then a full-mouth dental reconstruction will be performed to stabilize the occlusion. This orthodontic retraction could not have been performed without the assistance of osseointegrated implants.

Periodontist: Gary E. Renegar, DDS/*Orthodontist:* Richard D. Roblee, DDS, MS
Restorative Dentist: R. Berry Broyles, DDS

The four types of preparatory restorative therapy all use restorative principles, knowledge, and procedures to facilitate the planned definitive therapies in producing optimal and consistent dentofacial results, as well as to set up the dentition and supporting structures to allow for optimal definitive restorative therapy.

Preparatory restorative-type I therapy can facilitate all the various treatment modalities by maintaining the integrity of the teeth in a noninterfering way during definitive therapy. Preparatory restorative-types II, III, and IV therapies further facilitate the performance of specific definitive therapies to prepare for optimal definitive restorative therapy and/or to finish comprehensive care with optimal dentofacial results. The four types of preparatory restorative therapy are summarized below.

Type I: Prepares the teeth to withstand the stresses of the various planned definitive therapies without creating iatrogenic interference.

Type II: Facilitates the orthodontist and/or oral and maxillofacial surgeon in optimally positioning the teeth and their supporting structures.

Type III: Aids the periodontist in optimally preparing the periodontal tissues.

Type IV: Performed in cooperation with the implant surgeon to facilitate the proper placement of dental implants.

Fig 6-7 Summary of preparatory restorative therapy. Each type is discussed in more detail in this chapter.

In this instance, preparatory restorative therapy can be used to rebuild the tooth and allow a proper access opening to be made to facilitate ideal isolation with a rubber dam so that asepsis can be established during the root-canal procedures.

When definitive orthodontic, periodontic, or implant therapies are planned, preparatory restorative-type I therapy should be used to replace all broken-down and temporary restorations (placed as part of relief of pain or initial therapy) with either definitive intracoronal restorations or crown buildups (Fig 6-8). Definitive intracoronal restorations (made from amalgam, composite-resin filling, or glass ionomer material) can be performed on teeth which have cuspal integrity and have less than one-third of the occlusal width involved. These restorations should conform exactly to the anatomy of the remaining tooth structure to assist in the maintenance of periodontal health, as well as to allow the involved teeth to be ideally positioned and occluded if orthodontic therapy is planned. Overcontoured restorations can interfere mechanically with adjacent and opposing teeth during tooth movement (Figs 6-22a and 6-22b) and force the orthodontist to compromise the final relationships. In addition, undercontoured restorations can lead to interproximal and interocclusal instability of the final result.

If the tooth is severely broken down and the affected area of the occlusal surface is greater than one-third of the width, then the tooth should be provisionally restored with a material that will help prevent tooth fracture and recurrent decay during orthodontic, implant, or periodontal therapies. This provisional restoration will be used as a crown buildup during the definitive restorative therapy. When the cusp tips are still intact, a good provisional restorative material is reinforced glass ionomer[71] (Figs 6-8c and 6-8d). It is ideal because glass ionomer bonds to tooth structure,[72] possibly adding strength to the weakened tooth, and releases fluoride to help prevent demineralization[73] and recurrent caries. When the cusp tips are involved, a harder material, such as composite resin or a pin-retained amalgam, should be used to reestablish a natural tooth anatomy. It is important to have the coronal portion of the restoration approximate the natural anatomy of the tooth to assist in periodontal maintenance, and when orthodontic therapy is planned, to facilitate proper positioning of the root to allow the eventual placement of a noncompromised definitive restoration. Periapical radiographs are very helpful in determining the angulation of these broken-down teeth when restoring proper coronal anatomy.

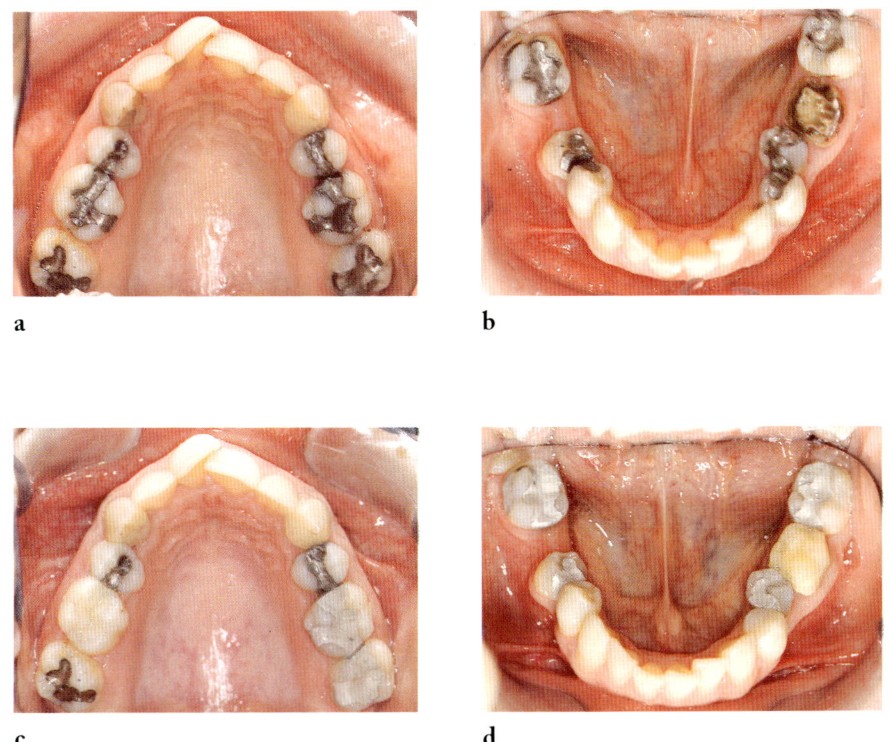

Fig 6-8 Preparatory restorative-type I therapy.

a, b Occlusal intraoral views of IDT patient with numerous carious lesions, broken-down teeth, and large restorations.

c, d Occlusal views after preparatory restorative-type I therapy has been completed to prepare the teeth for periodontic and orthodontic therapies. Conservative definitive restorations may be performed at this time, but more extensive definitive restorations (such as crowns or fixed partial dentures) should be postponed until after the final dental, periodontal, and skeletal relationships are completed.

Definitive fixed prosthodontic procedures (crown and bridge) should rarely be placed prior to periodontal, implant, and/or orthodontic therapies for a variety of reasons. Optimal margin placement of these restorations frequently cannot be determined until after definitive periodontal therapy has been completed and the tissues are fully healed. Also, easily removable provisional restorations can frequently be used to facilitate various procedures during periodontal therapy by increasing accessibility. With implant therapy, necessary fixed prosthodontics on the remaining dentition can be more ideally constructed when placed in conjunction with implant prosthetics after the dental implants have been placed and allowed to osseointegrate. Definitive crowns and fixed partial dentures should not be made before orthodontic therapy, because they will be constructed to the preorthodontic malocclusion. This can force a compromise in the orthodontic positioning of the restored teeth and their occlusal relationship, or necessitate replacement of the restoration(s) if the associated roots are positioned properly. When fixed prosthodontics are to be placed after orthodontic therapy, the roots should be ideally positioned for health of the supporting tissue and for placement of optimal restorations. After orthodontic therapy is completed, definitive restorative therapy should be used to perfect the coronal morphology of broken-down teeth to help ensure optimal function, stability, periodontal health, and esthetics in the final result.

Provisional (temporary) full-coverage acrylic-resin restorations should also be avoided before orthodontic therapy unless absolutely necessary, because provisional fixed prosthodontics can be the source of complications during orthodontics due to dislodging and breakage. Ideally, the provider should perform a crown buildup that attempts to replicate natural tooth morphology. If a provisional restoration must be used, it needs to follow the axial inclinations of the root with proper coronal shape and size (Fig 6-8d) so the ultimate root position, after orthodontic therapy, will be ideal. The fabrication and maintenance of provisional restorations are discussed in preparatory restorative-type III therapy. When provisional restorations are used for preparatory restorative therapy types I, II, or III, they must be securely cemented to minimize dislodgement of the provisional restoration and to prevent decay and sensitivity of prepared teeth during definitive therapy. This can be accomplished by roughening the internal surface of a properly constructed provisional (ideally by sandblasting), thoroughly cleaning and drying the preparation, then cementing with a polyacrylic resin cement that adheres to enamel and dentin.[74]

Preparatory restorative therapy types II, III, and/or IV may be performed simultaneously with type I or at various other times in the definitive-therapy phase of IDT as necessary to best facilitate the planned definitive therapies. These three other types of preparatory restorative therapy are discussed in detail later in this chapter, in conjunction with the major therapy that each facilitates.

Neoplasm

Treatment of benign or malignant tumors that occur in the oral and maxillofacial area[75] may create minor or major functional and/or esthetic deformities. The extent of these deformities depends on the type and nature of pathology, the size of the neoplasm, the reoccurrence tendency, the structures involved, and therapeutic management. Reconstructive management following neoplasm removal is similar to that of traumatic injuries. The main difference between neoplasm therapy and traumatic-injury therapy is that trauma is usually an emergency and treatment must be initiated at the initial appointment as part of relief of pain. Because of this, it is often difficult to perform a comprehensive evaluation and treatment plan when treating traumatic injuries, and this may lead to significant problems during reconstructive procedures in definitive therapy. Even though neoplasm removal must frequently be done expeditiously, more time is initially available, compared to traumatic injuries. These patients should quickly be taken through the interdisciplinary diagnostic and treatment-planning process and the neoplasm removed as part of the preparatory therapy with the ideal reconstructive procedures already outlined. This gives the surgeon valuable information about the treatment objectives so that he or she can modify the surgery to allow for optimal postoperative reconstruction.

Reconstructive management of neoplasm therapy is different from traumatic-injury therapy when the neoplasm is metastatic and the patient has had or needs radiation therapy to oral and maxillofacial structures. In these patients, extensive dentofacial reconstruction may be contraindicated because radiation therapy may significantly compromise the blood supply. Even minor procedures on these patients can lead to development of osteoradionecrosis, which could destroy large areas of bone and soft tissues. All necessary endodontic, periodontal, restorative, and surgical preparatory therapies should ideally be completed before these patients begin radiation therapy.

Miscellaneous

There are many other types of preparatory therapy that may need to be performed to optimize definitive therapy and its long-term results. For example, identification and management of functional airway obstruction may be important to the quality of treatment outcome. Nasal airway obstruction (caused by hypertrophied turbinates, deviated septum, adenoids, etc) may be a causative or contributory factor in the development of dentofacial deformities, periodontal disease,[76] sinus disease, and dental and skeletal instability after dentofacial therapy. Obstruction of the nasal, nasopharynx, and/or oropharynx may also cause sleep disturbances, snoring, and sleep apnea.[77] Identification and correction of these obstructions will create more normal airway functions that can enhance dentofacial growth in growing individuals, aid in controlling periodontal disease, improve stability of results after dentofacial therapy, and possibly enhance overall health.[78] Surgical correction of airway dysfunction should be accomplished during preparatory therapy. Occasionally, orthognathic procedures are planned; these surgeries can be performed simultaneously to reduce the number of surgeries. Orthognathic surgery is known to be a highly effective treatment for obstructive sleep apnea syndrome (Fig 6-9).[78]

Case Summary

Patient: M.D. is an 18-year-old male with a history of TMJ problems, including closed lock and pain related to the TMJ disorder. He complains of difficulty chewing, difficulty breathing through his nose, myofacial pain, headaches, and mild sleep apnea symptoms.

Abbreviated Problem List

- Anterior vertical maxillary excess and slight posterior vertical maxillary deficiency
- Transverse maxillary deficiency
- Anterior-posterior mandibular deficiency
- Significant infraorbital hypoplasia
- Class I canine on the right and Class II end-on on the left
- Anterior open bite
- Anterior interarch tooth-size discrepancy of 4 mm with lower anterior teeth being excessive
- Left posterior crossbite
- Bilateral TMJ articular disc dislocation with reduction, but with a history of closed lock
- Impacted maxillary and mandibular third molars
- Minimal attached gingiva in the mandibular anterior area
- Hypertrophied turbinates
- Deviated nasal septum

Treatment Plan

Interdisciplinary Dentofacial Therapy

- Preparatory Dentoalveolar Surgical Therapy
  - Surgical removal of impacted mandibular third molars
- Preoperative Orthodontic Therapy
  - Align and level the maxillary arch in segments
  - Align and level the mandibular arch; morphologic air-rotor stripping (MARS) on mandibular anterior teeth and premolars to adjust for the tooth-size discrepancy and to prevent the incisors from flaring forward
- Orthognathic Surgical Therapy
  - Multiple maxillary osteotomies to advance and expand the maxilla and move the anterior portion superiorly to level the occlusal plane
  - Bilateral mandibular ramus osteotomies to advance the mandible and rotate it counterclockwise
  - Bilateral TMJ articulator disc repositioning and ligament repair
  - Bilateral infraorbital augmentations with porous block hydroxyapatite
  - Removal of maxillary impacted third molars
  - Augmentation of genioplasty with porous block hydroxyapatite
  - Bilateral inferior turbinectomies and nasal septoplasty to open the nasal airway
  - External rhinoplasty
- Postoperative Orthodontic Therapy to refine and retain occlusion

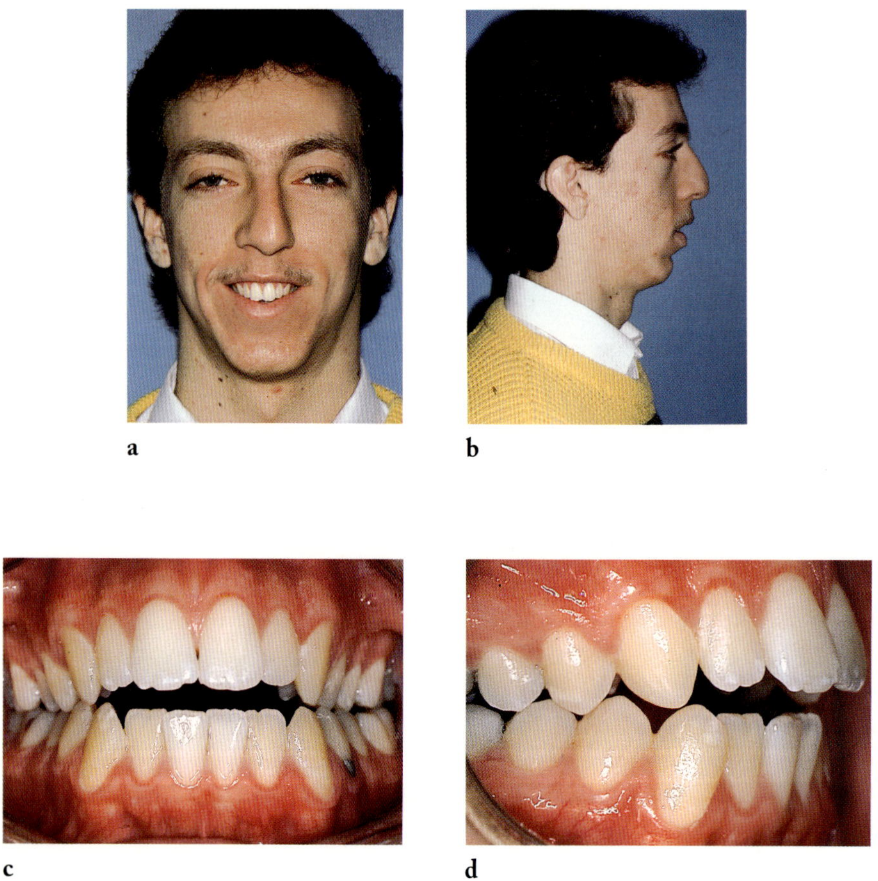

Fig 6-9

a, b This 18-year-old male has vertical maxillary excess, A-P and transverse maxillary deficiency, A-P mandibular deficiency, and A-P microgenia. There is a significant external and internal nasal deformity, and he has mild sleep apnea symptoms, as well as bilateral TMJ problems.

c, d Patient has an anterior open bite and transverse maxillary deficiency with posterior crossbites.

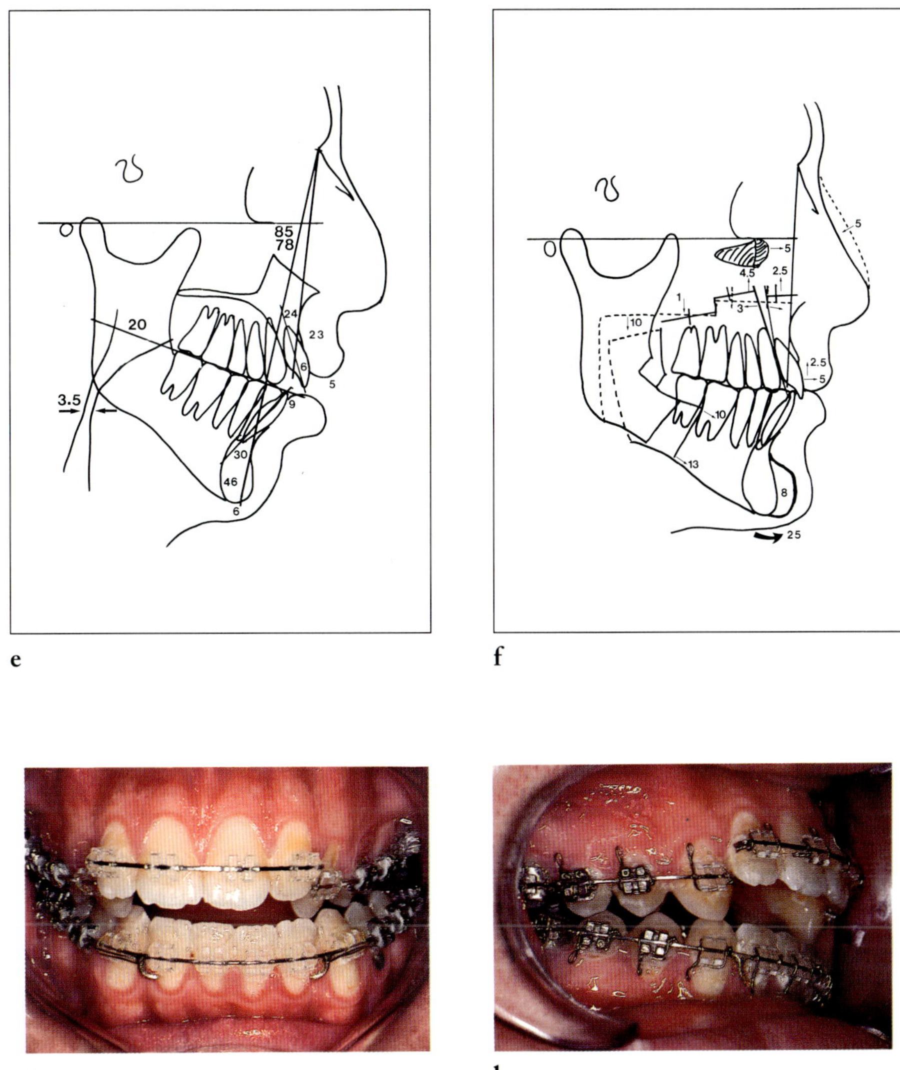

g

h

Fig 6-9 (continued)

e Cephalometrically, this patient has A-P maxillary and mandibular deficiency, vertical maxillary excess, and increased occlusal plane angulation of 20°. Note the decreased oropharyngeal airway and the nasal deformity.

f The surgical treatment objective (prediction tracing) illustrates the changes to be made, including a maxillary advancement of 5 mm and superior repositioning of 2.5 mm, infraorbital augmentations, mandibular advancement, genioplasty with pogonion coming forward 25 mm, and a simultaneous rhinoplasty. The articular discs were also planned to be put back into position at the same surgical procedure.

g, h The orthodontic setup prior to surgery used segmentalization of the maxillary archwire to prevent inappropriate extrusion of the maxillary teeth. A solid archwire can be used, but appropriate compensating steps are necessary to prevent tooth extrusion, which can lead to relapse in the final result.

Fig 6-9 (continued, opposite page)

i to l Facial photographs of the patient taken at 42 months postoperative. Notice the improved facial esthetic balance.

m Superimposition of pretreatment cephalometric (dotted line) and 42-month follow-up evaluations (solid line) demonstrates the functional and esthetic changes achieved. Sleep apnea has been eliminated and the TMJ problems corrected. The occlusion now remains very stable.

Orthodontist: Richard McLaughlin, DDS/*Oral and Maxillofacial Surgeon:* Larry M. Wolford, DDS

Discussion

This case illustrates how numerous problems can sometimes be addressed in one surgery. The counterclockwise rotation of the maxillomandibular complex is a very stable procedure when properly performed. Performing simultaneous TMJ and orthognathic surgery may allow correct repositioning of the articular disc and establishment of balance to the joints, occlusion, and musculoskeletal system in one surgery. However, it requires outstanding surgical skills and techniques to successfully perform these procedures together. The TMJ surgery is traditionally done at a separate operation during initial TMD therapy, but if circumstances are such that it is done simultaneously with orthognathic surgery, the TMJ surgery should be performed first. Rhinoplasties are most predictably performed as a secondary surgical procedure during adjunctive facial cosmetic surgery, unless the patient so requests to do it simultaneously to avoid an additional surgery. This patient has complete elimination of myofacial pain, headaches, and sleep apnea symptoms, in addition to benefitting from a good functional and esthetic result. This case also exemplifies how closely the orthodontist and orthognathic surgeon must work together to help each other consistently obtain optimal results.

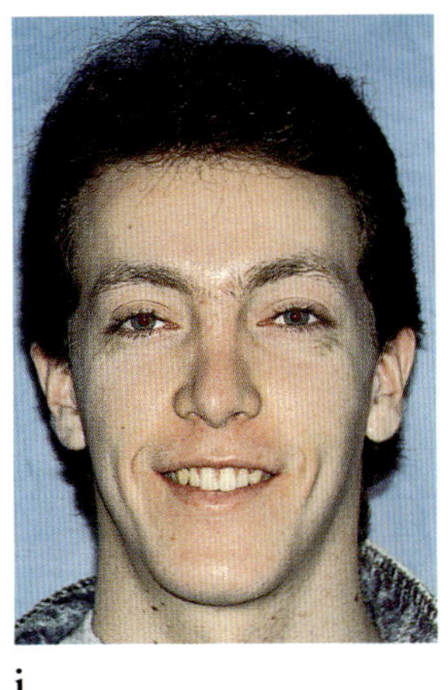
i

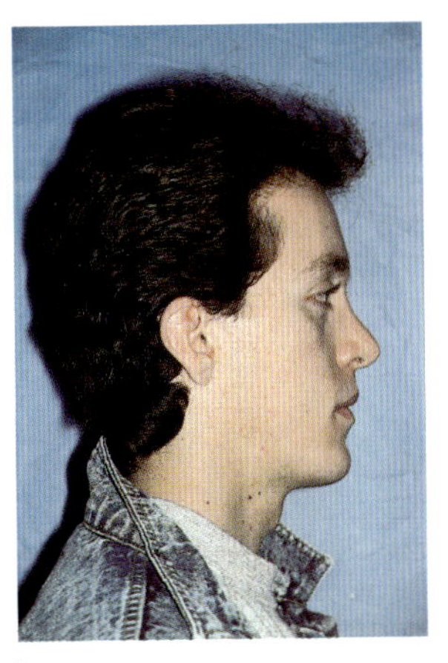
j

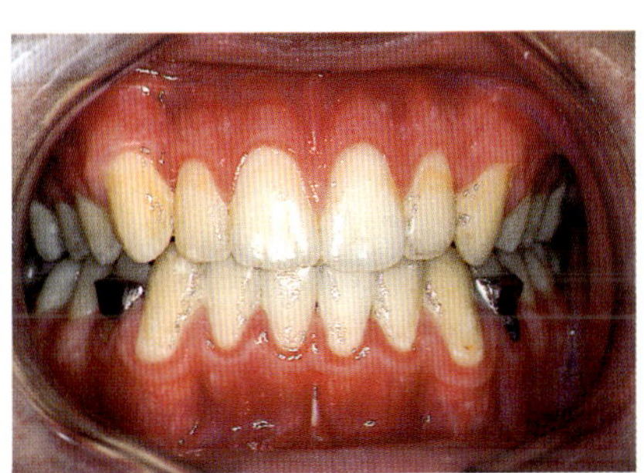
k

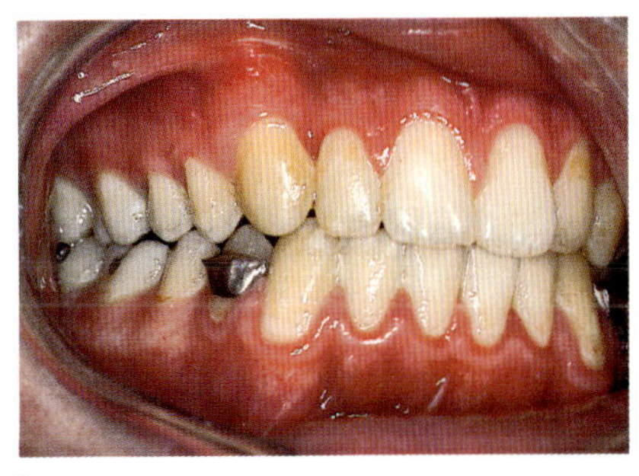
l

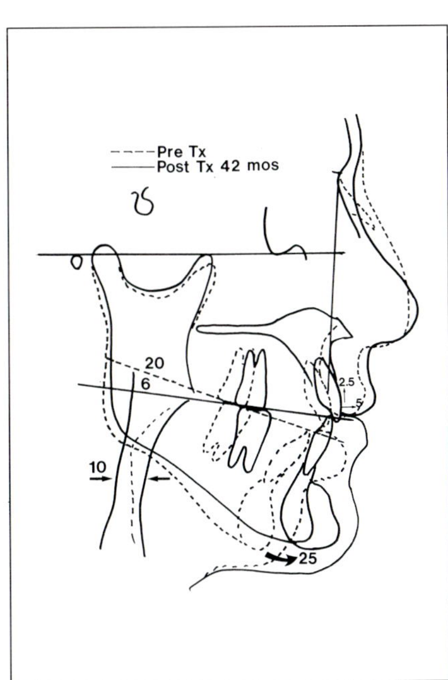

m

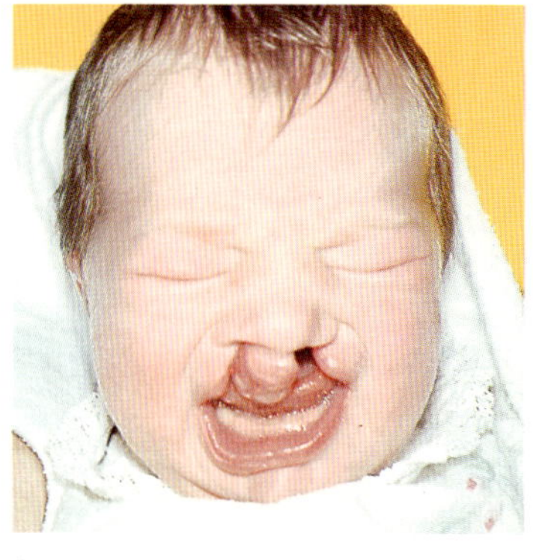

a

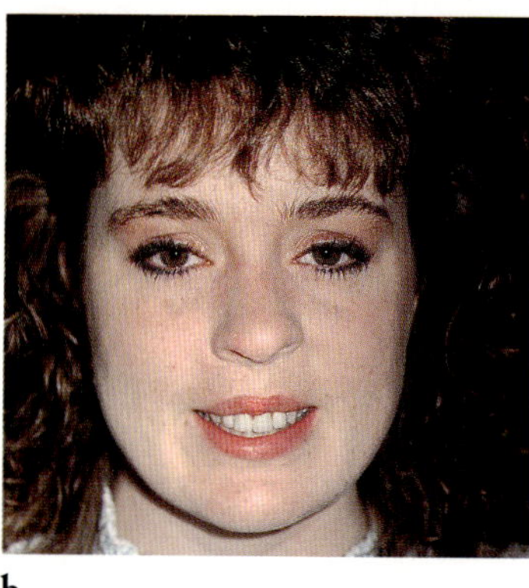

b

Fig 6-10 a, b Before and progress photographs of a patient being treated for severe cleft lip and palate deformities. These types of deformities make up some of the most challenging and most rewarding cases that an interdisciplinary team will encounter. Even severe dentofacial problems such as these can be handled under the same interdisciplinary philosophy presented in this text. However, it must be expanded to encompass several different phases of therapy before a definitive reconstruction can be made. (Reprinted with permission from Berkowitz S. The Cleft Palate Story. Chicago: Quintessence, 1994:4, 96.)

Other preparatory therapies that may be needed include procedures necessary to prepare the patient with cleft deformities or other congenital dentofacial deformities for definitive dentofacial reconstructive procedures. These deformities make up some of the most challenging and some of the most rewarding cases that an interdisciplinary team will encounter (Fig 6-10). Several different stages of preparatory therapy may be required by the various team members before a definitive reconstruction can be initiated. These types of deformities can be handled within the context of the IDT flowcharts, but a detailed description of this management is beyond the scope of this text.

Definitive Orthodontic Therapy

Like the other disciplines in dentistry, modern science and technology has made many sweeping advances in orthodontic therapy. Once a specialty that dealt primarily with adolescent patients, orthodontics is now used to help improve the dental health and overall well-being of dentulous patients in virtually any age group. *Definitive orthodontic therapy* can be adjunctive or comprehensive in nature,[79] depending on the results needed to optimally complete dentofacial therapy. Adjunctive orthodontic treatment is usually limited in scope and deals with a particular portion of the occlusion. In contrast, comprehensive orthodontic treatment deals with the entire occlusal relationship of the dentition and should be performed by an orthodontic specialist with complete fixed appliances.[80]

Whether the definitive orthodontic therapy is adjunctive or comprehensive in nature, the major goals should be the following.

1. Establish an acceptable functional occlusal relationship or set up the potential to establish one through restorative procedures.
2. Position teeth to accept more ideal and conservative restorative procedures.
3. Improve health, stability, and maintenance of supporting structures by:
   - **a.** positioning teeth in proper relationship to supporting structures;
   - **b.** improving interproximal relationships;
   - **c.** leveling bone crests between the teeth
   - **d.** improving crown-to-root ratios (in conjunction with occlusal reduction and/or restorations);
   - **e.** allowing occlusal forces to be transmitted through the long axis of teeth.
4. Set up dentition for and finalize occlusion after orthognathic surgery.
5. Enhance dental and dentofacial esthetics.

Adjunctive orthodontic procedures are aimed at improving specific occlusal relationships as part of an overall treatment plan usually involving major components of periodontal and restorative therapy.[79] For example, adjunctive orthodontic therapy may be performed to rapidly extrude an endodontically-treated single tooth that was fractured or decayed at or below the level of the bone, so that the tooth can be restored without violating the "biologic width" (Fig 6-11).[81] Another example of adjunctive orthodontic therapy is the uprighting of a tipped molar to improve periodontal health and to improve the molar position for use as a fixed partial denture abutment. Adjunctive tooth movement can be accomplished with removable appliances, partial fixed appliances (Fig 6-11), or even provisional restorations (Fig 6-12), and can often be performed by the restorative or periodontal team members as part of their therapy. Fixed appliances are often necessary to obtain predictable tooth positioning.

Comprehensive orthodontic therapy is much broader in scope than adjunctive therapy. It involves the entire dentition and its supporting structures, altering the overall occlusal relationship. Many tremendous advances have been made in comprehensive orthodontic techniques and materials[82] that enable the orthodontist to predictably treat a broad range of dentofacial problems. Orthodontic appliances have been revolutionized since the advent of composite-resin bonding. Even the stigma associated with adults wearing braces has been all but eliminated with the development of bonded metal brackets, tooth-colored brackets,[83] and lingual brackets (Fig 6-13). Similar advancements have been made in virtually all aspects of orthodontic therapy.

Orthodontic therapy primarily aligns teeth, but it is also critical in the proper alignment of the skeletal structures in the middle and lower face. In the nongrowing adult patient, the orthodontist must usually work with the orthognathic surgeon to correct skeletal discrepancies, but in the growing juvenile or adolescent patient, the orthodontic team member can make significant changes through dentofacial orthopedics to nonsurgically alter skeletal relationships.[84] Properly timed arch-development orthopedic procedures can help prevent the need for future dental extractions and/or orthognathic surgery (Fig 6-14). Even sagittal Class II (Fig 6-14) and Class III (Fig 6-15) therapies can be addressed orthopedically when properly timed in growth and development[84] to help prevent the necessity of future surgical intervention to correct the problems.

In more traditional orthodontic therapy, orthodontists are shifting away from routinely extracting premolars in their therapy, even though it has been proven that, when properly performed, this is not a factor in initiating temporomandibular disorders.[85,86] Non-extraction orthodontic therapy should only be performed when the configuration of the skeletal base will allow proper orthodontic alignment of the teeth within the supporting structures. When non-extraction and/or nonsurgical orthodontic therapy is performed and proper alignment of the dentition in its supporting structures is not possible, disastrous consequences can occur (Fig 2-2). As already discussed, orthopedic procedures by orthodontic team members can greatly assist non-extraction therapy in a growing individual (Figs 6-14 and 6-15). In an adult dentition with mild to moderate crowding, non-extraction orthodontic therapy can often be performed in conjunction with procedures such as air-rotor stripping (ARS)[87,88] to properly align the teeth (Fig 6-16). ARS has been shown not to have a negative effect on the teeth and supporting structures when properly performed.[89,90] For this reason, a better term for it could possibly be morphologic air-rotor stripping (MARS), because the final anatomy and surface texture should closely resemble the pre-treatment anatomy surface texture.[91] Situations still arise however, when dental extractions and/or orthognathic surgery must be performed in growing and nongrowing patients to allow proper alignment of the dentition within the supporting structures and face (Fig 6-17). These treatment modalities should be considered optimal for these patients.

The orthognathic surgeon can be a tremendous asset to the orthodontist when treating a nongrowing individual with significant skeletal discrepancies. When orthognathic surgical procedures are planned, orthodontic therapy will usually consist of two stages. The first stage is to decompensate any teeth that are compensating for the skeletal discrepancies and ideally set up the arches to accept the optimal surgical skeletal repositioning. The second stage is used to finalize and perfect the occlusal relationship subsequent to the orthognathic procedures.

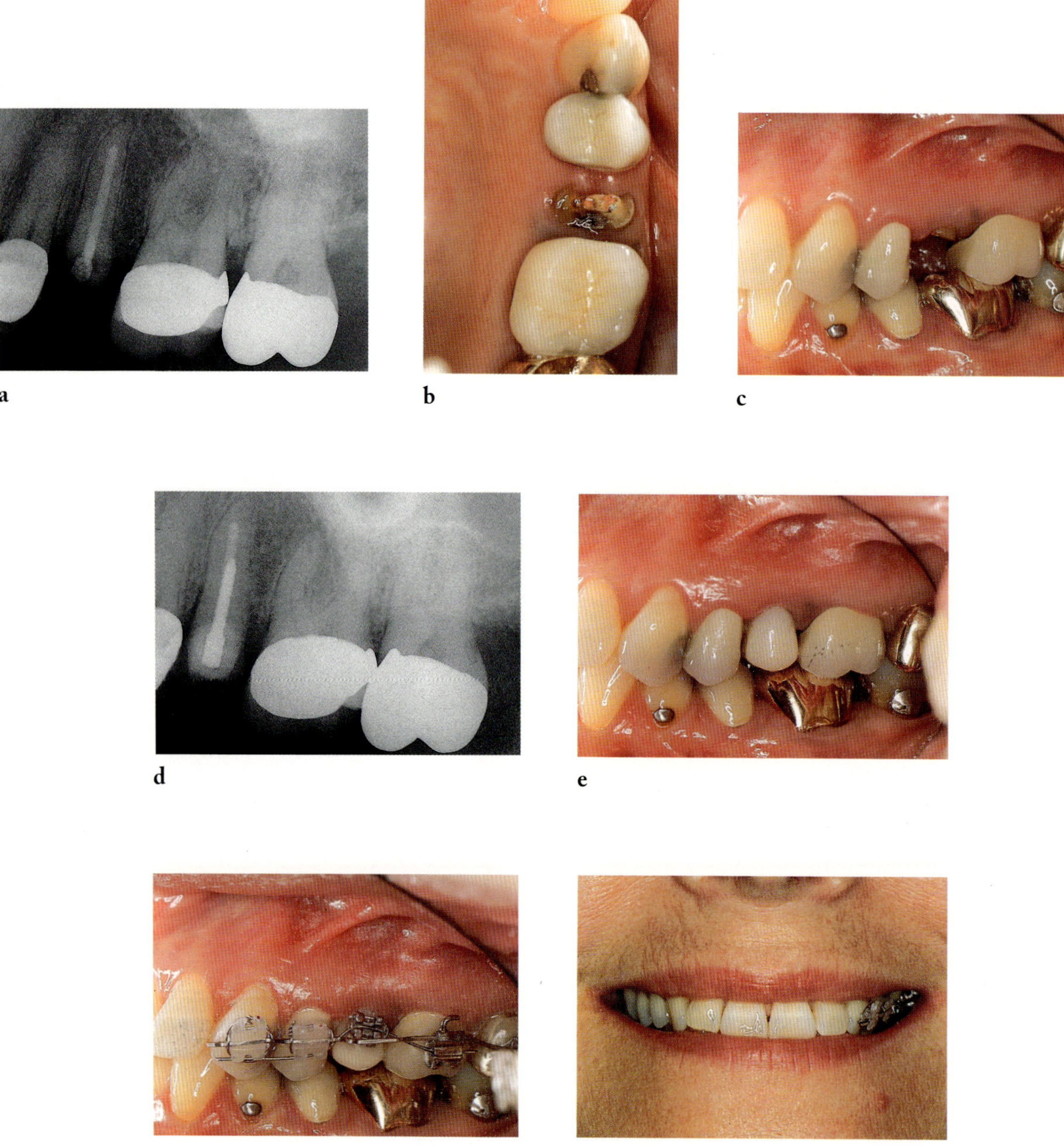

Fig 6-11 Adjunctive orthodontic therapy.

a to c Initial radiograph and photographs of left maxillary second premolar that decayed underneath an existing crown and fractured off to the level of the osseous tissue. This tooth is not restorable in its present relationship without violating the biologic width.

d, e Progress radiograph and photograph after preparatory endodontic and preparatory restorative therapies were performed by the endodontist to prepare the tooth for definitive orthodontic and restorative therapies.

f, g Progress photographs after initial orthodontic appliances were placed. Note how esthetics were maintained while extensive anchorage was used to rapidly extrude the broken-down tooth.

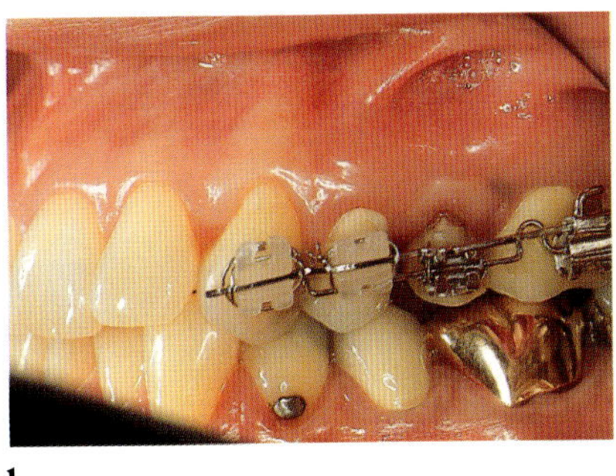

h

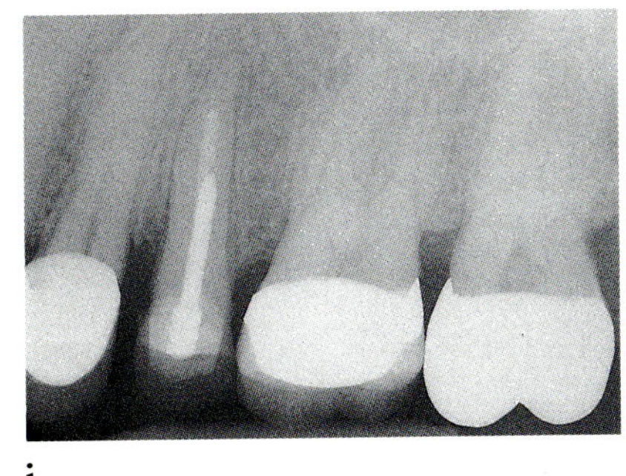

i

Fig 6-11 (continued)

h Six-month progress photograph after extrusion had been completed and tooth had been stabilized for a minimum of 3 months to allow maturation of the supporting tissues.

i Postextrusion and postmaturation radiograph illustrating improved relationship of the tooth to its supporting structures. The fractured tooth can now be optimally restored without violating the biologic width. Some minor osseous recontouring may be indicated after the maturation to remove any lipping of osseous structures that occurred as a result of the rapid extrusion.

Endodontist (post and core only): James M. Tinnin, DDS, MSD/*Orthodontist:* Richard D. Roblee, DDS, MS
Restorative Dentist: David Grace, DDS

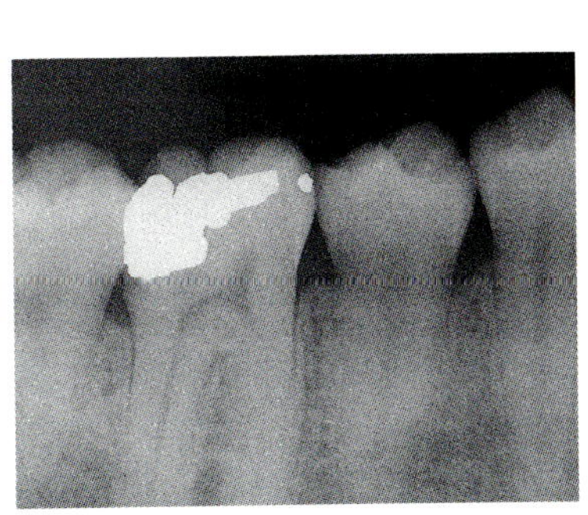

a

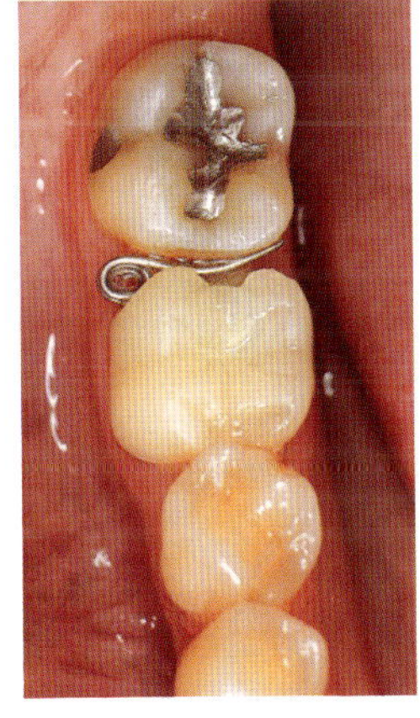

b

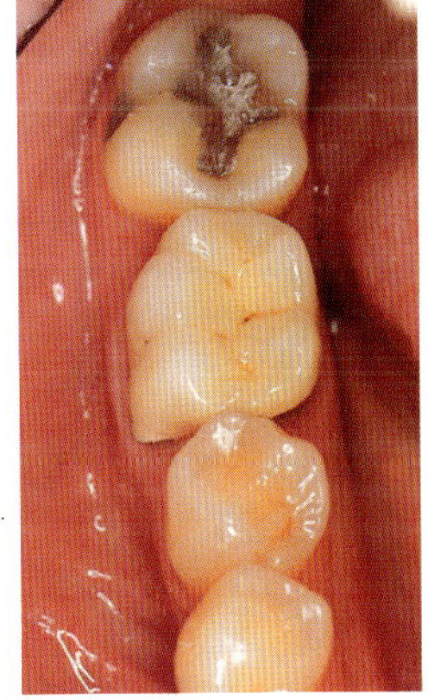

c

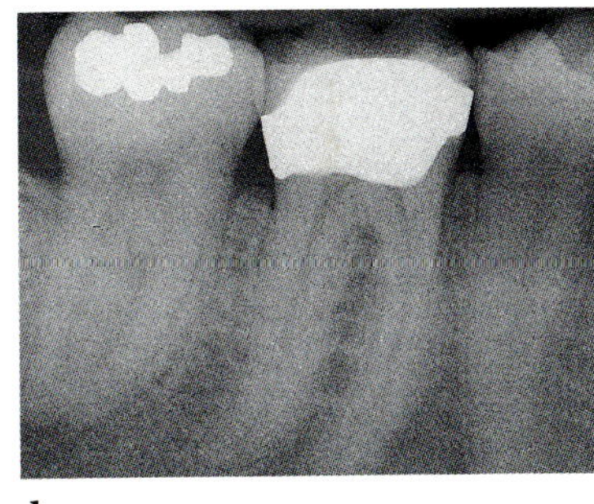

d

Fig 6-12 Adjunctive orthodontic therapy using provisional restorations.

a Initial radiographic appearance of severely broken-down mandibular first molar with recurrent decay. Mandibular second molar has drifted into the broken-down area, making optimal restoration of the first molar impossible due to root proximity and lack of proper space to allow draw of the proposed full-coverage restoration without significantly recontouring the mesial surface of the second molar.

b Occlusal view of the first molar after an acrylic-resin provisional restoration was placed with uprighting spring embedded into the distal aspect.

c Final occlusal view of full-coverage restoration after second molar was uprighted into proper position.

d Final radiographic appearance illustrating optimal interproximal relationships.

Restorative Dentist: Richard D. Roblee, DDS, MS/*Laboratory Technician:* Jeffery Singler, CDT

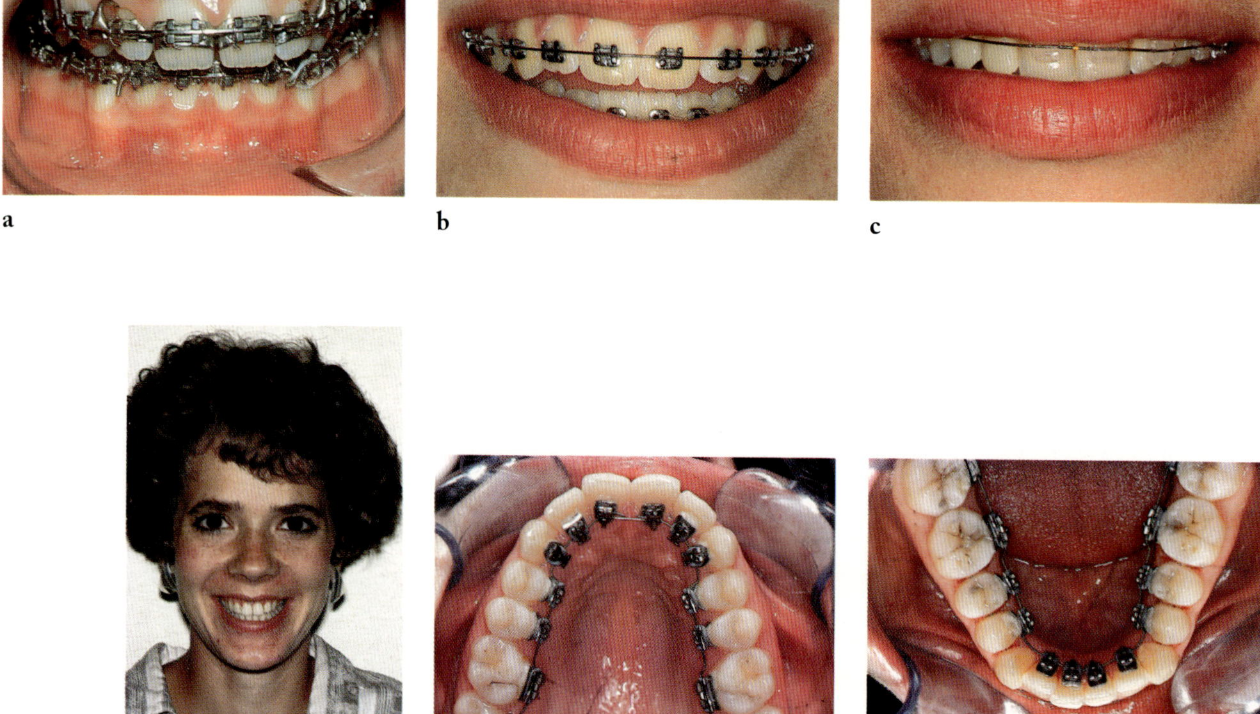

Fig 6-13 Orthodontic appliances have been revolutionized since the advent of composite-resin bonding. When orthodontic therapy is suggested, many people think of the appearance of banded appliances, as in *a*. However, these views are unfounded since the development of modern esthetic appliances (*b* to *f*). The stigma associated with adults wearing braces can be greatly reduced or eliminated with today's orthodontic appliances.

a Typical appearance of orthodontic therapy before bonded brackets were developed.

b Bonded metal "minibrackets."

c Tooth-colored orthodontic brackets.

d to f Smiling and occlusal views of lingual orthodontic appliances.

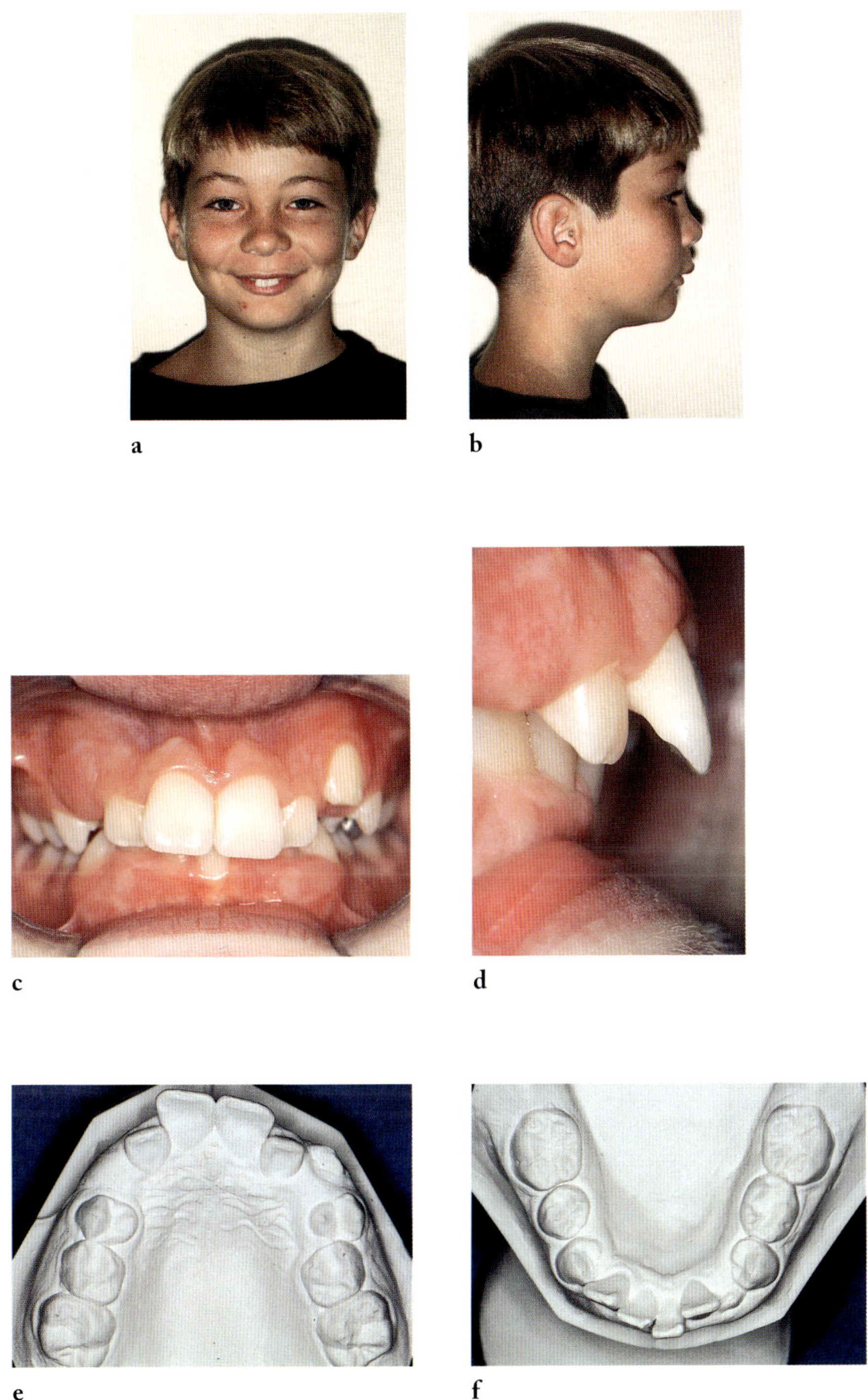

Fig 6-14 Orthopedic/orthodontic correction of severe dental and skeletal malrelationships.

a, b Initial facial views illustrating "buck-tooth" appearance and Class II skeletal relationship with maxillary dentoalveolar protrusion and retrognathic mandible.

c to f Initial intraoral views (*c* and *d*) and models (*e* and *f*) of Class II dental relationship with constricted dental arches, excessive vertical and horizontal overlap, and severe maxillary and mandibular crowding. Note completely blocked-out mandibular right canine.

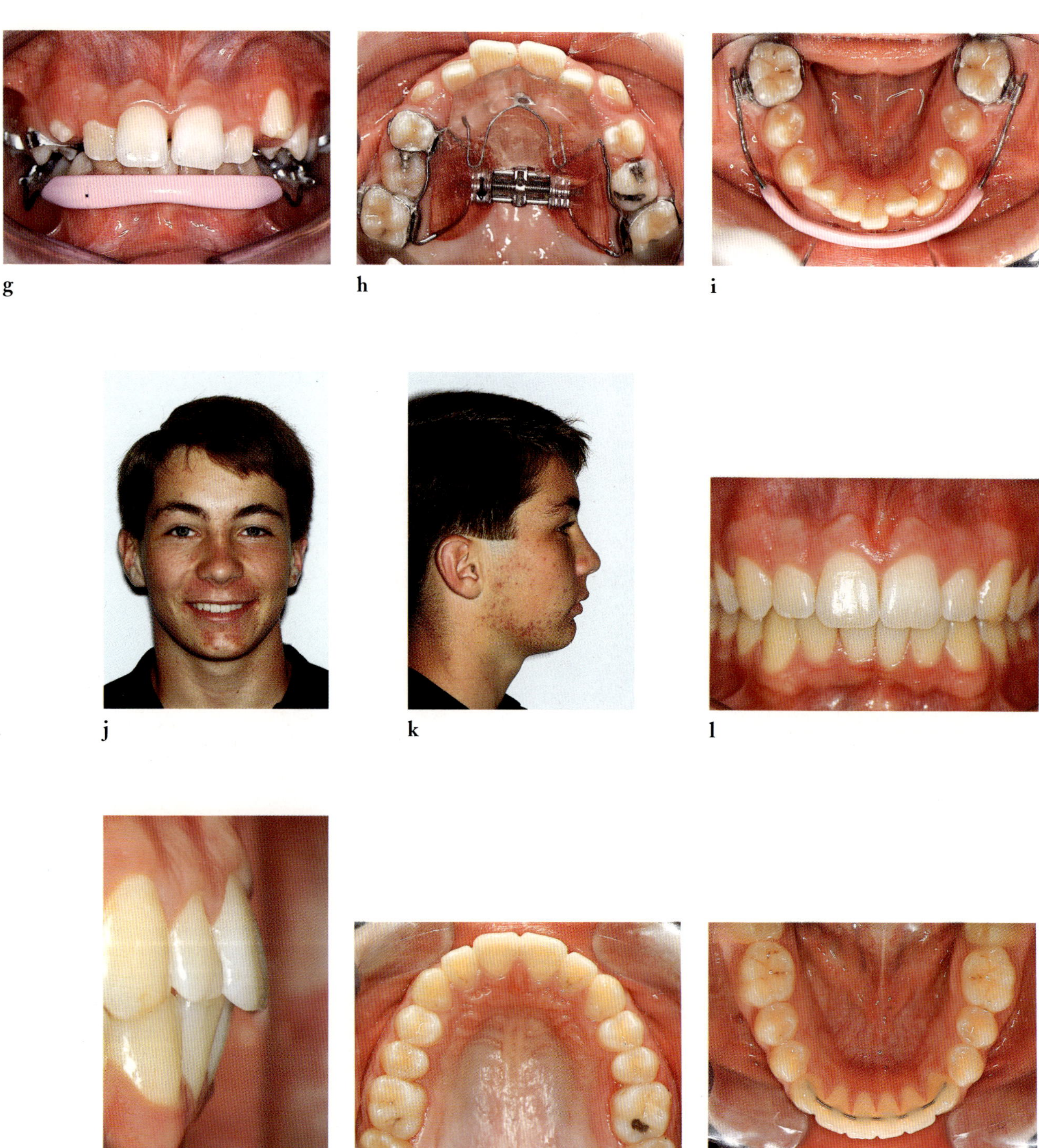

g h i

j k l

m n o

Fig 6-14 (continued)

g to i Progress intraoral views of orthopedic phase of therapy. The maxillary arch was developed using a rapid palatal expander and the lower mandibular arch was developed using a lip bumper. The Class II dental and skeletal discrepancies were addressed with a high-pull headgear and maxillary anterior biteplane.

j to o Intraoral and extraoral views after completion of orthopedic and orthodontic correction. Note complete ideal correction of all dental and skeletal discrepancies and malrelationships. Without orthopedic therapy and proper timing during growth and development, this case probably would have required dental extractions and possibly even orthognathic surgery to correct.

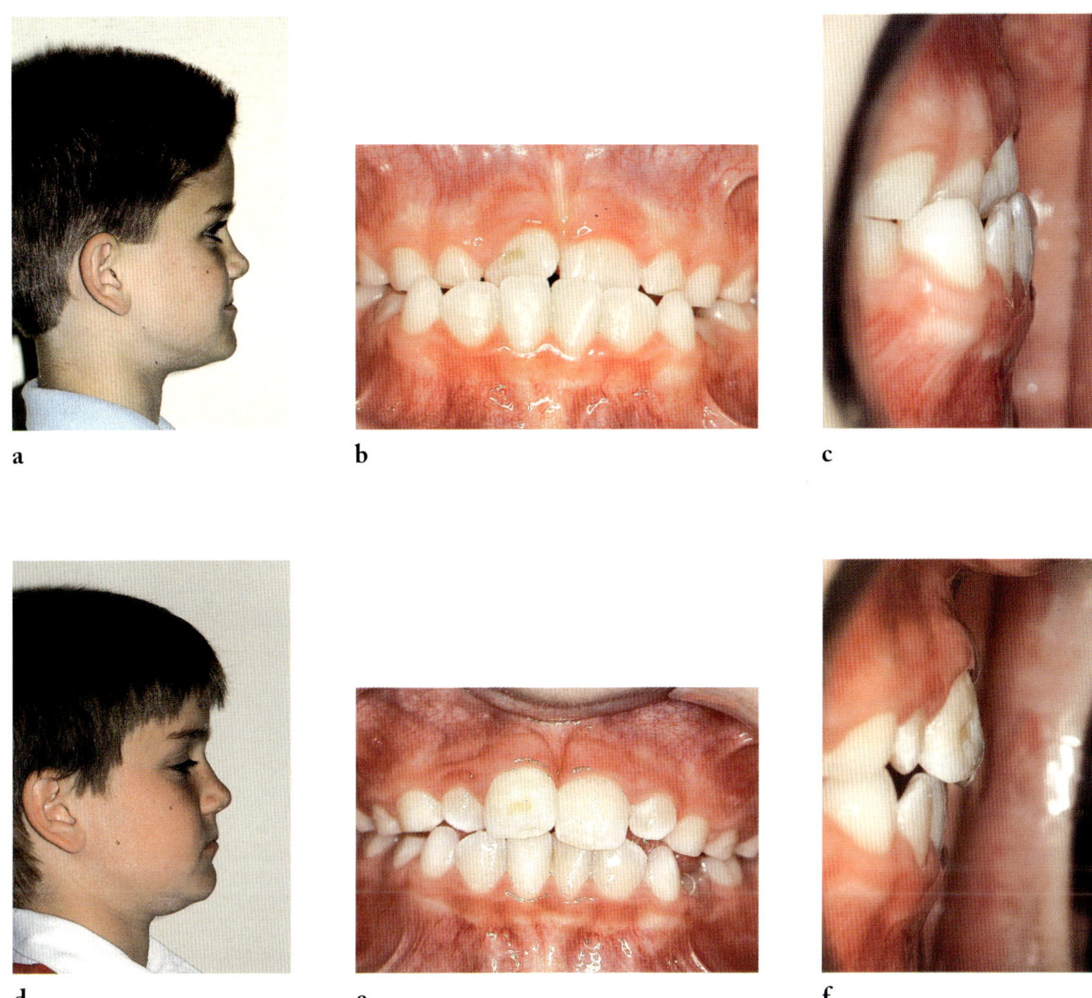

Fig 6-15 Orthopedic correction of Class III skeletal discrepancies.

a to c Initial facial and intraoral appearance of 10-year-old male with dental crowding, constricted maxillary arch, and Class III dental and skeletal relationships due to retrusive maxilla. He was treated with orthopedic appliances to correct only the underlying skeletal discrepancies. This therapy lasted for 1 year and consisted of a rapid palatal expander (for transverse maxillary correction) and a reverse-pull face mask (for A-P maxillary correction).

d to f Final facial and intraoral appearance 6 months after completion of orthopedic therapy. Note the tremendous improvement in the facial profile and dental relationships and the reduction of dental crowding in the maxillary arch. Through proper diagnosis and treatment of skeletal discrepancies at the ideal time during growth and development, future extraction and/or orthognathic surgical procedures can often be prevented.

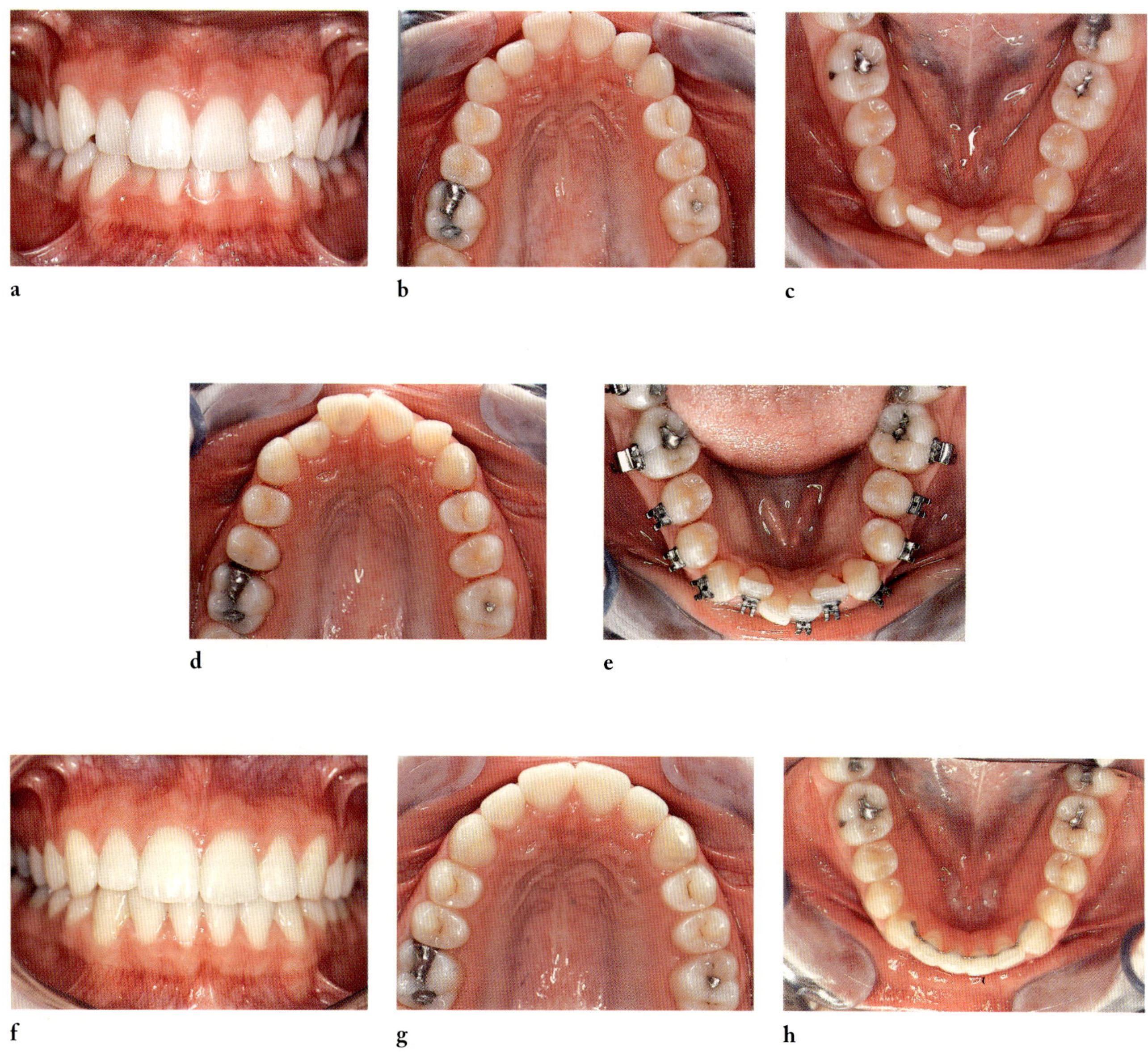

Fig 6-16 Non-extraction orthodontic therapy of an adult dentition with moderate dental crowding.

a to c Initial photographs of adult with Class I dentition with moderate maxillary and mandibular crowding.

d, e Progress occlusal views immediately following morphologic air-rotor stripping (MARS) and before any active tooth movement was initiated. Note the extensive amount of space gained through this procedure. Also note how the morphology of individual teeth was maintained. No MARS was performed in the anterior dentition to maintain optimal esthetics in that highly visible area.

f to h Final views illustrating complete resolution of dental crowding and the proper alignment of dentition within supporting structures. Non-extraction therapy should be used in a crowded dentition only if the teeth can be positioned properly in the supporting structure without causing any deleterious side effects to periodontal health, stability, and dentofacial esthetics.

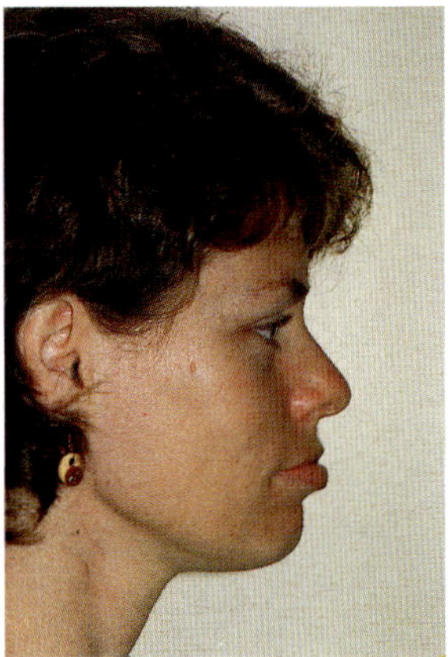

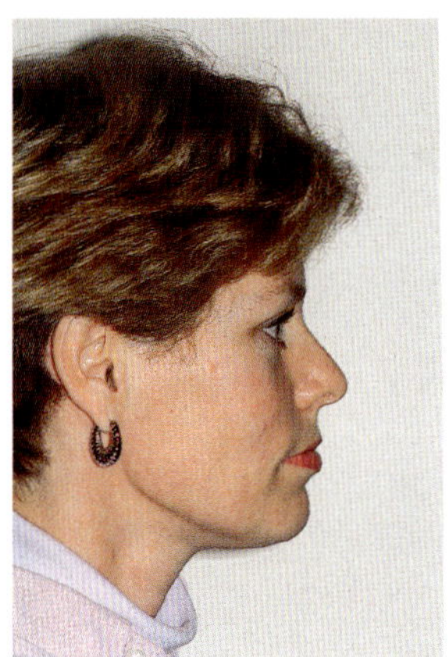

Fig 6-17 Before and after lateral facial views illustrating the profound effect extraction therapy can have on dentofacial appearance. The patient initially had severe bimaxillary dentoalveolar protrusion with lip incompetency, which was corrected by orthodontic extraction therapy. Orthodontic extraction therapy is often an important part of comprehensive dentofacial care. It is frequently indicated for certain dentofacial problems to promote optimal esthetic results while minimizing iatrogenic periodontal problems (see Fig 2-2) and dental instability caused by not positioning teeth properly in their supporting structures.
Orthodontist: Richard D. Roblee, DDS, MS/*Restorative Dentist:* Harvey Smith, DDS

An important point to remember in any orthodontic therapy, especially in comprehensive dentofacial therapy in which the patient frequently has a compromised periodontal situation, is to proceed with orthodontics as quickly as physiologically possible using appliances that have light forces[92] and that minimize the mechanical and chemical (through decreased plaque accumulation) irritation to supporting tissues. It has been shown that there is a significantly greater loss of attachment in orthodontic treatment longer than 24 months when compared to patients treated for less than 24 months.[93] Also, orthodontic bands extended subgingivally may be a periodontal irritant (Fig 6-18).[94] In an adult, these bands may promote negative changes in the sulcular ecosystem similar to those seen with improper fitting subgingival crown margins.[95–97] This change in the sulcular environment can make it more acceptable to periodontopathic microorganisms that may eventually cause inflammation, loss of attachment, and bone loss.[98] These problems can be significantly reduced by using bonded brackets on molars instead of bands.[98] If orthodontic bands must be used, the gingival portion should be trimmed if necessary to minimize subgingival extension and subsequent irritation.

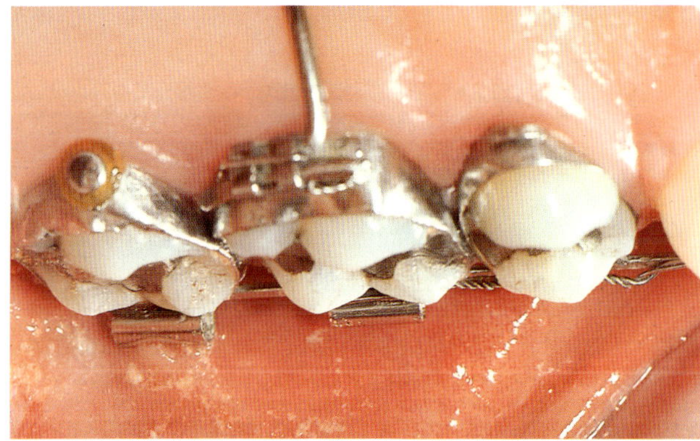

Fig 6-18 A clinical view of an adult whose orthodontic bands extend into the gingival crevice, with subsequent marginal inflammation. To control inflammation during orthodontic therapy, optimal oral hygiene must be maintained and bonded appliances used whenever possible. If orthodontic bands must be used, the gingival portions should be well-contoured and trimmed so that they do not extend subgingivally.

Whenever possible, it is desirable to use indirect bonding procedures[99,100] that allow precise placement and bonding of orthodontic brackets to the teeth with minimal flash of the composite-resin bonding material (Fig 6-19). This makes it possible to carry out orthodontic treatment with less periodontal irritation[101] because bracket placement and the composite-resin bonding material can be better controlled.

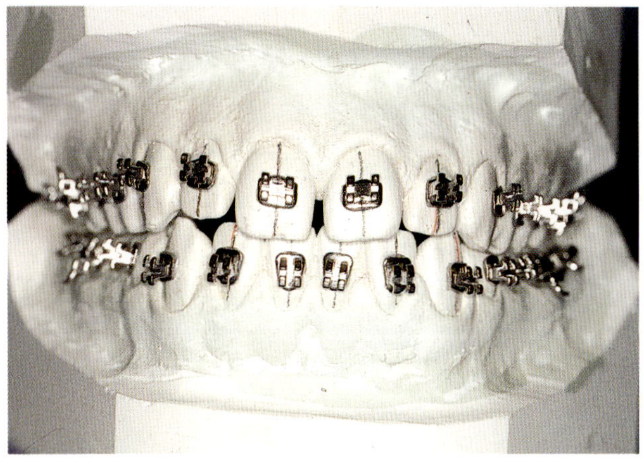

a

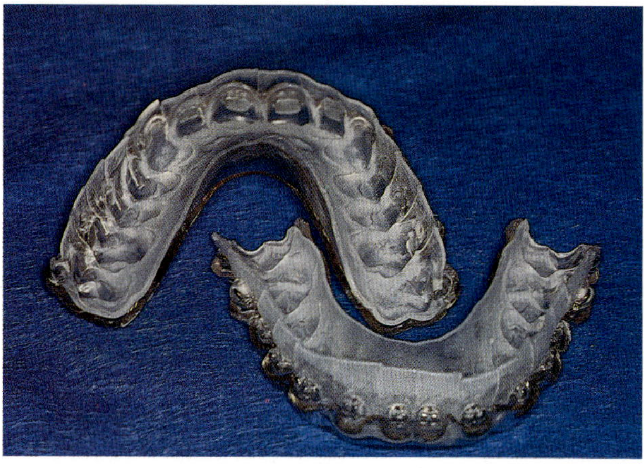

b

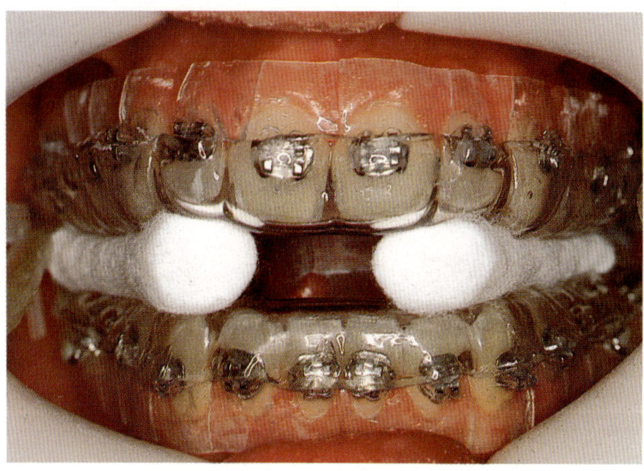

c

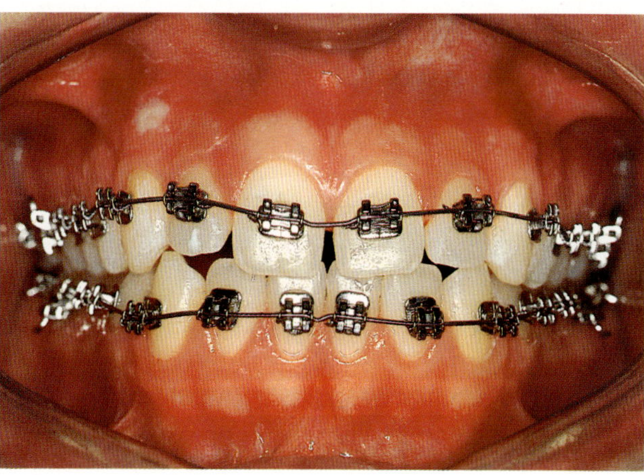

d

Fig 6-19 Indirect bonding of orthodontic appliances.

a Orthodontist indirectly positions brackets onto a stone model, which allows better placement than when performed directly in the mouth.

b, c Transfer trays are constructed, allowing the brackets to be transferred to the mouth in exactly the same relationship to the teeth as they were on the model. A heavily filled composite resin is used to place the brackets on the model and creates a custom pad, as seen in *b*. An unfilled resin is then used to bond the custom pads to the teeth, which allows for easy cleanup of the excess unfilled resin after the bonding is completed.

d Progress view immediately after indirect placement of orthodontic brackets. Note ideal bracket position and cleanup without residual composite-resin flash, typically seen when brackets are placed directly in the mouth. Properly performed indirect bonding can lead to more efficient orthodontic therapy with better overall results in a shorter period of time, and with less gingival irritation compared to directly placing the appliances in the mouth.

Uncontrolled composite-resin material can lead to severe periodontal irritation over the course of orthodontic therapy. The indirect bonding of orthodontic brackets has also improved the accuracy of their placement[101] compared to placing them directly in the mouth. Indirect bonding allows the operator to position the brackets ideally on a stone model, then transfer that bracket position to the teeth (Fig 6-19). Since most modern orthodontic brackets now have a prescribed amount of torque, in-out, and tip built into the bracket[102] to reduce wire bending, treatment will proceed more quickly and efficiently when brackets are placed as ideally as possible in relationship to each individual tooth. This concept of indirect bonding of appliances can be extended by the use of an instrument that actually measures the teeth on the stone model and allows the placement of the brackets in the most ideal position possible (Fig 6-20). This instrument enables the orthodontist to customize the tipping of and vertical forces on each tooth according to the specific treatment needs of that malocclusion. This takes the previously described concept of prescription appliances a step further, and is often referred to as "prescription orthodontics." When a bracket is placed in an improper relationship, that tooth will be moved to an improper relationship, and bends will have to be made in the wire to correct the problem. Proper bracket placement can easily reduce the treatment time of definitive orthodontic therapy by 6 months or more, compared to improper bracket placement. This is especially true when proper bracket placement is combined with superelastic nickel-titanium wires and springs that can supply continuous light forces over very large deflections without permanent deformation (Fig 6-19d).[103,104]

Lindhe and Svanberg[50] have shown that dogs have more rapid periodontal pocket formation when a traumatic occlusion is present with inflammation, compared to the presence of inflammation alone. Since this probably also applies to humans, the orthodontist and the rest of the interdisciplinary team must be alert throughout orthodontic therapy for teeth which are in excessive traumatic occlusion with subsequent fremitus (functional mobility) or discomfort. Fremitus should be brought under control as soon as possible either by changing the orthodontic mechanics or by occlusal splint therapy. Trauma to the supporting tissues is also decreased by using minimal orthodontic forces.[105] Brown showed that when occlusal trauma and inflammation are controlled during orthodontic tooth movement, bone loss can also be controlled.[106]

It is important that the restorative dentist, prosthodontist, periodontist, and oral and maxillofacial surgeon monitor the progress of orthodontic treatment if part of the orthodontic therapy is to prepare the dentition for their future therapy. No

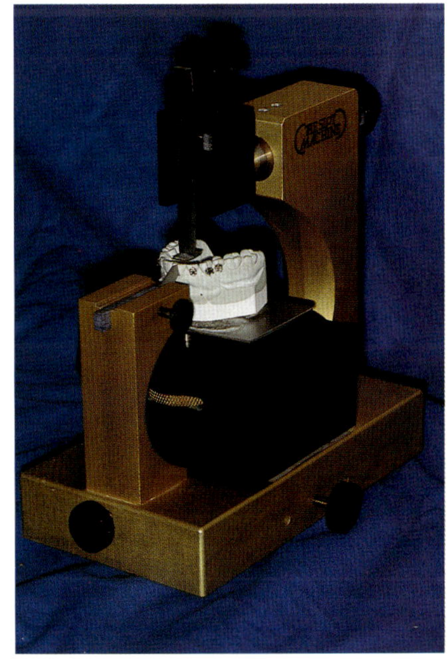

Fig 6-20 The concept of indirect bonding of orthodontic appliances can be taken a step further by using instruments such as the Creekmore Slot Machine. This instrument allows the desired three-dimensional relationship of the individual teeth to be programmed into the bracket placement when using the straight-wire orthodontic philosophy. This programming is often referred to as "prescription orthodontics" and can be a tremendous asset during orthodontic therapy; especially with complex adult mutilated dentitions in which the normal morphology of the teeth has been destroyed.

one team member knows more about what is needed for a particular aspect of the therapy than the specific team member whose expertise is in that area. That provider should help the orthodontist decide the position of the teeth for that therapy. The orthodontist, with his or her expertise, then has to determine if the tooth positions desired by the other team members can be attained within the physiological parameters of the supporting structures. All too often the orthodontist is forced to make treatment decisions concerning the positioning of teeth for periodontal, restorative, and surgical therapies when he or she obviously cannot be an expert in all areas. Only through team monitoring can all orthodontic treatment objectives of the interdisciplinary dentofacial therapy be optimally fulfilled before the appliances are removed.

Through team monitoring and interaction, the total orthodontic treatment time can be reduced. This is accomplished by the team members interacting with pertinent information and deciding what compromises might be made by the orthodontist in tooth position that can be compensated for prosthetically, periodontally, or surgically. These compromises should not affect the function, periodontal health, esthetics, or longevity of the result. Without this interaction, many cases would be orthodontically overtreated to ideals that would have no significant positive impact on the eventual treatment result[107] except to significantly lengthen the time needed to attain it.

In addition to a negative influence on periodontal health, a prolonged orthodontic phase can also have a significant negative psychological impact on patients, which may lead to frustration and subsequent loss of motivation and cooperation. In contrast, a shortened orthodontic phase can have a tremendous positive psychological impact on patients because they see improved dentofacial results even sooner than they had originally thought (Fig 6-23).

An example of this type of compromise between the orthodontic and restorative therapies would be a maxillary second molar that is planned to function as a terminal abutment. The molar root may be in proper position buccolingually and mesiodistally, but is rotated approximately 90 degrees. Since the tooth is going to have a full-coverage restoration on it anyway, it may make little sense to correct the rotation and lengthen treatment if the occlusion can be optimally restored and periodontal health maintained in the final restoration without the correction.

The compromises in orthodontic therapy discussed here should be compensated by compromises in the other disciplines' therapies to produce optimal results expeditiously. As discussed previously, these beneficial and positive compromises are called interdisciplinary compromises. It is often necessary for the different providers to communicate during active orthodontic therapy in order to give feedback as to the type and degree of compensation each member can allow to correct a specific problem. Without this interaction, one area may have to compensate to a degree that is not compatible with long-term health, function, and stability (Fig 2-3). In addition to shortening treatment time and preventing unnecessary compromises, the team interaction of interdisciplinary compromises promotes creative solutions to complex problems that otherwise would provide less-than-optimal results (Fig 5-3).

It is imperative that there is smooth progression from orthodontic therapy into the definitive periodontal and restorative phases. If the transition is not well-planned, it can lead to lengthened treatment times, confusion, orthodontic relapse, and less-than-optimal results in the remaining therapies. Retention is another very important aspect of the final stages of definitive orthodontic therapy, which will be discussed later in this chapter.

Preparatory Restorative-Type II Therapy

Preparatory restorative-type II therapy is an excellent example of how interaction between the different providers promotes optimal results. Whenever definitive restorative therapy is planned after definitive orthodontic and/or orthognathic surgical therapy, the restorative team member should interact with the orthodontist and oral and maxillofacial surgeon to provide information and services that can facilitate the attainment of the best dental and skeletal relationships and optimally set up for the future placement of any planned prosthodontics. Without

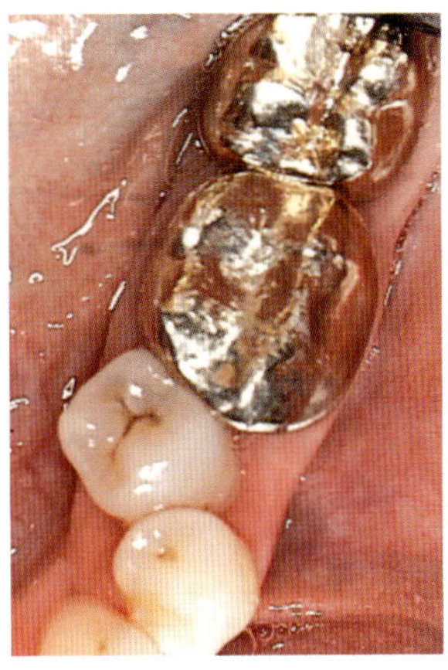
a

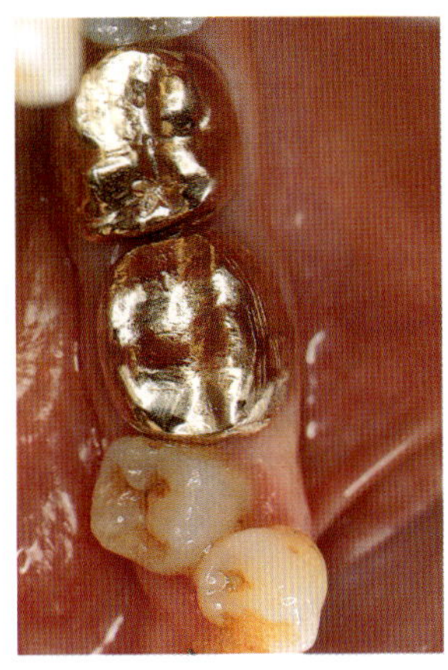
b

Fig 6-21

a Occlusal view of right mandibular first molar that was previously restored using unidisciplinary compromised therapy. Note how restoration is overcontoured buccolingually as well as mesiodistally. This quadrant cannot be properly aligned during orthodontic therapy with the restoration in this form.

b Occlusal view after preparatory restorative-type II therapy has been performed to reshape the restoration so that the tooth can be properly aligned to the adjacent dentition during orthodontic therapy. This restoration will be replaced to the new relationship after orthodontic therapy has been completed.

this assistance, the orthodontists and oral and maxillofacial surgeons may have to perform procedures and make treatment decisions for which they are not best qualified, and subsequently finish with less-than-optimal results for which the restorative team members may have to make detrimental compromises in their therapy.

Basic preparatory restorative-type II procedures are usually done in conjunction with preparatory restorative-type I therapy. These procedures usually consist of reshaping previously placed crowns and bridges as needed so that the anatomy better conforms to natural coronal anatomy in relation to its root structure. During unidisciplinary therapy, crowns and bridges are frequently constructed on and/or in relation to malaligned teeth. Because of this, compensations are usually built into the restorations in an attempt to better restore the malaligned relationships (Figs 2-1 and 6-22a). The reshaping described here is used to decompensate these restorations so that they will not interfere with orthodontic positioning of roots in their proper relationships. This reshaping includes coronal contours, overextended interproximal contacts, improper marginal ridge heights and contours, and irregular cusp tip positions (Figs 6-21 and 6-22). Panoramic and vertical bitewing radiographs are extremely useful in this decompensating process (Fig 6-22a). For example, if a second molar has been restored using unidisciplinary therapy after it tipped into the extraction site of a first molar, the mesial contact is usually overextended to close the space, and the mesial marginal ridge is overextended occlusally to reestablish and maintain occlusion with the opposing dentition (Figs 6-22a and 6-22b). These restorative compensations may help maintain stability in the dental arches; however, it is less than ideal for the long-term health of the supporting tissues associated with the tooth. If this compensated restoration were left unaltered during orthodontic therapy, the root could not be ideally positioned because of occlusal and proximal interferences with the anatomical compensations (Fig 6-22c). To properly position the tooth orthodontically, the restoration must be decompensated through reshaping or by removing the restoration and replacing it with a provisional restoration which better conforms to natural coronal anatomy and the axial inclination of the root.

Some reshaping of teeth and provisional restoration placement cannot be ideally performed until after some tooth movement has been performed, due to previous tipping, extrusion, and inadequate inter-

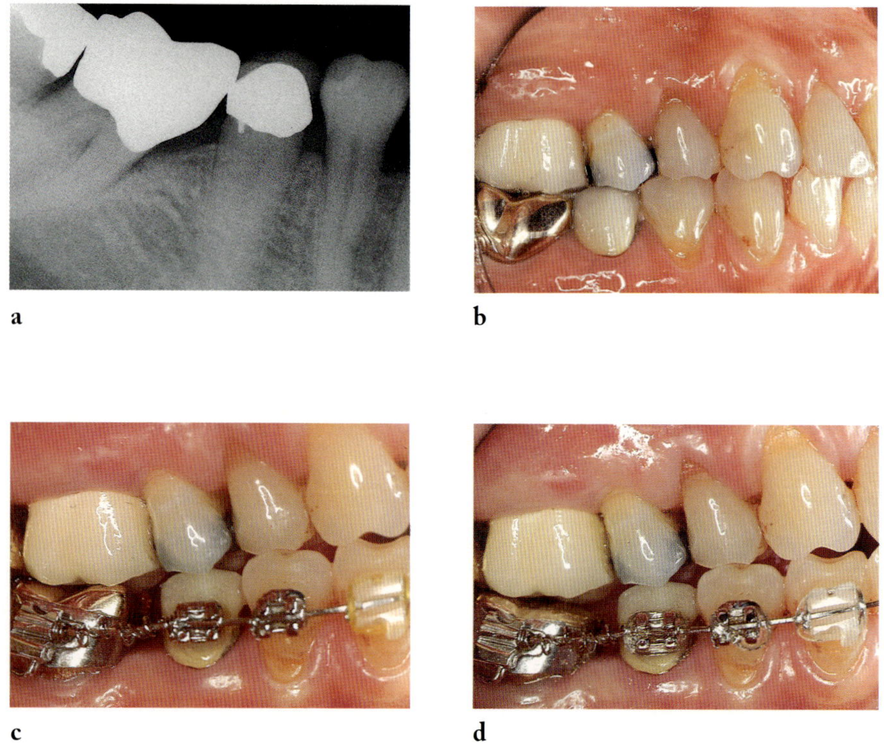

Fig 6-22

a, b Initial radiograph and intraoral view of right mandibular second molar restored with unidisciplinary compromised therapy to compromise for its tip relationship to the previous first molar extraction site. Note how the mesial contact and mesial marginal ridge have been overextended in an attempt to reestablish a stable intra-arch relationship. This compromised therapy does not address the problems associated with the supporting tissues around the tooth and may in fact exacerbate these problems.

c The overcontoured and overextended relationships of the crown prohibit proper orthodontic uprighting due to occlusal interferences with the mesial marginal ridge.

d Preparatory restorative-type II therapy was performed to decompensate the restoration and allow proper uprighting of the tooth. Note that the occlusal surface has been reduced on the mesial aspect of the crown. The first-molar extraction sites will be reopened and an ideal three-unit bridge placed following orthodontic therapy. This decompensating process of the restorations can be performed before definitive orthodontic therapy in conjunction with preparatory restorative-type I therapy, or it can be performed during active tooth movement.

proximal spaces. This preparatory restorative therapy will be performed at the optimal time during definitive orthodontic therapy as part of preparatory restorative-type II therapy.

Advanced preparatory restorative-type II procedures are usually performed at many different stages in the orthodontic therapy. They are indicated whenever postorthodontic restorative procedures will alter the shape, size, or number of natural teeth, or will replace previous unidisciplinary compromised restorations. When it comes to establishing new shapes and sizes of teeth to better conform to the patient's facial form, smile, and personality, the restorative team member is usually the most qualified and experienced. Preparatory restorative-type II therapy allows the restorative team member to determine and illustrate the three-dimensional shapes and sizes of his or her final restorations so that the orthodontist and surgeon can precisely position the teeth and/or skeletal components in the proper relationship to accept optimal definitive restorations. This will be performed at different stages in the orthodontic therapy, because tooth movement is usually necessary to make room for these three-dimensional changes in tooth size. During this stage, the restorative dentist or prosthodontist should perform restorative procedures that will enable the orthodontist to perform optimal tooth movement while maintaining and gradually improving the esthetic environment (Fig 6-23). This aspect helps promote the dentofacial counseling philosophy by providing positive reinforcement for the patient, because he or she is continuously seeing esthetic enhancements.

The restorative team member has at his or her disposal several different modalities to assist the orthodontist. One of the most basic is the sectioning of fixed partial dentures after the orthodontist has placed orthodontic brackets (Fig 6-23g). This frees the abutment teeth so that they can be more optimally positioned. The loose pontic(s) can then be attached on the arch-wire to maintain esthetics (Fig 6-23h). Another useful service is the selection and customizing of denture teeth to illustrate the optimal shape and size of the future restorations. The orthodontist can measure these denture teeth to get information necessary to precisely position the natural teeth so that they will accept the future optimal restorations (Fig 2-5f). The restorative team member can perform adjunctive diagnostic procedures, such as a diagnostic waxup, after the orthodontist feels that the teeth are close to their proper positions, to further illustrate the final changes so that the orthodontist can make any necessary final adjustments (Fig 2-5g). Denture teeth can also be placed onto the arch-wire when replacing missing teeth (Fig 4-3). These teeth will not only give the orthodontist the actual size of the eventual bridge pontic(s) so that he or she can properly position the abutment teeth, but will also elevate esthetics and provide positive reinforcement for the patient.

The restorative team member and orthodontist can be very creative in this therapy. The restorative dentist or prosthodontist can actually simulate ideal tooth shapes and sizes during definitive orthodontic therapy by using provisional restorations, direct-addition dental materials, or enameloplasty. The orthodontist can then position these provisionally restored or altered teeth as if they were the final restorations. When teeth are going to be enlarged, the orthodontist will usually have to first reposition the teeth to create space. Then the restorative dentist or prosthodontist can construct provisional restorations or add to the teeth to illustrate what he or she feels are the optimal shapes and sizes (Fig 6-23j). This completely eliminates guesswork by the restorative and orthodontic team members. Frequently, the opposite is true, and natural teeth or previously placed restorations are too large or overcontoured. In these instances, the restorative team member can reshape the natural teeth (enameloplasty) (Fig 6-24) or restorations in conjunction with preparatory restorative-type I therapy or construct smaller, more ideally shaped provisional restorations to allow precise orthodontic positioning.

Preparatory restorative-type II therapy can also assist the oral and maxillofacial surgeon in repositioning dentulous and edentulous jaws to allow optimal prosthetic rehabilitation.[108] This preparatory restorative therapy is usually performed with the construction of surgical stints, occlusal rims, and waxups to simulate optimal prosthetic relationships to the edentulous ridges, and to develop the proper vertical dimension. Existing dentures can frequently be modified to provide the same information described above.

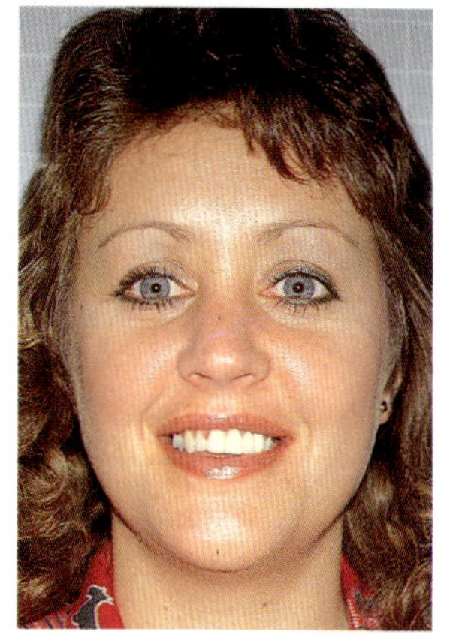
a

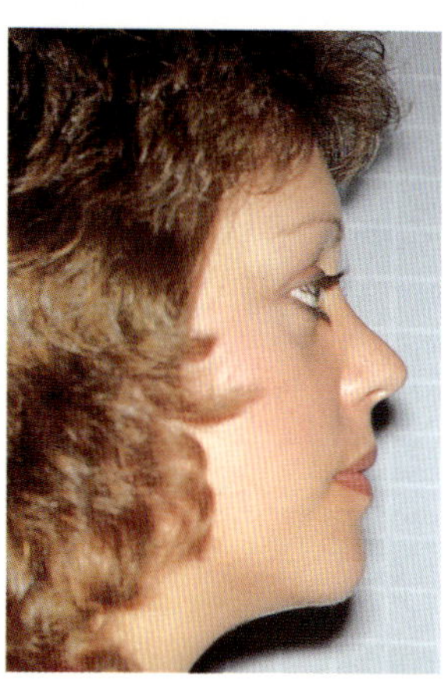
b

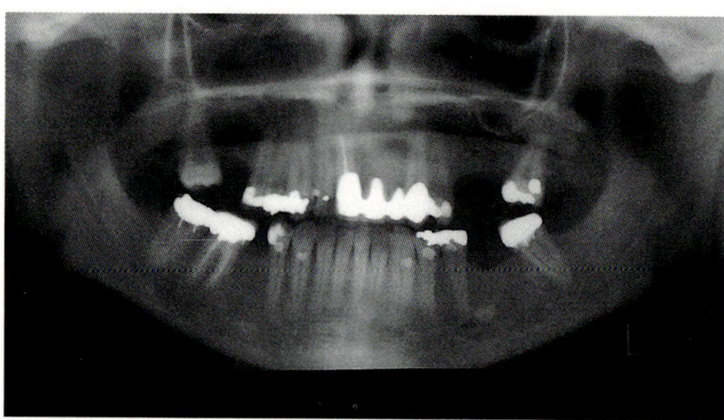
c

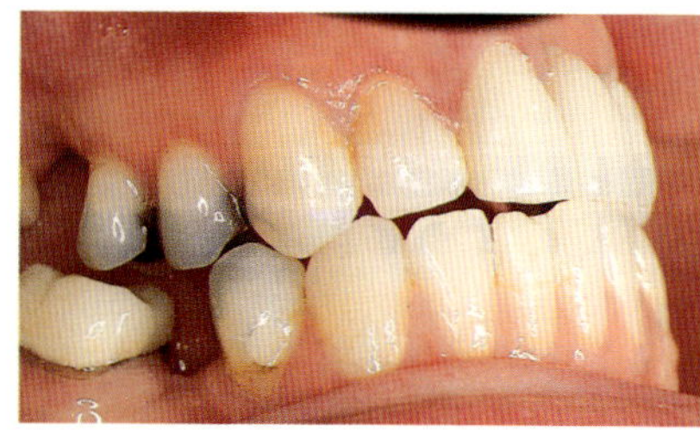
d

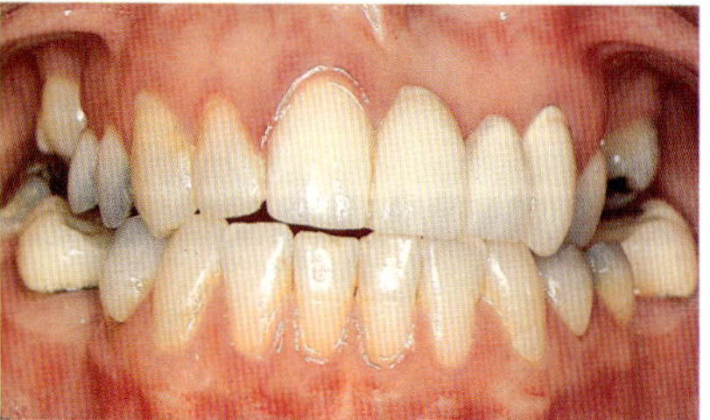
e

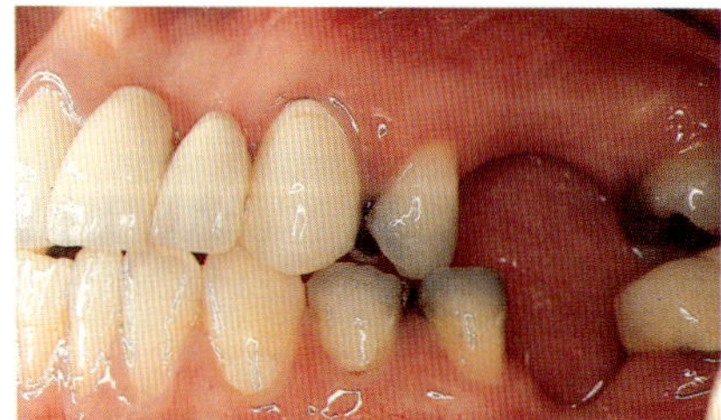
f

Fig 6-23 30-year-old female reported for dental therapy with chief concern of "I want my teeth to look better." She had been receiving unidisciplinary therapy to this point.

a, b Facial photographs illustrating good facial symmetry and proportionality. Maxillary dental midline is approximately 3 mm to the left of the skeletal midline.

c to f Initial radiographic and intraoral appearance illustrating a mutilated dentition with numerous missing teeth, compromised restorative dentistry, and a transverse skeletal deficiency in the maxillary arch. Definitive orthodontic and periodontal therpaies were planned to align the dentition and supporting structures for an optimal full-mouth reconstruction. Preparatory restorative-type I therapy was performed to prepare the teeth for definitive orthodontic and periodontal therapies; full-mouth orthodontic appliances were also placed.

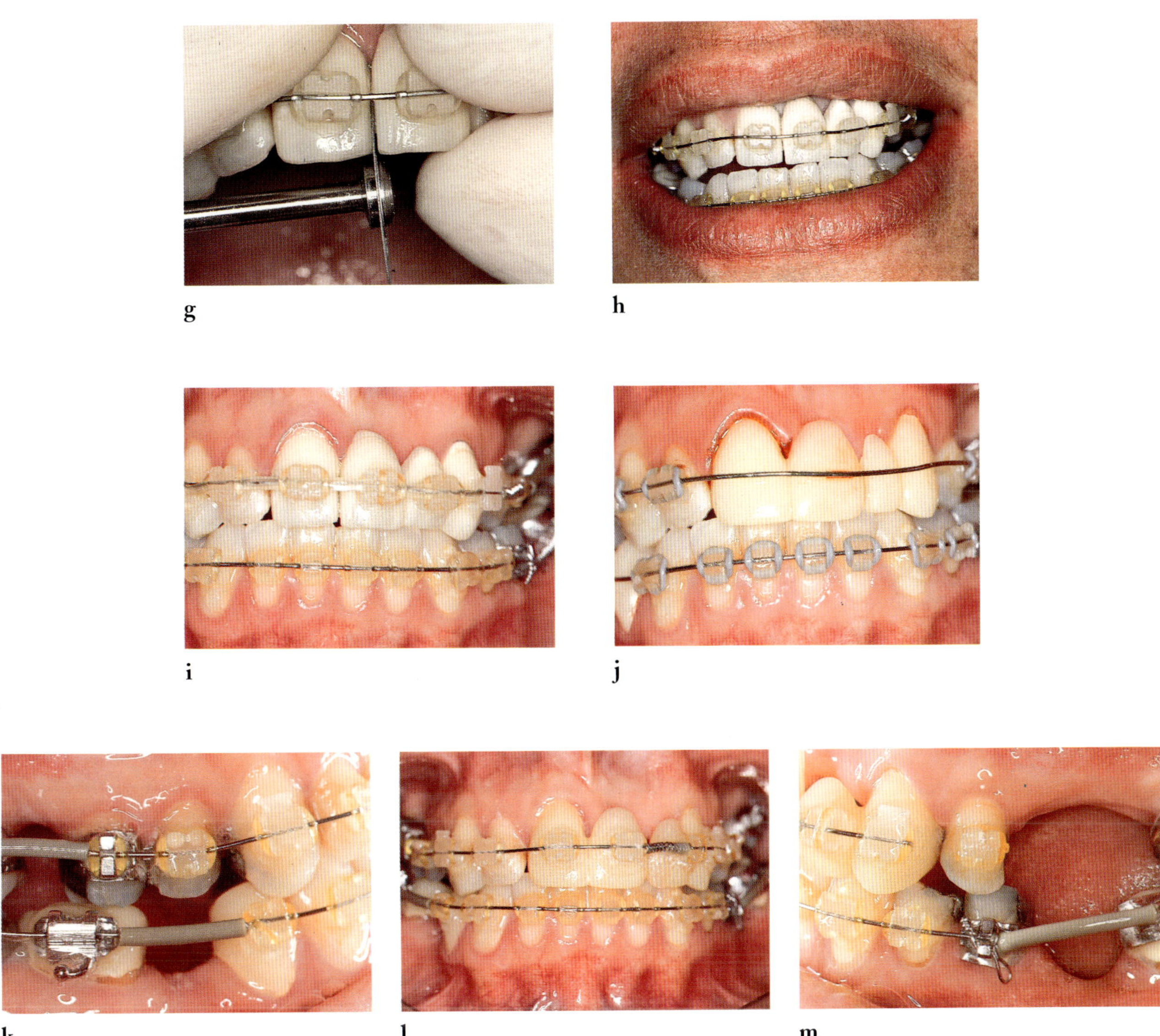

Fig 6-23 (continued)

g The restorative dentist sectioned the fixed partial denture (preparatory restorative-type II therapy) to allow optimal orthodontic positioning of abutment teeth 11 and 23.

h The loose pontic teeth 21 and 22 were fixed on the archwire to maintain esthetics while the long axis of the abutment teeth were being optimally related to their supporting structures.

i, j After 3 months of definitive orthodontic therapy, the long axis of the abutment teeth had already been properly positioned. The restorative dentist removed the compromised restorations on teeth 11 and 23 and the overcontoured crown on tooth 46. Optimal provisional restorations that exactly simulated the desired contours of the final definitive restorations were constructed (preparatory restorative-type II therapy). Pontic tooth 21 is connected to tooth 11 and pontic tooth 22 is connected to tooth 23. The two central incisors were constructed to esthetically blend in with the patient's smile and facial form. Only the distal half of the lateral incisor pontic fit into the space at this time, due to the increased width of the provisional centrals. The orthodontist can now correctly position the maxillary dental midline without having to guess about the contours of the final restorations.

k to m Intraoral appearance 8 months into treatment. As the maxillary dental midline was corrected and the pontic space was opened between teeth 21 and 22, the orthodontist gradually added acrylic resin to a mesial aspect of tooth 22. This maintained esthetics during correction of the maxillary dental midline. Orthodontic therapy was now complete in the maxillary arch, with the exception of increasing the pontic space between teeth 15 and 17.

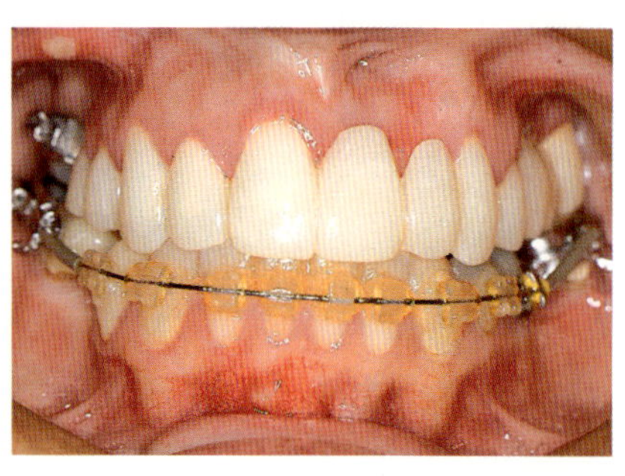

n

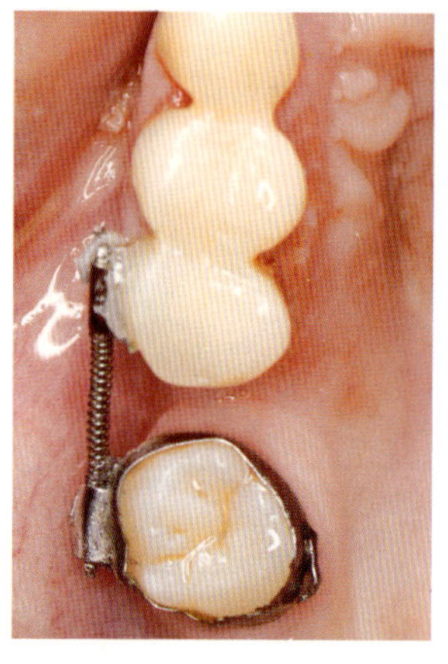

o

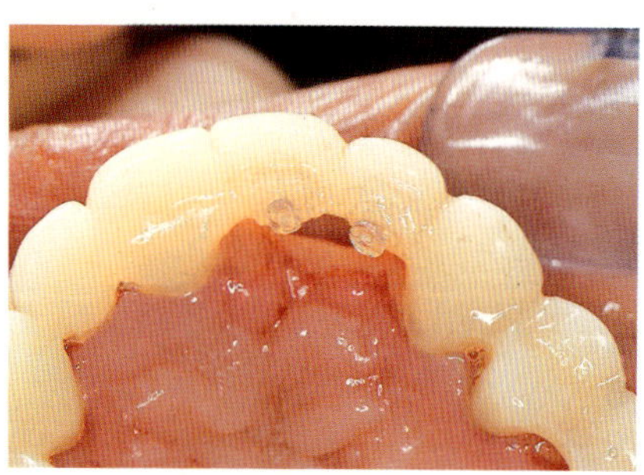

p

q

Fig 6-23 (continued)

n to p Instead of waiting for orthodontic therapy to be completed on the lower arch and on tooth 17, provisional restorations were constructed on the maxillary arch so that the patient could start enjoying the esthetic improvements. Orthodontic therapy was continued fully on the lower arch and partially on the upper arch to properly position tooth 17. In addition, the restorative dentist used the provisional restorations to illustrate the ideal cervical contours of pontic teeth 21 and 22 desired in the definitive restorations. This enabled the periodontist to use these provisional restorations as a template for ridge augmentation procedures in the anterior edentulous area (preparatory restorative-type III therapy). The restorative dentist also placed buttons on the lingual of the provisional restorations to give added stability to the periodontal pack.

q Orthodontic therapy was now completed, with the exception of tooth 17. Appliances were removed from the mandibular arch and a clear plastic stent was placed to esthetically maintain tooth positions until definitive restorative therapy is performed. Definitive restorative therapy will begin after the position of tooth 17 has been orthodontically corrected and ridge augmentation procedures are completed.

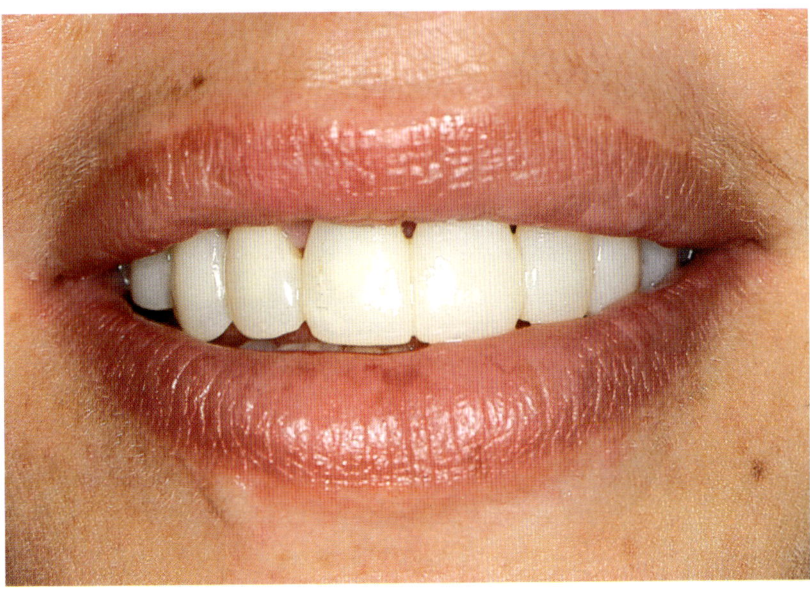

r

Fig 6-23 (continued)

r Smiling photograph illustrating the esthetic enhancements interdisciplinary therapy provided even before placement of definitive restorations. This case illustrated many important aspects of interdisciplinary therapy. First of all, it illustrates how the interdisciplinary treatment planning and communication can minimize unplanned compromises by the various team members and reduce the necessity of some extensive procedures without affecting the long-term prognosis. The team decided that the patient's transverse skeletal deficiency in the maxillary arch could be treated without significantly affecting the long-term prognosis by slightly compromising the orthodontic and restorative therapy to compensate for the discrepancy between the two arches. This case also illustrates how the different team members working together can help each other in attaining optimal and predictable results. Optimal communication and teamwork allowed therapy to progress as expeditiously as possible. One provider did not have to wait for the previous provider to complete his aspect of therapy before initiating his own therapy. Finally, effective interdisciplinary communication and therapy can help motivate patients by allowing them to enjoy esthetic improvements as early in treatment as possible. This is an excellent example of how the restorative dentist or prosthodontist can provide valuable services and information through preparatory restorative therapy-types I, II, and III to assist the orthodontist and periodontist in optimally performing their therapies.

Orthodontist: Carlos Navarro, DDS, MSD/*Restorative Dentist:* Richard D. Roblee, DDS, MS
Periodontist: Edward P. Allen, DDS, PhD

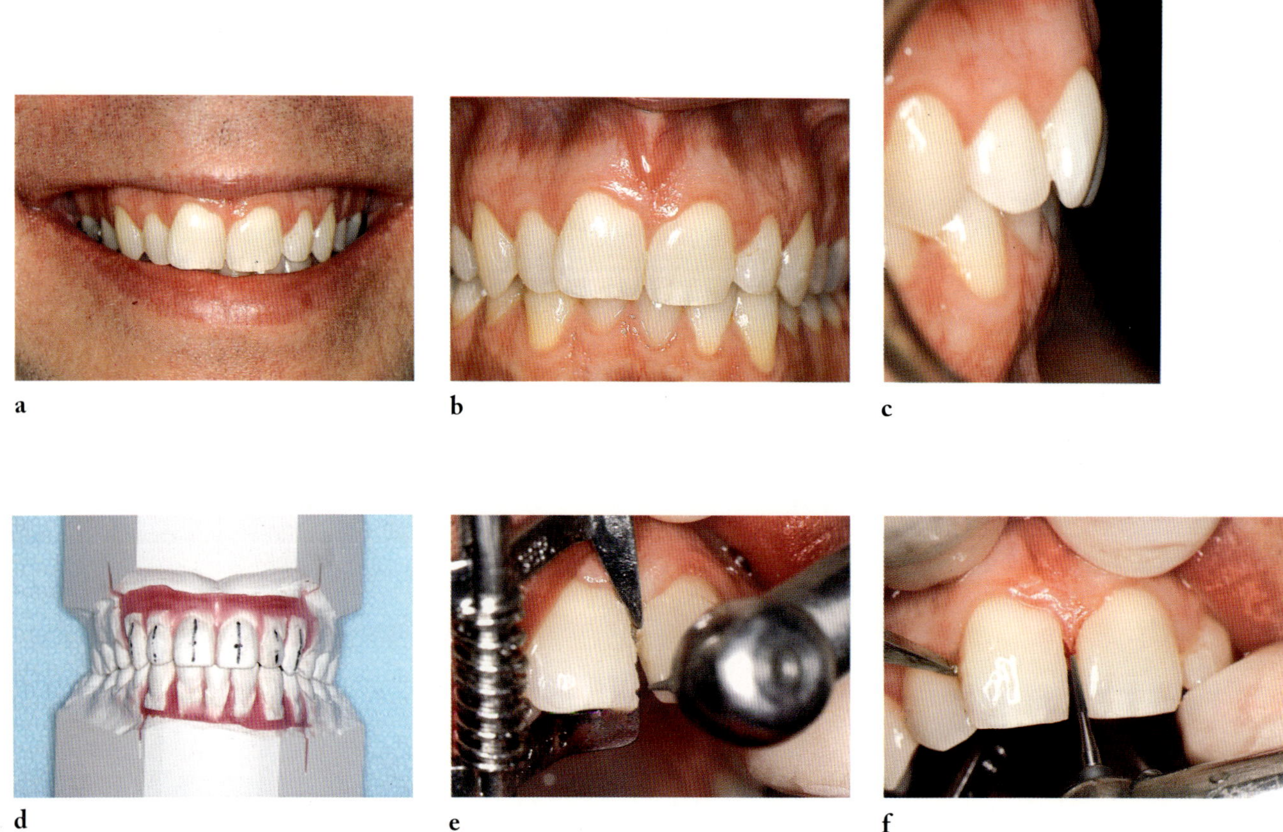

Fig 6-24 F.W. is a 35-year-old male who had previous unidisciplinary orthodontic therapy as an adolescent, with both maxillary first premolars and one mandibular central incisor extracted. His chief concern was that he thought his front teeth were too big and that they were tipping backwards.

a Initial smiling view illustrating the appearance of large central incisors that are out of proportion with the face and dentition.

b, c Initial intraoral appearance of anterior dentition which shows intra-arch tooth-size discrepancy between maxillary and mandibular anterior teeth due to large maxillary central incisors and a missing mandibular central incisor. In an attempt to adjust for this discrepancy, the maxillary anteriors were tipped backwards during the previous unidisciplinary orthodontic therapy. Note instability of interincisal relationship, with maxillary anteriors being retroclined and crowded. These problems have led to a traumatic functional relationship with subsequent incisor wear.

d An adjunctive diagnostic procedure of an orthodontic setup was performed and periapical radiographs were made to determine if reshaping the maxillary anterior teeth could create enough space to compensate for the missing mandibular incisor. It was determined that 6.5 mm could be gained by reshaping, which was enough to compensate for the missing lower incisor while creating a more esthetic appearance of the maxillary anterior teeth. The exact dimension of tooth structure necessary to be removed from each proximal surface was determined and recorded.

e Preparatory restorative-type II therapy. The restorative dentist used information gained through the adjunctive diagnostic procedure to make appropriate-depth cuts in all proximal surfaces of the maxillary anteriors to precisely indicate the ideal amount of tooth structure to be removed from each surface.

f The proper amount of tooth structure was removed, and the teeth were then shaped, smoothed, and polished to maintain a natural morphology for each tooth.

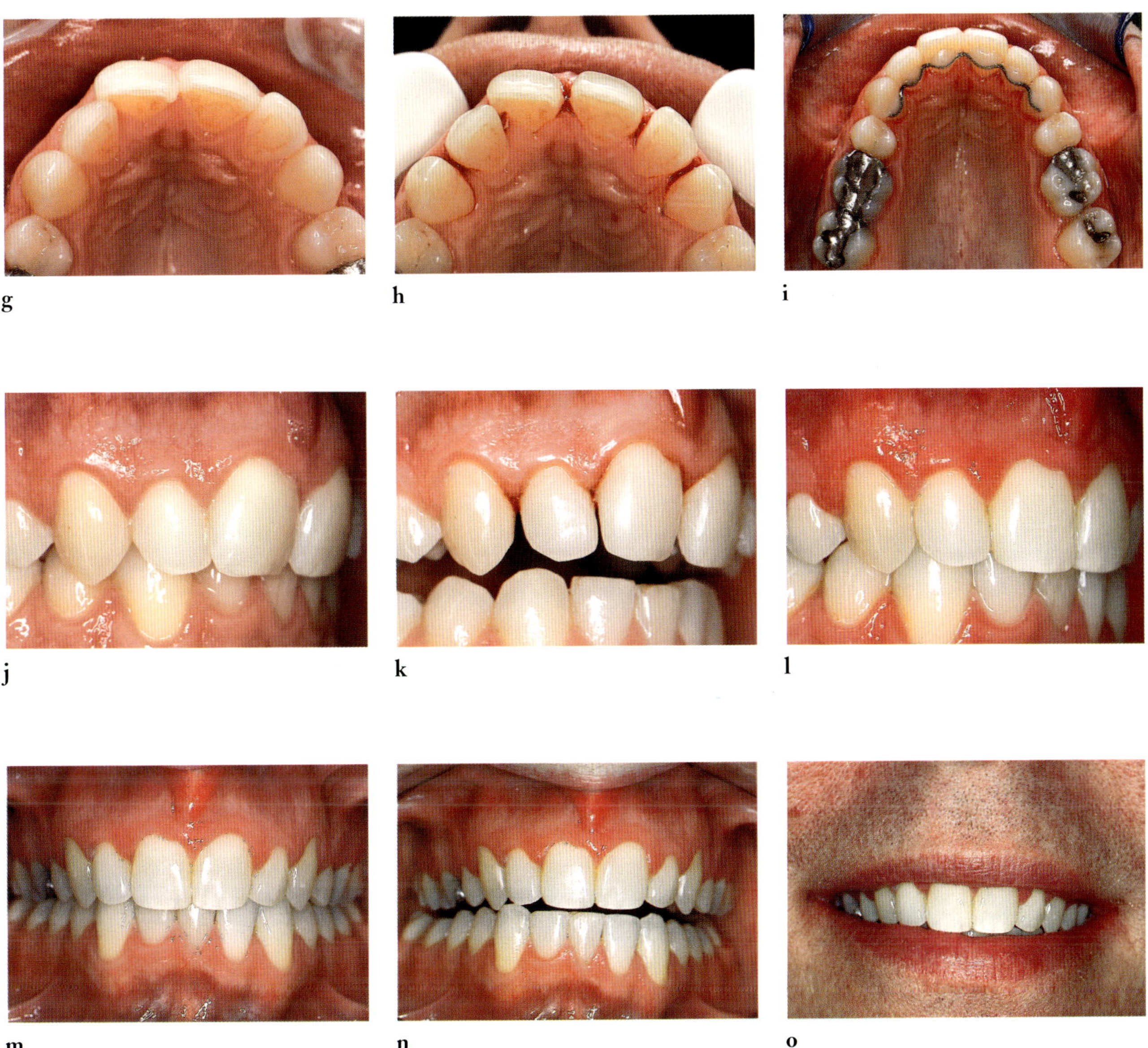

Fig 6-24 (continued)

g to i Initial, post-reshaping, and final occlusal views of maxillary arch. These photographs illustrate the extent of the reshaping performed and the good alignment attained.

j to m Initial, post-reshaping, and final intraoral views illustrating that the morphology of the maxillary anteriors was retained in the reshaping process, even though extensive amounts of tooth structure were removed. This also illustrates the good anterior interincisal relationship attained, and the extent to which the maxillary central incisor roots were torqued palatally to attain a more stable interincisal relationship.

n An ideal functional occlusion was established with anterior guidance and posterior disocclusion in all excursive movements.

o Final smiling photographs illustrating balance and proportionality of the anterior dentition after extensive recontouring procedures. This case illustrates how creative treatment planning by an interdisciplinary team can turn problems (large central incisors) into advantages to solve other problems (interarch anterior tooth-mass discrepancy due to extracted mandibular incisor). Even though 6.5 mm were gained by reshaping the maxillary anterior dentition, no posttreatment problems (such as sensitivity or caries) have occurred. Extensive periapical radiographs were taken of the anterior dentition during the diagnostic and reshaping procedures to help ensure intraenamel reshaping. Also, no anesthetic was used during the reshaping procedures so that the patient could report sensitivity if a surface was being overreduced.

Orthognathic Surgical Therapy

Orthognathic surgical therapy combines the diagnosis and treatment techniques of oral and maxillofacial surgery and various other dental and medical disciplines to correct musculoskeletal, dentosseous, and soft tissue deformities of the jaws and associated structures.[109–111] Deformities of the dentofacial structures can occur unilaterally or bilaterally, involve either one jaw or both, and involve all three planes of space: vertical, horizontal, and antero-posterior.

Many significant and exciting advances have been made in orthognathic surgical techniques during the past 10 years.[109,110,112–117] These advances enable the interdisciplinary dentofacial team to predictably treat most minor and major dentofacial deformities with unsurpassed results (Fig 6-25). At the same time, these improvements also make orthognathic surgery considerably easier for patients to undergo.

Probably the most significant advancement has been the development of rigid fixation with bone screws and plates.[118] Rigid fixation firmly stabilizes the jaws in a predetermined position so patients can open their jaws immediately after surgery. Rigid fixation, when properly performed, significantly decreases the risks and complications of surgery, improves the predictability of results, and improves long-term stability.[118]

There are five basic therapeutic goals for orthognathic surgery:

1. Correct functional deformities (ie, establish normal mastication, speech,[119] respiratory function, etc).
2. Provide optimal dentofacial esthetic results.
3. Provide long-term orthodontic and surgical stability.
4. Set up dentosseous structures for optimal fixed or removable prosthodontic procedures.
5. Decrease treatment time with proper treatment planning.

Thorough diagnostic and treatment-planning procedures are especially important for interdisciplinary cases requiring orthognathic surgery because of the magnitude of its impact on dentofacial structures. During preoperative clinical examinations, as in any facial examination, the patient should be examined either in a standing position or sitting in a straight-backed chair. The patient must be evaluated in centric relation, with the teeth lightly touching and the lips relaxed. The head should be oriented so that the clinical Frankfort horizontal (a line from the superior aspect of the tragus of the ear through the bony infraorbital rim) is parallel to the floor. The face must be evaluated in all three dimensions from the frontal and lateral views.

Additional attention should be given to these patients during the diagnostic phase of IDT in evaluations of speech, audiometric, psychological, neurological, medical, tongue, intranasal, TMJ, and other functions. Proper orthognathic surgery planning requires panographic and lateral cephalometric radiographics. Other specialized imaging techniques may also be indicated, such as PA cephalograms, tomograms, CT scans, MRIs, etc. The diagnostic findings from this specialized evaluation and data collection and any adjunctive diagnostic procedures are incorporated into the overall interdisciplinary problem list and discussed during team conferences (as described in Chapters 4 and 5) before the optimal orthognathic surgical procedures are planned.

During preoperative orthodontics, the orthodontist should properly align the teeth over the basal bone of the upper and lower jaws, or segments thereof, so that the oral and maxillofacial surgeon can optimally reposition the jaws and/or other facial structures as dictated by the existing deformities and therapeutic goals.

Case Summary

Patient: A.C. is a 22-year-old female who was dissatisfied with the function and esthetics of her previous unidisciplinary compromised orthodontic therapy.

Chief Concern: "I want to know if my teeth can be fixed."

Abbreviated Problem List

- Retrusive maxilla and mandible
- Low mandibular plane angle with decreased lower face height
- Bimaxillary dentoalveolar retrusion
- Previous orthodontic therapy with extraction of three premolars
- Severely retroclined maxillary and mandibular anterior teeth
- Dentoalveolar extrusion in maxillary and mandibular anterior segments with 110% vertical overlap
- Traumatic anterior dental coupling with severe incisal wear

Treatment Plan

Interdisciplinary Dentofacial Therapy

- Preoperative orthodontic non-extraction therapy to decompensate dentition
    - Reopen previous premolar extraction sites
- Orthognathic Surgery
    - Maxillary advancement
    - Mandibular advancement and rotation
    - Genioplasty
- Postoperative Orthodontic Therapy
    - Finalize occlusion and prepare dentition for restorative therapy
- Periodontal Therapy
    - Esthetic gingival recontouring of teeth 11 and 21
    - Soft tissue alveolar-ridge reduction in edentulous areas to create more vertical room for pontics
- Definitive Restorative Therapy
    - Fixed partial dentures to replace missing premolars 15, 34, and 44
    - Bonded ceramic restorations for teeth 11, 12, 21, and 22
    - Esthetically recontour mandibular incisors to compensate for wear
- Retention
    - Maxillary centric-relation nightguard
    - Mandibular spring retainer

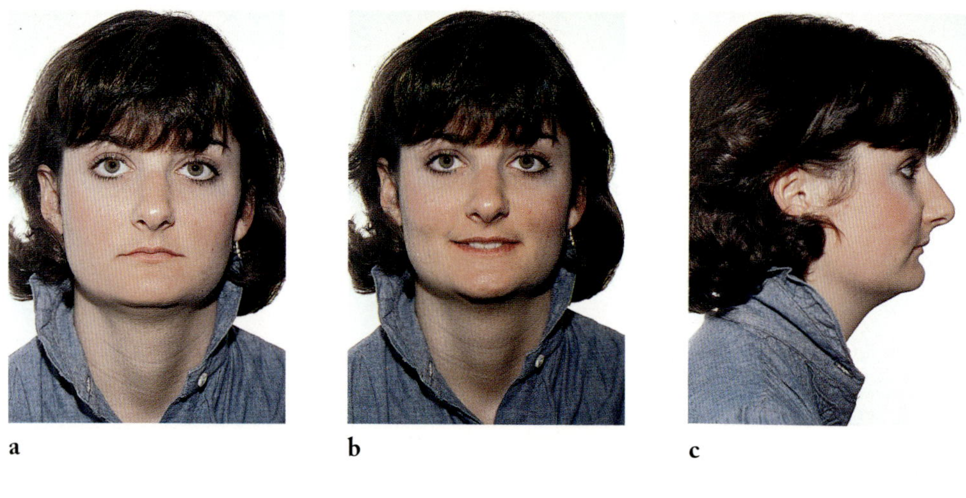

a b c

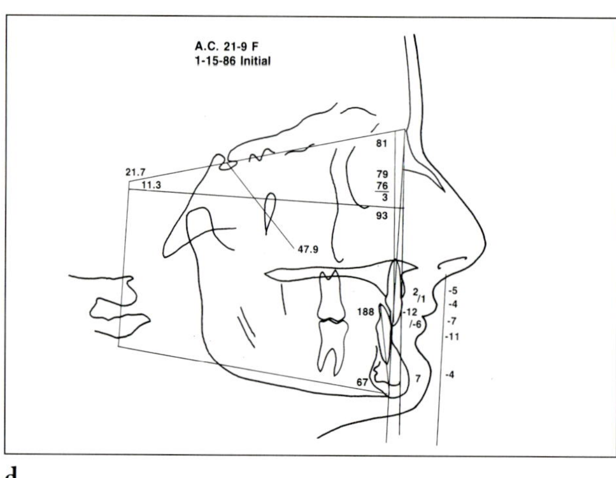

d

Fig 6-25 A.C. is a 22-year-old female who wants to improve dental function and appearance.

a, b Initial frontal view of face illustrating square facial form with decreased lower face height.

c Initial lateral facial view with maxillary and mandibular skeletal deficiencies, insufficient lip support, and a strong chin.

d Initial cephalometric analysis.

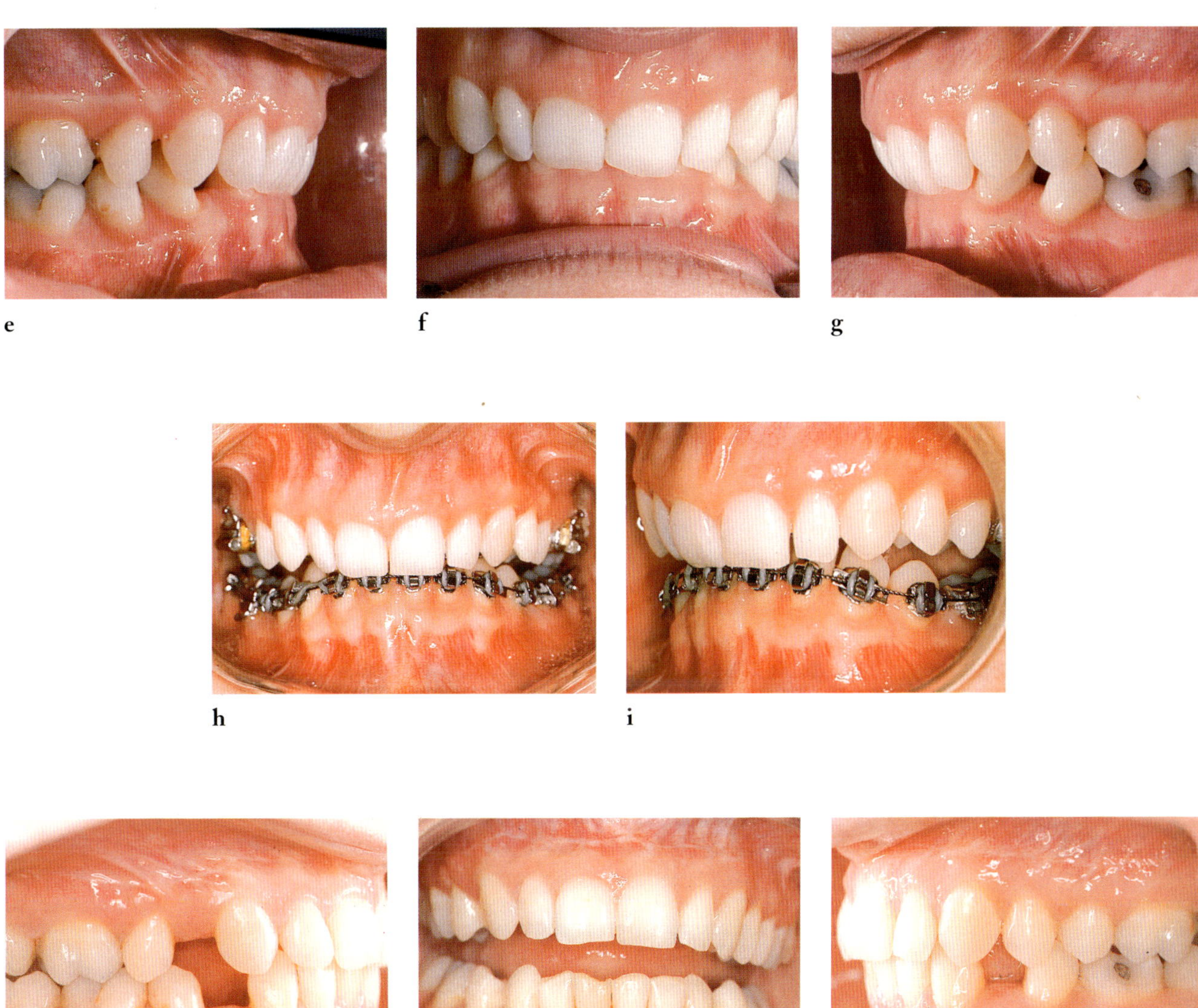

e f g

h i

j k l

Fig 6-25 (continued)

e to g Initial dental views illustrating the results of previous unidisciplinary compromised orthodontic therapy. Three premolars had been extracted and the maxillary and mandibular anterior components had been tipped lingually, causing a traumatic anterior relationship with excessive vertical overlap and subsequent severe incisal wear.

h, i Preoperative orthodontic therapy was used to position dentition in supporting structures to facilitate optimal surgical repositioning of the skeletal components. Lingual orthodontic appliances were used on the maxillary arch to address the patient's special considerations of low self-image and high esthetic concerns. The patient eventually gained confidence in herself and the interdisciplinary team, and allowed placement of labial orthodontic appliances to expedite treatment.

j to l Dental views following orthodontics and orthognathic surgery. Dental relationships have been tremendously improved. For numerous reasons, including limited treatment time, the orthodontist and restorative dentist had to reach an interdisciplinary compromise and finish orthodontics with less-than-ideal space for pontic teeth 14, 34, and 44, with teeth 15, 35, and 45 tipped distally.

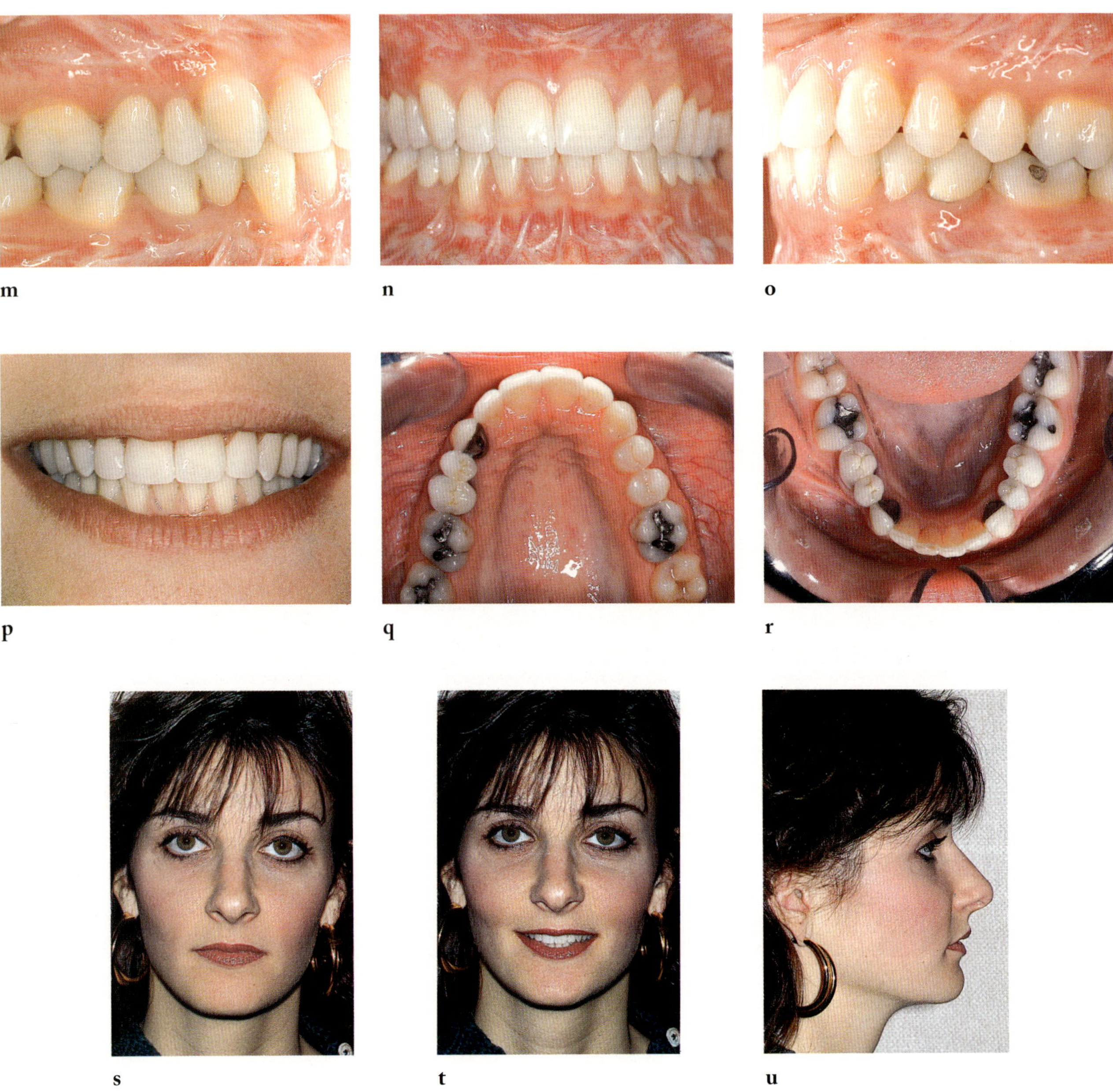

Fig 6-25 (continued)

m to r Final dental views following completion of periodontal plastic surgery and definitive restorative procedures. Esthetic gingival recontouring was performed on teeth 12 and 21 and bonded ceramic restorations were placed on teeth 11, 12, 21, and 22. Creative restorative procedures were performed to esthetically fill the small edentulous spaces and maintain esthetics of the anterior abutments. To accomplish this, the edentulous ridges were recontoured to create more vertical room and three fixed partial dentures were placed using resin-bonded metal wings with retention pins on the lingual of anterior abutments to maintain esthetics of the natural labial tooth structure.

s to u Final facial appearance following interdisciplinary dentofacial therapy. Orthognathic surgical procedures were performed to advance the maxilla and mandible and to increase lower face height.

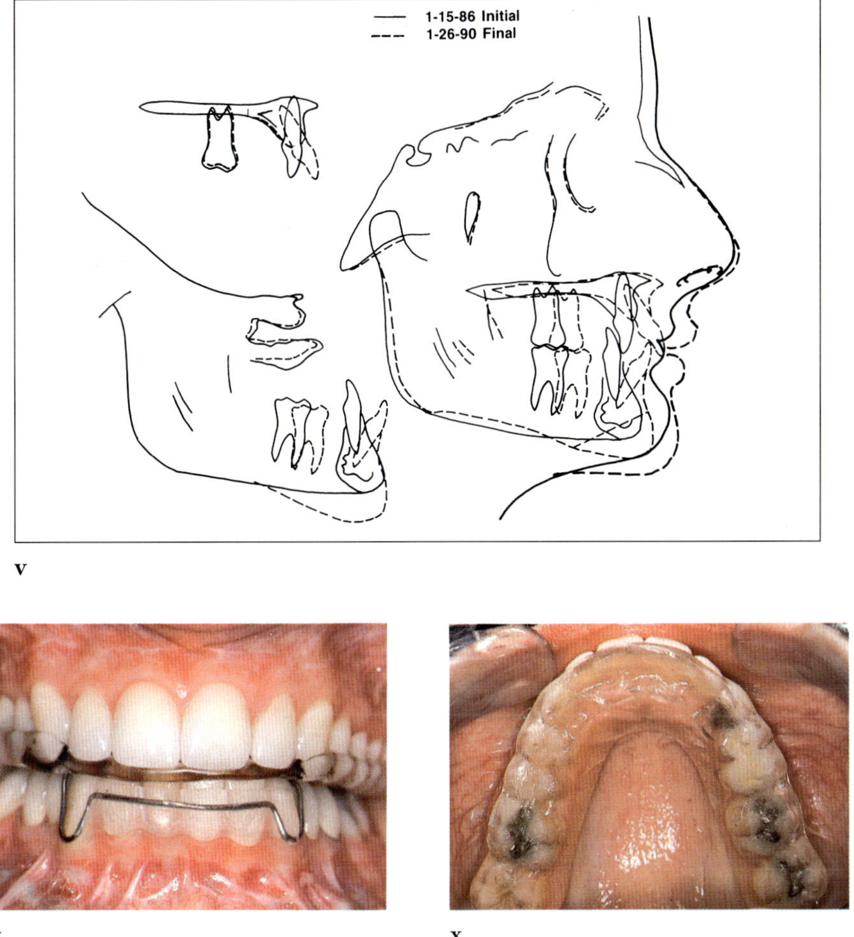

v

w

x

Fig 6-25 (continued)

v Initial and final cephalometric superimposition.

w, x Six months posttreatment. Dental changes were retained with a mandibular spring retainer and a maxillary centric-relation nightguard. A maxillary Hawley appliance was worn full-time for 4 months to allow postorthodontic occlusal settling. An equilibration was then performed and the nightguard constructed for long-term retention and TMD maintenance.

Orthodontist: C. Moody Alexander, DDS, M.S/*Oral and Maxillofacial Surgeon:* Larry M. Wolford, DDS
Restorative Dentist: Richard D. Roblee, DDS, MS/*Laboratory Technician:* Jeffrey Singler, CDT

Discussion

Many significant and exciting advances have been made in orthognathic surgical techniques that enable an interdisciplinary team to predictably treat dentofacial deformities with unsurpassed quality. This case exemplifies quality comprehensive therapy using orthognathic surgical therapy, as well as the differences between shortsighted unidisciplinary therapy and optimal interdisciplinary therapy. Interdisciplinary therapy was used to correct this patient's dentofacial problems that had been compounded by the previous unidisciplinary therapy.

Preoperative Orthodontics

Orthognathic surgical procedures usually take place somewhere in the middle of orthodontic therapy. These orthodontic procedures usually take from 3 to 12 months to complete. The preoperative orthodontic goals generally include the following.

1. Align, level, and correct rotations of teeth within their respective arches or arch segments.
2. Adjust for tooth-size discrepancies between the mesiodistal width of the maxillary and mandibular anterior teeth and premolars.
3. Diverge tooth roots adjacent to planned vertical interdental (between roots) bone cuts.
4. Use stable, predictable orthodontic mechanics.

Active preoperative orthodontics should be completed and stabilized for at least two months prior to surgery.

The surgical procedures to correct the existing musculoskeletal deformity must be carefully selected to provide the best functional and esthetic result, as well as provide long-term stability. The same level of interaction should take place between the oral and maxillofacial surgeon and orthodontist as was illustrated between the restorative dentist and orthodontist in preparatory restorative-type II therapy. The oral and maxillofacial surgeon will thus be able to maximize the surgical correction. As previously mentioned, the restorative dentist or prosthodontist can also provide valuable information and restorative procedures through preparatory restorative-type II therapy to assist the oral and maxillofacial surgeon in ideally planning and performing these surgeries, and set up the dentosseous structures so that future restorative procedures can be performed optimally.

In addition to continuous team monitoring during preoperative orthodontics, both surgeon and orthodontist should perform dentofacial reevaluations; one should make progress records (panoramic radiograph, lateral cephalometric radiograph and analysis, and hand-held dental casts.) These reevaluations and records should be done at least once, with ample time remaining in the preoperative orthodontic treatment so that the orthodontist can use the information acquired in the procedures to make final preoperative adjustments in the orthodontic therapy. In cases in which future restorative procedures are planned, the restorative dentist or prosthodontist should be included in this reevaluation process. After preoperative orthodontic therapy is completed and prior to surgery (within one week), final preoperative records (cephalometric radiograph and analysis, panoramic radiograph, dental models, face-bow mounting, photographs, and, ideally, TMJ tomograms) are made and evaluated. The adjunctive diagnostic procedures of cephalometric predictions (Fig 6-26g) and model surgery (Fig 5-5a) must also be performed at this time. The new cephalometric prediction tracing is created to establish the final desired functional and esthetic result. Accurate model surgery is performed on dental casts centrically mounted on an anatomical articulator to accurately determine the specific movements required to achieve the optimal jaw and occlusal relationship.

Orthognathic Surgical Procedures

There are a wide variety of surgical procedures and philosophies available to correct dentofacial deformities. Advanced techniques[109–117] eliminate the need to wire the jaws together so patients can have some immediate jaw function after surgery. In most cases, these patients have fully resumed their preoperative activity by 4 months postoperatively; however, the complete healing process may take 9 to 12 months. This section will describe some of the basic surgical procedures used on some of the more common types of dentofacial deformities.

Antero-posterior (A-P) Deformities

The most common procedure to correct A-P deformities of the mandible is the bilateral mandibular ramus sagittal split osteotomy,[114,116] which allows lengthening or shortening of the mandible and application of bone screws for rigid fixation (Fig 6-9). The chin can also be augmented or reduced (genioplasty) in A-P dimension (Fig 6-9). The maxilla can be advanced forward or set backward with the Le Fort I maxillary osteotomy procedure[115,117] and rigidly stabilized with bone plates and screws (Figs 6-9 and 6-25).

Vertical Deformities

If the maxilla is too long vertically, it can be shortened by removing bone from the maxillary walls and repositioning the maxilla upward (Figs 6-9 and 6-26). If the maxilla is too short vertically, it can be lowered and bone or synthetic bone placed in the bony gap created, using bone plates for stabilization.[115] If the mandible is too long or short vertically, appropriate changes can be made usually by vertically shortening or lengthening the chin (Fig 6-25).

Transverse Deformities

The transverse dimensions of the maxilla and mandible are often incompatible, resulting in lingual or buccal crossbites. Either jaw may require one or more interdental cuts (between teeth) to expand or narrow one or both jaws to correct the transverse differences (Fig 6-9).

Combined Deformities

Frequently, patients' problems include two or more of the above stated conditions affecting both jaws. With careful planning and appropriate surgical techniques, both jaws can be safely and predictably repositioned in one operation. When indicated, this could provide an optimal functional and esthetic result (Figs 6-9, 6-25, and 6-26).

Coexisting TMJ Problems and Dentofacial Deformities

Coexisting TMJ problems may be indicated for surgical correction. Usually, it is best to manage the TMJ problem at a separate operation prior to the orthognathic surgery during initial TMD therapy, but both are occasionally done simultaneously (Fig 6-26).

Nasal Surgery

Nasal septoplasty and partial inferior turbinectomies can be performed to improve the functional nasal airway at the same time as the orthognathic surgery. External nasal surgery (rhinoplasty) is preferably done at a second operation during adjunctive facial cosmetic surgery, but it can be done at the same time as the orthognathic surgery (Fig 6-9).

Other Surgical Procedures

Occasionally, orthognathic surgeries are performed that do not require preoperative orthodontic assistance. These cases are usually preprosthetic in nature and are used to orthognathically reposition partial or completely edentulous arches. When appropriate, other surgeries, such as dental implant placement, gingival grafting, third molar removal, cosmetic procedures, etc, may be performed in conjunction with orthognathic surgery to reduce the number of operations and anesthetics, as well as to shorten the overall treatment time. Impacted third molars can either be removed during the orthognathic surgery or be removed a minimum of 9 to 12 months prior to orthognathic surgery as part of preparatory dentoalveolar surgical therapy. Other cosmetic procedures that may be requested include cheek augmentation, other facial augmentations, removal of fatty tissue (lipectomy), face-lift (rhytidectomy), eyelid surgery (blepharoplasty), forehead/brow lift, etc. In some cases, the cosmetic procedure can be performed at the same time as the orthognathic surgery; it may also be performed at a second surgery during adjunctive facial cosmetic surgery. Many feel that these esthetic procedures can be more predictably performed during a second surgery, after the effects of the orthognathic surgery are fully realized.

Postoperative Orthodontics

Postoperative orthodontic therapy is used to finalize and perfect the dental occlusion relative to the new skeletal relationships. Orthodontic appliances are usually activated again anywhere from 4 to 8 weeks postoperatively if rigid skeletal fixation is used. The teeth, and to a limited extent the osseous segments, can be moved more rapidly during the first 4 to 5 months following surgery. Because of this rapid movement, the orthodontist can complete in 1 to 2 weeks as much as can normally be done in 4 to 6 weeks. The final positioning of the teeth generally requires from 3 to 12 months of postoperative orthodontic treatment, but may require more time.

Case Summary

Patient: C.T. is a 27-year-old female evaluated 4 years after a motor vehicle accident, in which she sustained facial trauma. She had a left mandibular subcondylar fracture, comminuted fracture of the right condylar head and neck, symphysis fracture, loss of a portion of the anterior maxilla, and loss of seven maxillary teeth. The fractures were reduced as best as possible. Later, she had open joint surgery on the right TMJ, and osseointegrated implants were placed in the maxilla to enable her to wear an upper prosthesis.

Chief Concerns: (1) Establish a functional bite relationship; (2) eliminate severe pain problems and headaches.

Abbreviated Problem List

- Anterior vertical maxillary excess
- Posterior vertical maxillary deficiency
- Transverse maxillary asymmetry with the right side 3 mm higher than the left side
- A-P mandibular deficiency
- Right ramus vertical deficiency
- Right TMJ severe osteoarthritis with condylar displacement, secondary to previous trauma
- Mandible is shifted 5 mm to the right side
- Class I malocclusion
- Missing teeth 11, 12, 13, 14, 15, 21, 22, 23, and 31
- Numerous failing root canals in maxillary posterior area
- Ankylosed mandibular right central incisor
- Severe myofacial pain on right side of face
- Headaches

Treatment Plan

Interdisciplinary Dentofacial Therapy

- Initial TMD therapy to improve comfort during preoperative treatment phase
- Re-treat failing endodontically treated teeth
- Preoperative orthodontics
- Orthognathic surgery
    - Multiple maxillary osteotomies to advance, superiorly reposition the anterior portion, and level the arch by downgrafting the posterior right side
    - Left mandibular ramus osteotomy to advance it
    - Right mandibular advancement and TMJ reconstruction, using a total-joint prosthesis
- Postoperative orthodontics to refine occlusion and setup dentition for restorative therapy
- Restorative dentistry to finalize dental occlusion and dentofacial esthetics

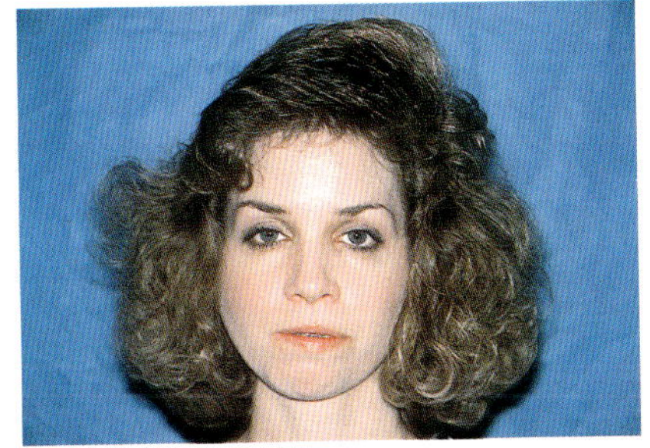
a

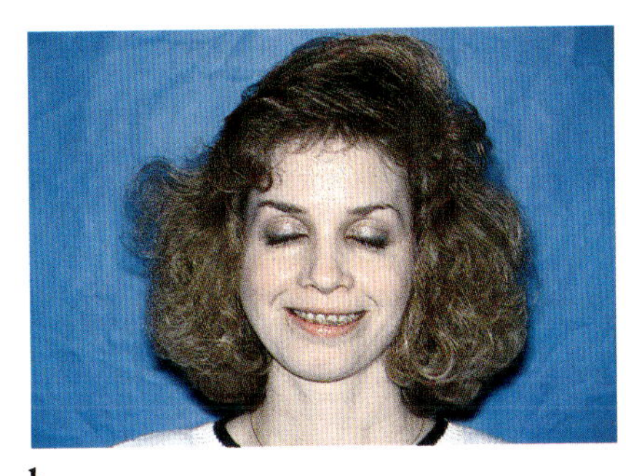
b

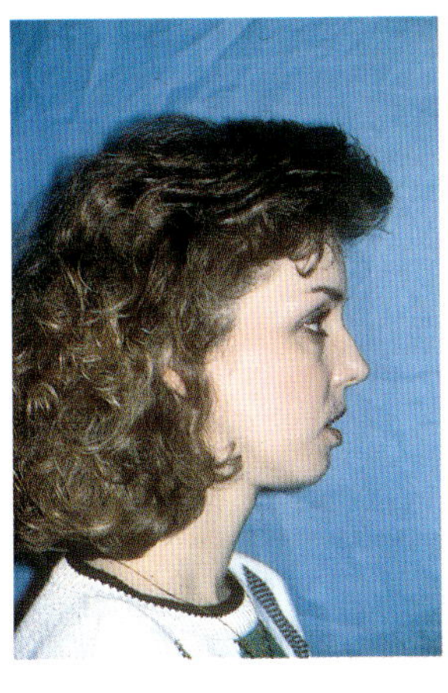
c

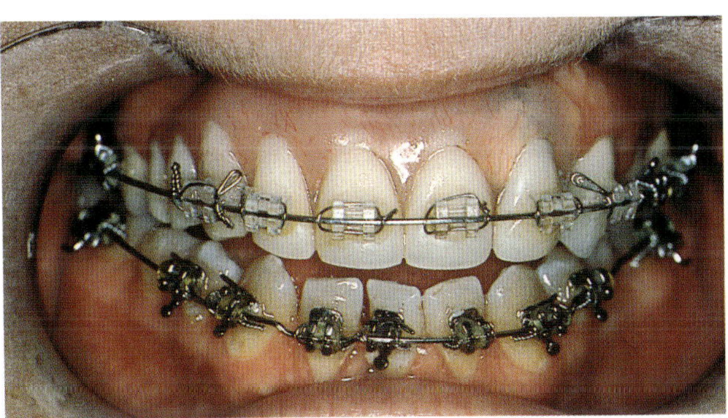
d

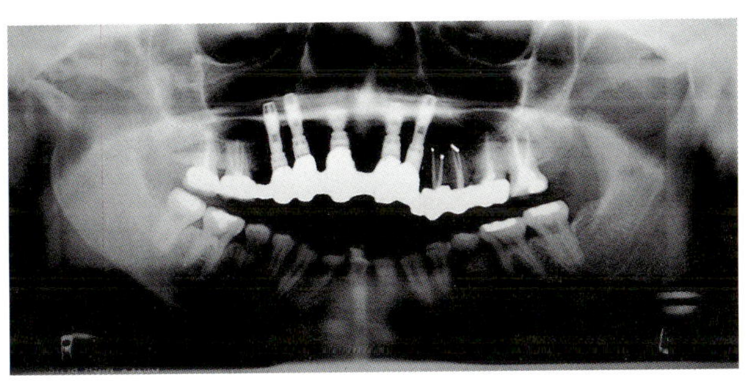
e

Fig 6-26

a, b Preoperative facial views demonstrate vertical maxillary excess and facial asymmetry.

c Preoperative lateral facial view showing excess in lower third of face and retruded chin position.

d Preoperative intraoral view. Anterior open bite is present, as well as a cant to the maxilla, with the right side about 3 mm higher than the left side. Patient is missing seven anterior teeth, but has a provisional prosthesis placed over osseointegrated implants; the prosthesis extends from the left lateral incisor to the right second premolar. Patient is also missing the mandibular left central incisor, and the mandibular right central incisor is ankylosed.

e Preoperative panoramic radiograph demonstrates the fractured and partially resorbed right condyle, as well as the presence of osseointegrated implants in the anterior maxilla.

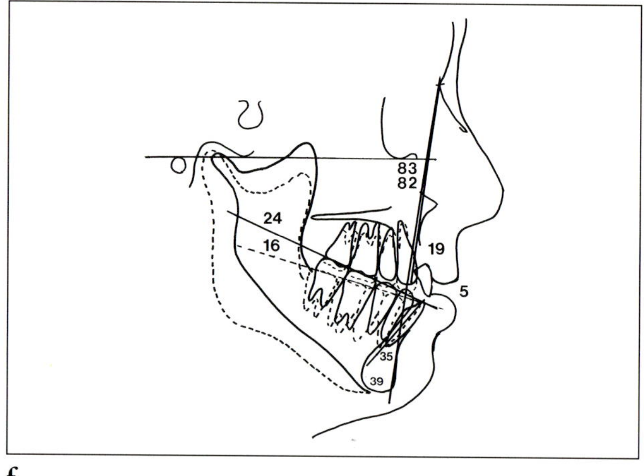

f

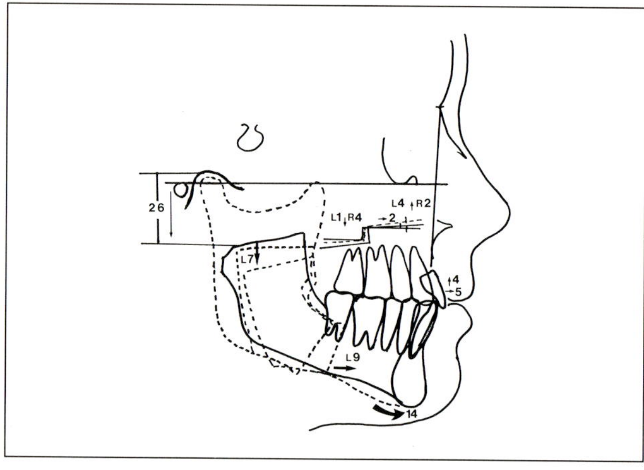

g

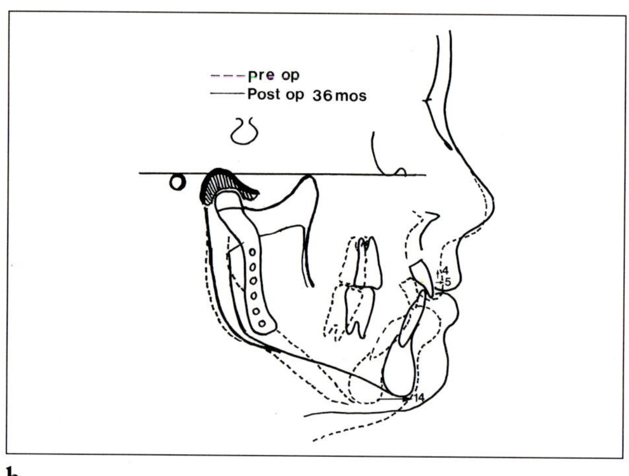

h

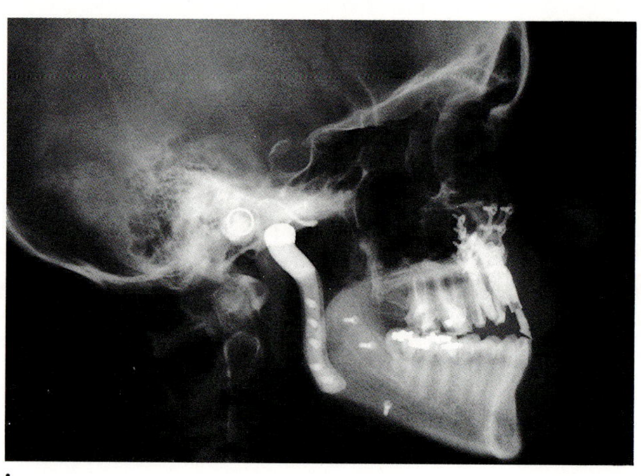
i

Fig 6-26 (continued)

f Cephalometrically, the patient demonstrates A-P maxillary and mandibular deficiency, as well as increased occlusal plane angulation of 24° on the right side and 16° on the left side. Vertical maxillary excess is also present. Note the difference in vertical height of the inferior borders of the mandible.

g Adjunctive diagnostic procedure. A surgical treatment objective (STO) was designed to advance the maxillary incisors 5 mm and superiorly 4 mm, and level the transverse occlusal plane. With the sagittal split, the left mandible will advance 9 mm. The Techmedica custom-made total-joint prosthesis (Techmedica Inc, Camaroailla, California) was used to lengthen the right ramus 26 mm and advance the mandible. Pogonion rotated forward 14 mm.

h The preoperative cephalometric study (dotted line) compared to the 36-month postoperative result (solid line).

i A postoperative cephalograph shows the total joint prosthesis. Note the osseointegrated implants and teeth prepared for the final restorations.

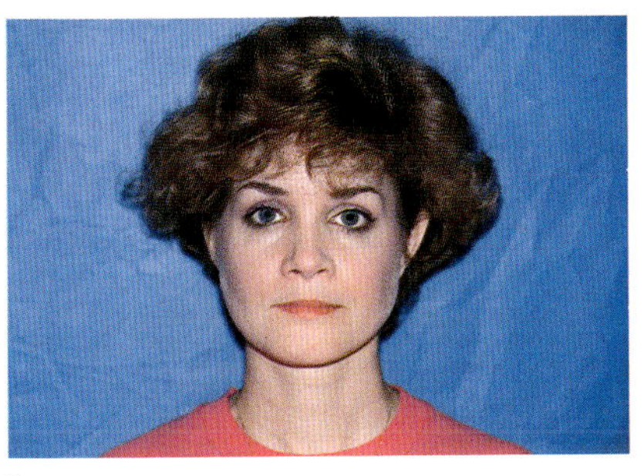
j

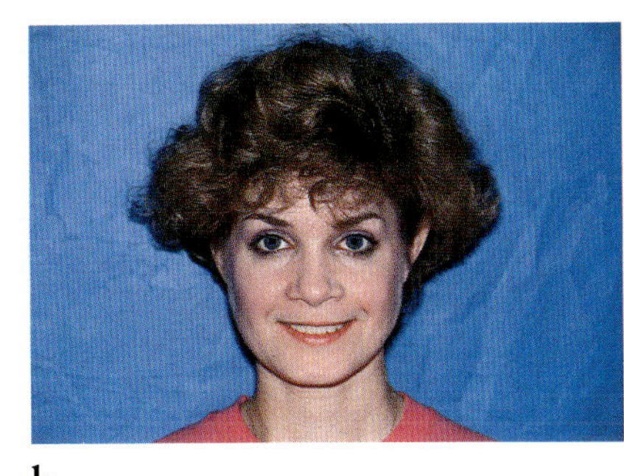
k

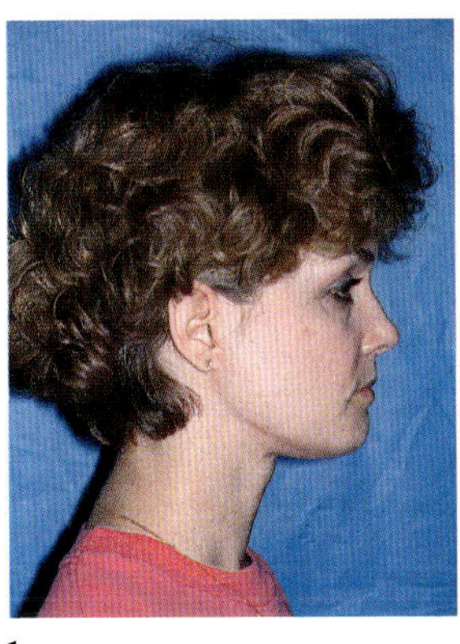
l

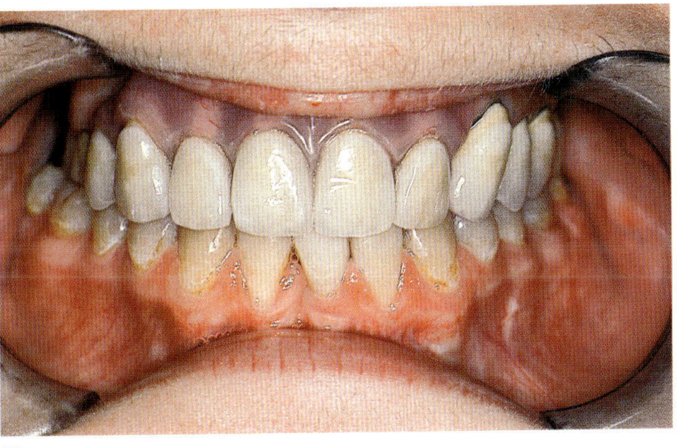
m

Fig 6-26 (continued)

j to m Facial and lateral facial views of the patient 36 months postoperative, showing significant improvement in facial balance and esthetics with good stable Class I canine occlusion.

Endodontist (re-treatment): James M. Tinnin, DDS, MS/*Implant Surgeon:* Robert Lewis, DDS
Oral and Maxillofacial Surgeon: Larry M. Wolford, DDS/*Orthodontist:* Richard D. Roblee, DDS, MS
Restorative Dentist (re-treatment): Frank Higginbottom, DDS

Discussion

This is a complex case involving a severe injury to the right TMJ and associated facial and functional imbalances. The above treatment plan provided excellent facial esthetics and total elimination of pain, while providing relatively normal jaw function, including a posttreatment incisal opening of 40 mm. The patient is now 3 years postoperative, with a very stable functional occlusion and good facial balance. This case also illustrates how osseointegrated implants can assist in restoring esthetics and function in patients who have significant deformities from trauma with loss of teeth and supporting structures.

Retention

Relapse has always been a complex problem in traditional orthodontic therapy, and it can even be more complex when orthognathic surgery and other definitive therapies are performed in conjunction with orthodontics. This increased complexity is due to the fact that the initial dentofacial problems are usually more severe. Preventing relapse can be further complicated by having several different providers treating different aspects of one overall therapy. However, relapse problems can be brought under control through team interaction about potential stability problems, followed by each team member performing and maintaining his or her therapy in a manner that helps prevent future relapse in the overall dentofacial result. In addition, interdisciplinary dentofacial therapy by its very nature promotes the optimal correction of problems while minimizing deleterious compromises; subsequently, IDT should attain more stable results than unidisciplinary or multidisciplinary therapy.

For example, in IDT, teeth are more likely to be ideally positioned in their supporting structures with skeletal problems being corrected surgically. This approach should be periodontally and dentally more stable than the unidisciplinary compromised orthodontic positioning of teeth to compensate for skeletal discrepancies.

The relapse of orthognathic surgical changes has been a major concern since these procedures were first performed. Many of the factors causing this relapse have now been overcome through a better understanding of the consequences of surgical changes in the condylar, muscular, and other soft tissue relationships.[120] This enhanced understanding has led to many significant improvements in orthognathic surgical techniques which have led to more predictable results.[121–124] One of the most important improvements is the use of rigid fixation[112,118,125] for skeletal stabilization. However, surgical relapse can still occur and should be diagnosed early so that corrective procedures can be performed.[127]

The most common relapse problems are usually related to orthodontic tooth movement. Its causes and prevention have been thoroughly addressed in several recent works.[128–131] The same philosophies for dental stability described in those works should be maintained here; however, traditional orthodontic retention appliances are not as effective in interdisciplinary therapy as in typical adolescent therapy.

The Hawley Appliance[132] (Fig 6-27), which is the standard retainer used in orthodontics, may be inappropriate for retention during definitive interdisciplinary therapy. More creative means of transitional retention are usually needed until all definitive therapies are completed. The goal of retention in interdisciplinary dentofacial therapy is to esthetically retain tooth position while allowing or even assisting the optimal performance of other definitive therapies.

After definitive therapies are completed, other factors, such as fixed prosthetics, will greatly aid retention. In addition, a good deal of orthodontic relapse is thought to be associated with the stretching of marginal gingival tissues when teeth are moved to set up an elastic pull back to the original preorthodontic position.[133] Many procedures in definitive periodontal therapy relieve these tissues and allow the fibers to reorganize and reduce relapse.[62] For these reasons, the timing and coordination of orthodontic, periodontal, and restorative therapies are very important in maintaining stability. Frequently, periodontal and restorative procedures are initiated during the latter stages of orthodontic therapy to aid retention procedures, as well as to shorten treatment time. Orthodontic appliances may even be left on after active tooth movement to act as full-time rigid retainers during periodontal therapy. If orthodontic appliances are removed, a clear, thin, full-coverage splint can be constructed to temporarily maintain tooth relationships (Fig 6-28). These full-coverage splints can be an esthetic, versatile, and inexpensive appliance for transitional retention of the dentition between definitive therapies.

When extensive prosthodontic procedures are to be performed, it is often advantageous for the restorative team member to remove orthodontic appliances at the same time he or she prepares the teeth for the restorations. This will prevent any chance of relapse between orthodontic and restorative therapies. If there is going to be a waiting period between these therapies, sectional archwires can be used to optimally retain fixed partial denture abutment teeth after orthodontic appliances are removed (Fig 6-29). When anterior teeth are missing, denture teeth can be added to the thin full-coverage splint or to a Hawley retainer to esthetically maintain spaces until the final restorative procedures are performed (Fig 6-30).

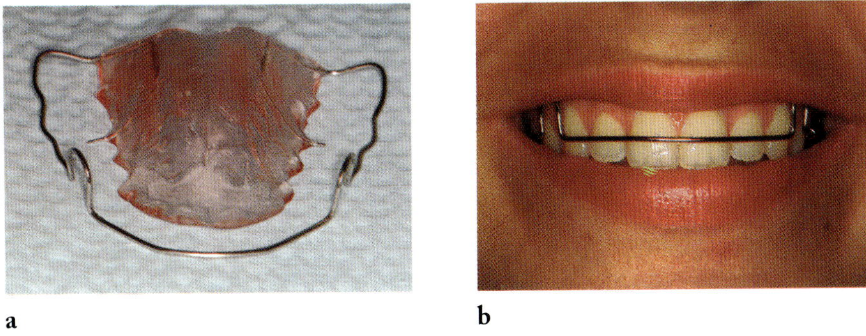

Fig 6-27a, b The Hawley retention appliance is the standard retainer used in traditional orthodontic therapy, but its uses may be somewhat limited in interdisciplinary therapy when extensive restorative procedures are going to be performed.

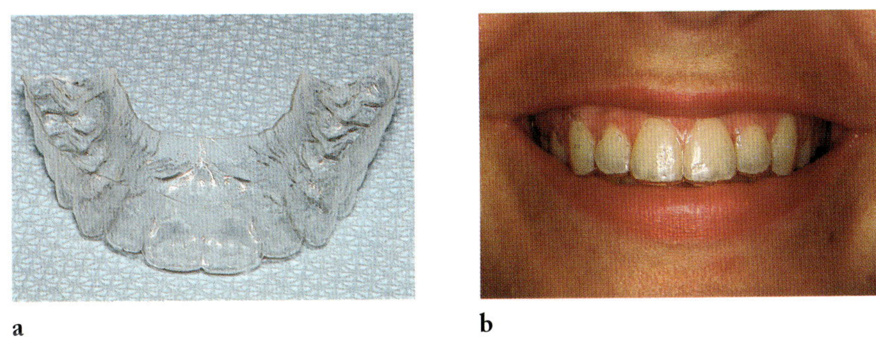

Fig 6-28a, b A clear, full-coverage splint can be an esthetic, versatile, and inexpensive appliance for transitional retention of the post-orthodontic dentition between definitive therapies. Long-term full-time wear of this appliance is not recommended.

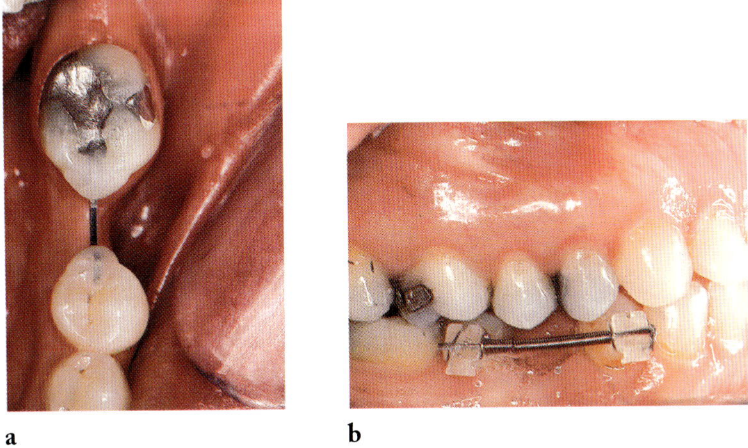

Fig 6-29 It is critical that retention is considered between the orthodontics and the various therapies to help assure that the teeth will not drift. Occlusal view *(a)* of a rectangular wire bonded to occlusal surfaces of two planned fixed partial denture abutment teeth which have been orthodontically positioned to an optimal relationship. Another excellent alternative *(b)* is for the orthodontist to leave selected orthodontic appliances in place for the restorative dentist to remove at the time of tooth preparation and provisional restoration.

Case Summary

Patient: D.W. is a 35-year-old male who received a traumatic blow to the mouth at age 15 and subsequently lost teeth 13 and 14 and a significant portion of the associated alveolar ridge.

Chief Concern: Stop tooth wear and improve appearance of smile.

Abbreviated Problem List

- Maxillary dental midline is 2 mm to left of skeletal midline
- Asymmetrical smile with left side superior to right side
- Dentoalveolar extrusion in maxillary and mandibular anterior segments
- Class III skeletal relationship with prognathic mandible and mandibular dentoalveolar retrusion
- Class III dental tendency
- Retroclined maxillary and mandibular incisors
- Severe alveolar-ridge defect in edentulous areas of teeth 13 and 14
- Asymmetrical gingival contours in maxillary anterior area
- Severe incisal wear

Treatment Plan

Interdisciplinary Dentofacial Therapy

- Initial TMD therapy using an occlusal splint with denture teeth
- Comprehensive orthodontic therapy to set up arches to allow optimal restorative procedures
  - Place denture teeth on archwire to replace missing teeth 13 and 14
  - Morphologic interproximal air-rotor stripping (MARS) on mandibular posterior teeth to correct interarch anterior-posterior discrepancy
  - Intrude maxillary anteriors and esthetically align gingival contours
  - Procline maxillary and mandibular anteriors for a more stable interincisal relationship after restorative therapy
  - Space maxillary anteriors interproximally and vertically to allow for most esthetic restorations with proper anterior coupling
- Definitive Implant and Periodontal Therapy
  - Implant placement in tooth positions 13 and 14 with hard and soft tissue regeneration and/or augmentation therapy
  - Periodontal plastic surgical procedures to esthetically recontour or add to gingival contours as necessary
- Definitive Restorative Therapy
  - Bonded porcelain jackets for teeth 11, 12, 21, 22, and 23
  - Implant crowns to restore teeth 13 and 14
- Maintain result with mandibular bonded lingual retainer and maxillary centric-relation nighttime splint

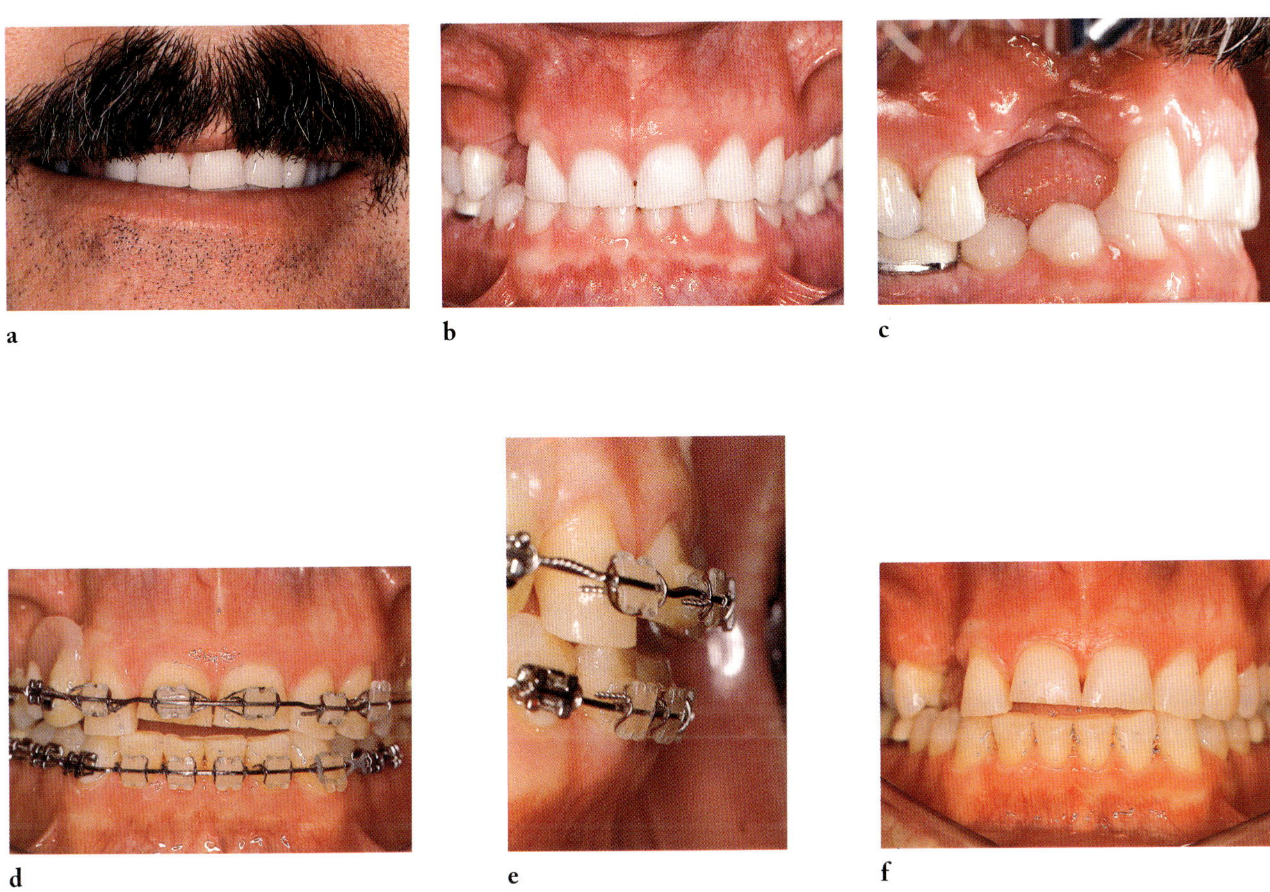

Fig 6-30

a Initial smiling appearance with asymmetrical smile and maxillary midline 2 mm to the right of skeletal midline.

b, c Initial intraoral views showing retroclined anterior dentition with severe wear and dentoalveolar extrusion. Also note severe buccal-lingual and vertical alveolar-ridge defects in edentulous area and Class III dental relationship.

d Intraoral progress view illustrating improved alignment of maxillary gingival contours and maxillary dental midline. Also note denture teeth with fibered acrylic resin added to the archwire to maintain esthetics throughout the orthodontic therapy (preparatory restorative-type II therapy).

e Lateral progress view of improved incisal inclinations.

f Postorthodontic intraoral appearance. The gingival contours around the remaining maxillary anterior teeth have been optimally aligned and an interincisal relationship has been established that will allow optimal restorative procedures with the proper gingival and incisal relationships. This patient is now ready for definitive implant, periodontal, and restorative therapies. The patient could not afford to pursue these therapies at this time, so retention procedures were performed to maintain the dental relationships until the remaining definitive therapies could be performed.

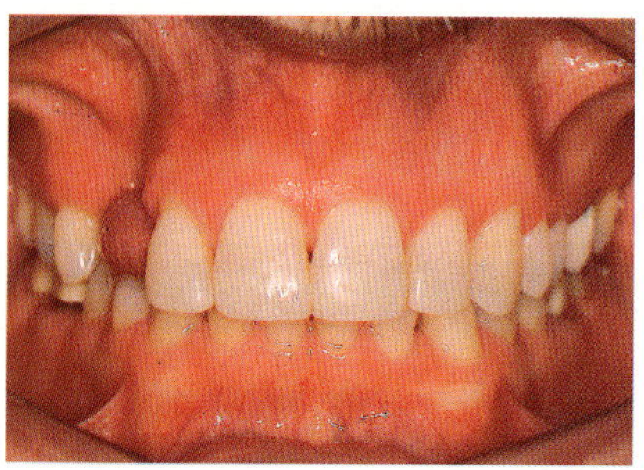
g

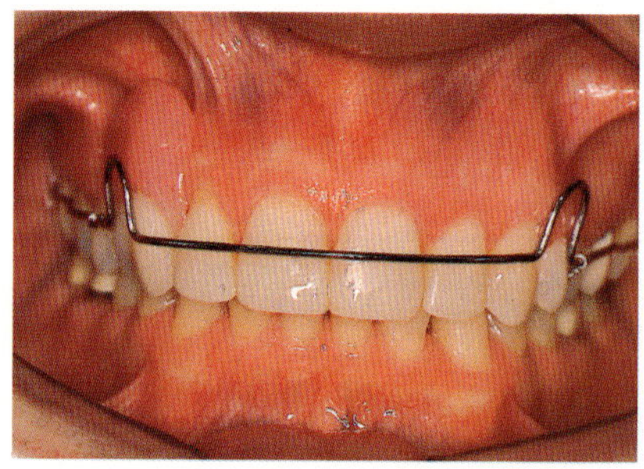
h

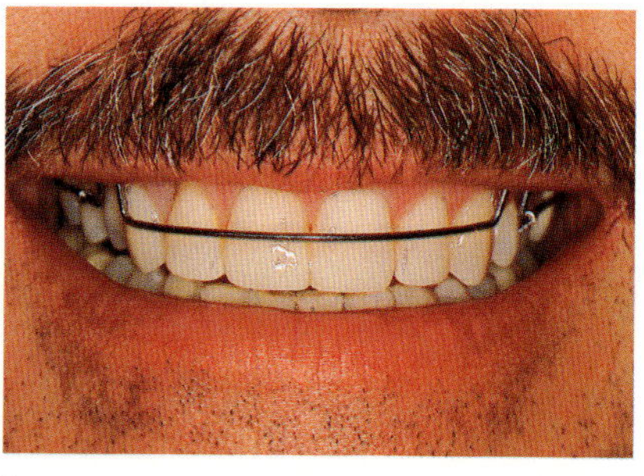
i

Fig 6-30 (continued)

g The four maxillary incisors were temporarily built up using composite resin to help stabilize the interincisal relationship and allow the patient to start enjoying the esthetic enhancement of his smile.

h, i A maxillary orthodontic retainer was constructed that included denture teeth and acrylic resin to esthetically fill the edentulous area while retaining the dental relationships. Patient is currently saving money for the remaining definitive therapy.

Discussion

This case illustrates optimal dentofacial treatment of several complicated dentofacial problems. It also shows how definitive therapy can be extended to accommodate the patient's financial needs without compromising esthetics or the final result. Several procedures were performed in the orthodontic retention phase so that the dental and periodontal relationships could be esthetically maintained until the definitive implant, periodontal, and restorative therapies could be initiated. The same retainer will also be used as part of preparatory restorative-type III and IV therapies to facilitate the various surgeons in properly placing the dental implants and performing the osseous and periodontal augmentations.

Provisional restorations can provide ideal retention after orthodontic tooth movement. Bonded lingual retainers are an effective means for esthetically holding mandibular anterior teeth during and after any remaining definitive therapies (Fig 2-5j). Bonded lingual retainers can also be useful in the maxillary arch (Figs 2-5j and 6-24i).

If retention is indicated after definitive therapy is completed, a Hawley retainer can be used. However, probably the most favorable retainer in these cases is a properly constructed occlusal splint[134] that is worn at night (Fig 6-25x). It will retain the teeth and at the same time direct all the occlusal forces in an axial direction to the teeth. This is much more favorable to the supporting structures than the potentially damaging lateral jiggling forces that a Hawley retainer may introduce.[135] By idealizing the occlusion, the occlusal splint is effective in controlling TMD symptoms. Its nighttime use can help maintain long-term health in the temporomandibular complex. It will also assist in maintaining the integrity of teeth, dental implants, and restorations by protecting them from the damaging affects of nocturnal bruxing.

Preparatory Restorative-Type III Therapy

Preparatory restorative-type III therapy can be performed in conjunction with preparatory restorative-type I therapy, or during or after the final stages of orthodontic therapy, if it is planned. It is similar to preparatory restorative-type II therapy in that the prosthodontist or restorative dentist uses it to convey information concerning future definitive restorative therapy. The difference is that this time it facilitates the periodontist (instead of the orthodontist or oral and maxillofacial surgeon) in optimally performing any necessary definitive periodontal therapies and in preparing the soft tissues to accept ideal definitive restorations. This preparatory restorative therapy is usually accomplished through fixed provisional restorations (Figs 5-3i, 5-3j, 5-3k, 6-23p, 6-23q, and 6-35f to 6-35 h); however, a removable provisional prosthesis can also be used (Fig 4-3). Adjunctive diagnostic procedures, such as a diagnostic waxup (Fig 2-5g), are often needed to determine the precise type and extent of periodontal plastic procedures.

Preparatory restorative-type III therapy can also greatly assist the periodontist in performing definitive periodontal surgery by enhancing access and maintenance through the easy removal of the provisional restorations (Fig 6-23p). These restorations can also provide for enhanced patient access for oral hygiene during maturation periods following periodontal procedures. In addition, provisional restorations can provide optimal postorthodontic retention or stabilize periodontally involved teeth throughout definitive periodontal therapy.

Provisional restorations at any stage in therapy should enhance proper oral hygiene and not detract from it (Figs 5-3m and 5-3n). They should have properly fitting margins that are highly polished to minimize irritation to the soft tissue. Facial and lingual contours must be properly constructed to further promote periodontal health.[136] The gingival embrasures should be open to allow proper access for hygiene. In this stage, all attempts should be made to construct provisionals with supragingival margins, because subgingival margins are a potential source of gingival irritation.[137] It is often advantageous to make the provisional margins slightly short and then cement them with a zinc oxide–eugenol periodontal dressing to further reduce gingival irritation. Properly contouring and fitting acrylic-resin provisional restorations will minimize associated gingival irritation and promote reversal of tissue changes previously caused by poorly contoured or defective restorations.[138]

Another important reason for providing good provisional therapy is that patients can visualize the final result, enabling them to provide positive or negative feedback. Provisional therapy can also add a positive psychological boost to patients by getting them out of the orthodontic appliances and allowing them to preview and enjoy the esthetic enhancement that their interdisciplinary dentofacial therapy can provide (Figs 6-23q and 6-23r). Provisional restorations may have to function for a period of 12 months or more, depending on the progress of the definitive orthodontic, periodontal, and restorative therapies. Higginbottom outlined a maintenance schedule for provisional restorations used for an extended period of time (greater than 2 months).[139] Since provisional restorations are made out of a relatively soft, flexible acrylic resin, they may have to be repaired and/or recemented from time to time. They should be evaluated every 2 to 3 months to check for washout of cement, wear, fracture, and other problems. If provisionals are not properly maintained, problems can arise, including recurrent decay from leakage and drifting of the dentition following acrylic-resin wear or fracture.

For all the reasons discussed above, provisional restorations are considered therapeutic, but they can also be a very important diagnostic tool. They can give invaluable diagnostic information when they are used to evaluate questionable teeth or changes in occlusion, function, phonetics, and esthetics. Provisional restorations can be used to exactly replicate and determine the prognosis of changes that are planned to be made in definitive restorative therapy. Excellent provisional restorations can be constructed either directly in the mouth by utilizing a template made from a diagnostic waxup of the desired results, or indirectly in the lab by making a shell of the proposed final contours and relining in the mouth. These template techniques will give the restorative dentist rough provisional restorations that he or she can finalize using the patient's lip support, smile, phonetics, facial form, and function to create an optimal dentofacial effect (Fig 2-5m). When properly used, provisional restorations can be a valuable diagnostic, as well as therapeutic, tool in the attainment of optimal interdisciplinary dentofacial results.

Definitive Periodontal Therapy

Definitive periodontal therapy can be performed to do any or all of the following: *(1)* promote an environment conducive to long-term periodontal health; *(2)* increase stability of the orthodontic result; *(3)* assist in the placement of optimal prosthetics; and *(4)* enhance dentofacial esthetics. The periodontal procedures necessary to address these indications frequently overlap. For simplicity, definitive periodontal therapy will be described in two major categories: osseous therapy and periodontal plastic surgery.

As previously discussed in the sections on preparatory periodontal therapy and retention, practically any periodontal procedure will usually enhance the stability of the orthodontic result through realignment of the periodontal tissues. The circumferential supercrestal fiberotomy (CSF),[140,141] gingivoplasty of excess gingival tissues between two orthodontically approximated teeth,[67] and a frenectomy[63] in the site of an orthodontic diastema closure are definitive periodontal procedures usually performed solely to enhance stability (Fig 6-31).[62] In most of the other periodontal procedures, enhancement of postorthodontic dental stability is a secondary effect. This enhancement of stability, and the fact that the configuration of mucogingival and osseous tissues change during tooth movement, are two main reasons why definitive periodontal therapy should be performed after definitive orthodontic therapy (if possible) rather than before. The above soft tissue procedures used to help control dental relapse should ideally be performed when necessary after active tooth movement is completed and 6 weeks or more before the orthodontic appliances are removed.[142] Occasionally, a gingival graft may be needed in addition to a frenectomy. Also, if there are no osseous problems, any other necessary soft tissue procedures should be completed prior to orthodontic appliance removal (Figs 2-5h and 6-31). This can assist in the maintenance of the orthodontic result by allowing the reattachment of fibers while the orthodontic appliances are maintaining tooth positions. It will also expedite the progress of the interdisciplinary therapy and shorten overall treatment time (Fig 6-23). The above periodontal procedures are not recommended during active movement of the teeth or in cases with moderate to severe gingival inflammation because of the unpredictability of regeneration of the epithelial attachment in such situations.[62]

Osseous Therapy

Osseous therapy involves many traditional periodontal procedures. In cases of periodontal breakdown, bone surgery should ideally not be performed until after definitive orthodontic therapy because proper orthodontic movement can minimize or negate the need for osseous therapy.[39] Patients who had areas with periodontal pockets preorthodontically should be reevaluated by the team periodontist postorthodontically to determine whether therapy is indicated. Before a final determination can be made, a maturation period must pass to allow proper bone fill in the areas of orthodontic movement. This maturation

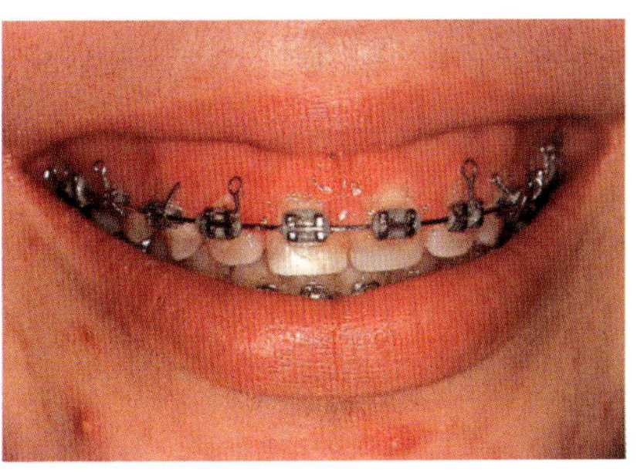

a

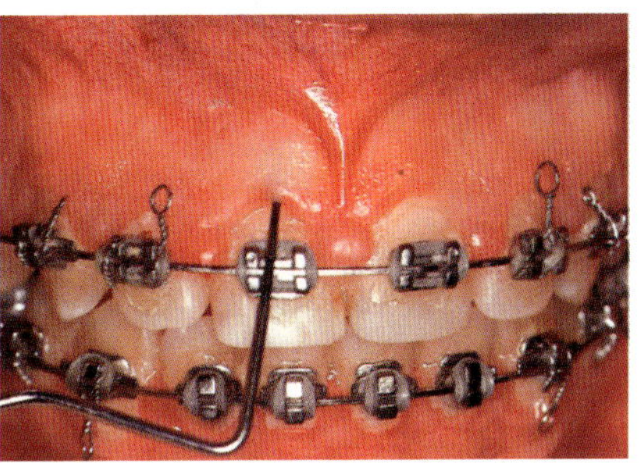

b

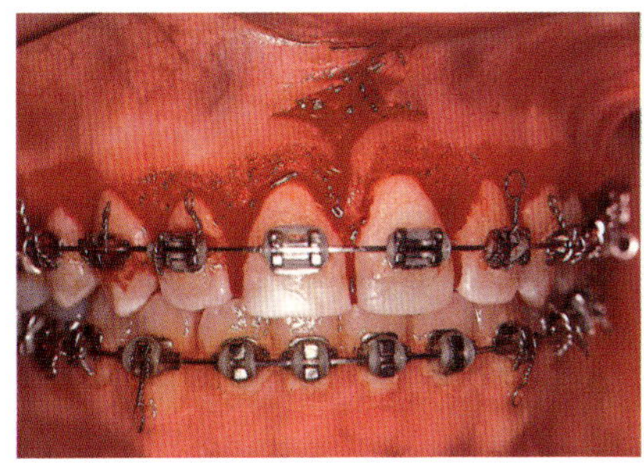

c

d

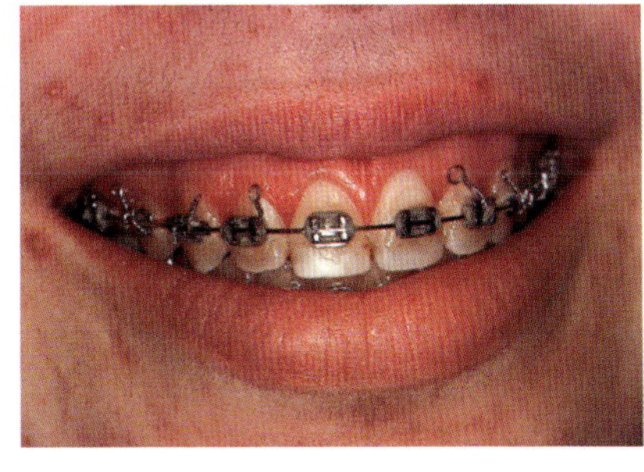

e

Fig 6-31 Gingivectomy and frenectomy.

a, b Excessive gingival display with enlarged papillae and an aberrant frenal attachment.

c Gingivectomy and gingivoplasty were performed to reduce the excessive tissues and expose the anatomic crowns. A frenectomy was also performed.

d, e Two months postoperative and prior to orthodontic appliance removal, the tissues appear normal in color and the smile is more esthetically pleasing. Performing soft tissue surgical procedures after active tooth movement is completed, and prior to appliance removal, can assist in maintaining tooth positions and expedite IDT.

Periodontist: Edward P. Allen, DDS, PhD

period should be a minimum of 6 months.[143,144]

During the maturation period, it is imperative that retention procedures are carried out along with supportive periodontal and dental therapy (SPT). Regularly scheduled SPT should be maintained and the patient's home care must be evaluated. It is also important that the occlusion be stabilized so that optimal periodontal healing can take place.

If osseous therapy is deemed necessary, there are two types of periodontal surgery available to address the problem: *(1)* resective and *(2)* regenerative. The overall goal of either type of surgery should be to stabilize the periodontium. Suprabony pocket probing depths of 5 to 6 mm or more found after initial periodontal therapy can often be treated with soft tissue procedures such as gingivectomies and apically positioned flaps.[48] Moderate chronic adult periodontitis is often treated by a flap approach, often with resective procedures entailing judicious reshaping of bone.[48] Also, the "biologic width"[145,146] must be preserved after restorative therapy. For this reason, crown-lengthening procedures involving bone removal occasionally need to be performed to provide sufficient tooth length to retain restorations without compromising the periodontium.

Deeper pocket-probing depths with vertical bone loss are usually treated with bone-regenerative procedures, including osseous grafting and guided tissue regeneration (GTR) using membranes.[49,144] GTR techniques can produce dramatic responses in specific types of defects, including deep proximal defects. Significant gains in both bone and attachment levels have been achieved; these gains have been shown to be stable for up to 5 years.[147] Since GTR has only been performed since the mid-1980s, long-term evaluations are not yet published. Teeth

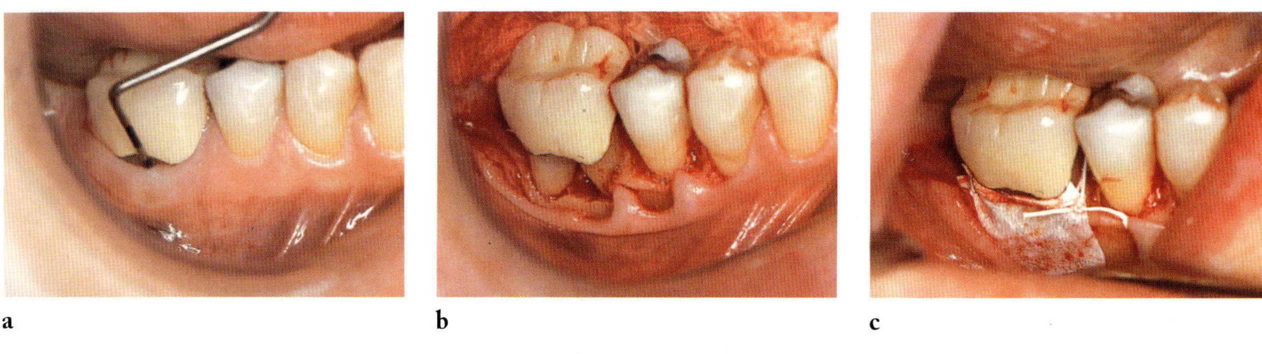

a b c

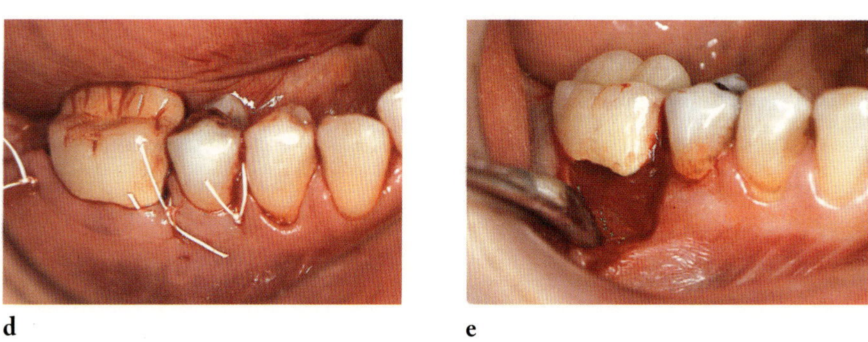

d e

Fig 6-32 Guided tissue regeneration (GTR)

a Periodontal probe in 6-mm Class II bifurcation.

b Full-thickness mucoperiosteal flap revealed loss of bone in the bifurcation.

c A Gore-Tex membrane was adapted over the bifurcation defect and sutured around the tooth.

d Flap closed with interrupted Gore-Tex sutures to completely cover the membrane.

e The membrane remained covered for 6 weeks postoperatively. A flap was reflected and the membrane removed; regenerated tissue had filled the bifurcation.

Periodontist: Edward P. Allen, DDS, PhD

that are essential to the total comprehensive treatment plan but that have severe loss of bony support should be evaluated by a periodontist for possible regenerative therapy. Often, periodontal defects resistant to conventional therapy can be successfully treated by GTR or bone grafting (Fig 6-32). The GTR technique has been especially useful and predictable when placing endosseous implants into a site with osseous defects such as fenestrations, dehiscenses, ridge defects (Fig 6-40), and occasionally for failed implants .[148] GTR and bone-regeneration techniques may also be useful when placing implants into immediate and recent extraction sites.[149,150] These definitive periodontal therapy procedures are performed in conjunction with implant surgical therapy to reduce the number of surgeries.

After definitive osseous procedures have been performed, another postoperative maturation period must take place before evaluation of the success of the therapy and judgement of the necessity of further osseous or soft tissue procedures. This maturation period should be a minimum of 3 months after resective surgery, and a minimum of 6 months after regenerative procedures.[144] The fact that a significant percentage of sites show an apical displacement of the marginal tissues of at least 2 mm between 6 weeks and 6 months after periodontal surgery suggests that in esthetically critical areas, restorations should be delayed until the site has demonstrated stability of the gingival margin.[151]

Periodontal Plastic Surgery

The scope of *periodontal plastic surgery* traditionally has been limited to treatment of insufficient dimensions of gingiva associated with frenal or muscle pull, inadequate vestibular depth, and gingival recession. The rationale and indication for treatment of gingival recession were discussed in the section on preparatory periodontal therapy. While gingival recession has been recognized as a perplexing problem for many years, successful root coverage by gingival-grafting or pedicle-flap procedures has been unpredictable until recently. New techniques and modifications of previous techniques now allow a high predictability of success as well as superior esthetics (Fig 6-33). In addition, new surgical procedures have allowed the periodontist to apply surgical therapy to embrace the treatment of esthetic problems such as excessive gingival display with insufficient clinical crown length, gingival asymmetry, flat marginal contour, improper relationship of gingival margins, loss of interdental papillae, and localized alveolar ridge deficiency.[64] Allen has described the esthetic objectives and periodontal surgical procedures for achieving enhanced dentofacial esthetics.[58]

Clinical crown lengthening is a useful but underused surgical procedure for esthetic enhancement in patients with incomplete exposure of the anatomic crowns and a high lip line, causing a "gummy smile." This is one of several areas where the periodontist can have a powerful impact on the final interdisciplinary result (Fig 6-34). While the crown-lengthening procedures may be done during preparatory periodontal therapy to facilitate orthodontic treatment, surgical crown lengthening for esthetics is generally performed after the completion of orthodontics. A period of 6 weeks to 6 months after orthodontics should elapse to allow for natural regression of enlarged tissues. During this time, good oral hygiene should be encouraged and supportive periodontal therapy provided as needed. Healing and maturation following crown-lengthening surgery is similar to resective surgery.

Abrams et al[152] reported that greater than 90% of periodontal patients with missing anterior teeth had edentulous ridge defects. These defects occur in both vertical and buccolingual dimensions. Surgical techniques such as subepithelial connective tissue grafts,[153,154] de-epithelized connective tissue pedicle grafts,[155] full-thickness onlay grafts,[156,157] and guided tissue regeneration,[158,159] have greatly enhanced the results and predictability of localized alveolar-ridge augmentation. These techniques, combined with the invaluable insight that preparatory restorative-type III therapy can provide (concerning the eventual restorative configuration), give the periodontist the capacity to develop an optimal ridge anatomy (in addition to optimal gingival relationships) so that the restorative dentist can place ideal uncompromised restorations (Fig 6-35). A maturation period of at least 2 months should elapse after soft tissue ridge-augmentation procedures and 6 months after guided tissue regeneration procedures are completed before any definitive restorative therapy is initiated.

Implant recipient sites also frequently have vertical and buccolingual defects that may require soft or hard tissue augmentation[160] before implant placement (Fig 6-39). Preparatory restorative-type IV therapy, in conjunction with the appropriate adjunctive diagnostic procedures, can greatly assist the surgeon in determining the configuration and type of augmentation necessary for optimal implant placement. These augmentation procedures should be performed as soon in treatment as possible (occasionally as part of preparatory periodontal therapy) to shorten treatment time, because augmentations and implants require extensive individual healing periods. A minimum of 30 days healing for soft tissue augmentations and 6 to 18 months healing for hard tissue augmentations (depending on the nature and extent of the graft) are required before implants can be placed. As described in the previous section on osseous therapy, it is possible in some cases to perform augmentation procedures simultaneously with implant placement to save time and reduce the number of surgeries.

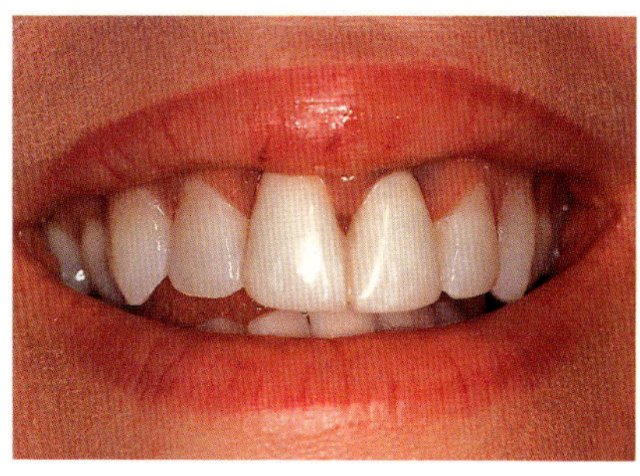

a

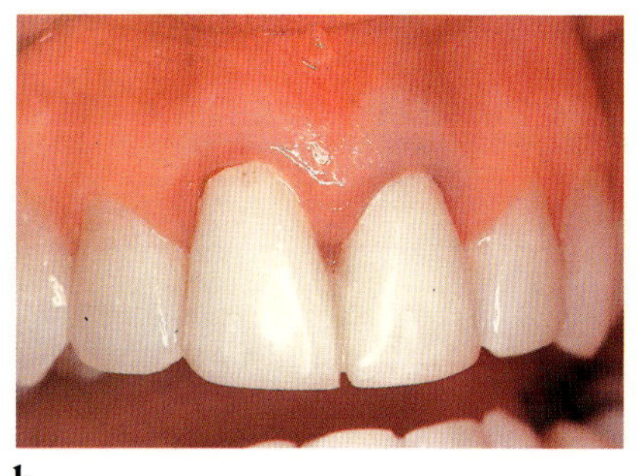

b

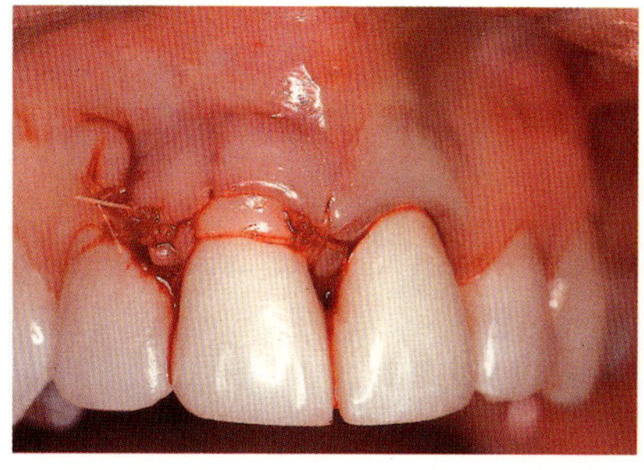

c

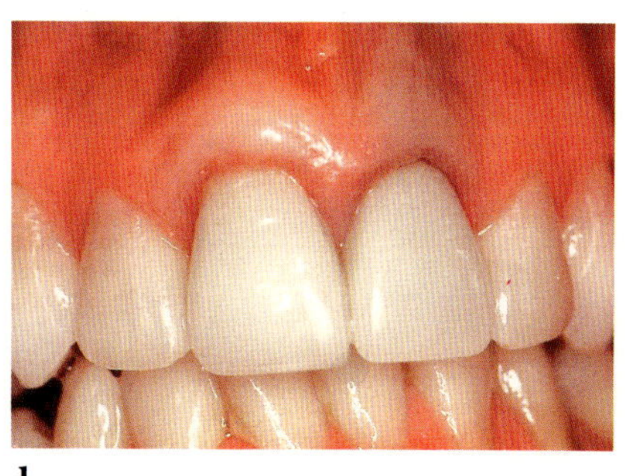

d

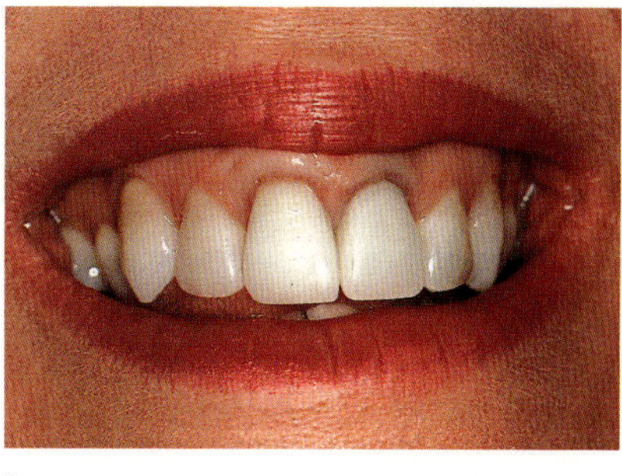

e

Fig 6-33 Connective tissue graft.

a, b Excessive length of maxillary right central incisor due to gingival recession. Provisional crowns have been placed on each central incisor.

c A connective tissue graft was used to reestablish the proper gingival level on the right central incisor and to correct the gingival asymmetry.

d, e One year postoperative and 6 months after new crowns had been placed, normal gingival contour and color and enhanced esthetics have been achieved.

Periodontist: Edward P. Allen, DDS, PhD

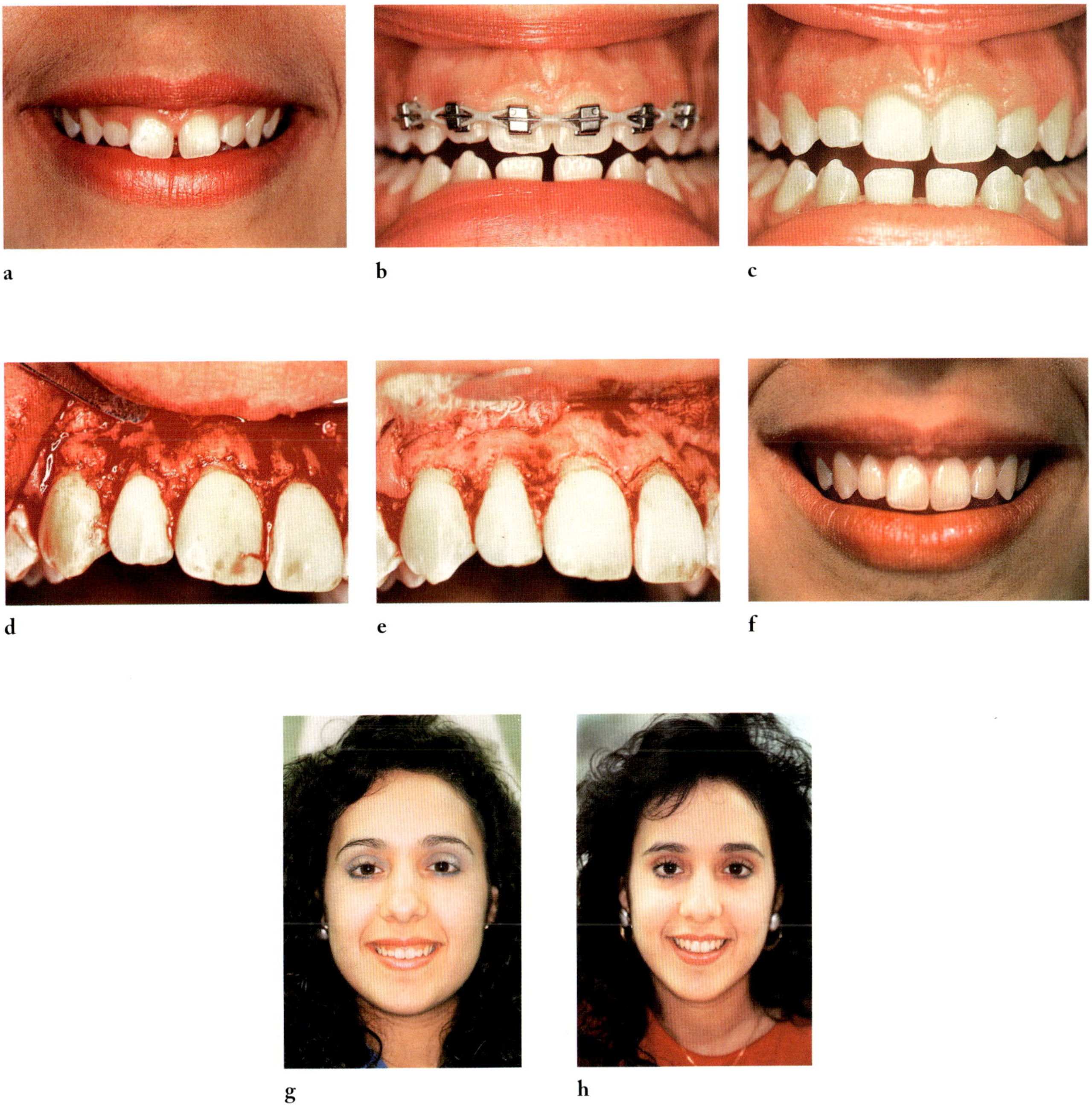

a b c

d e f

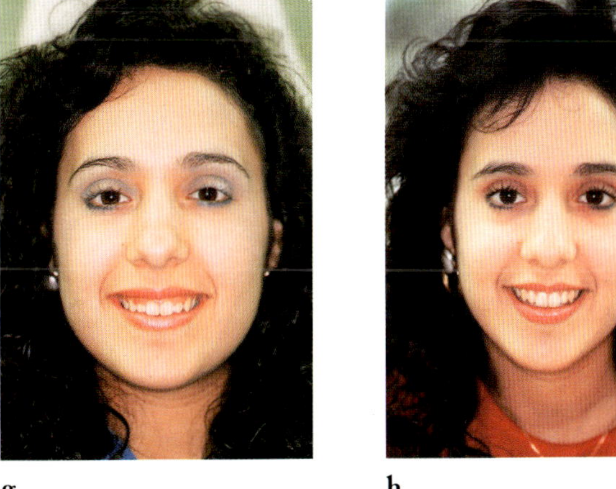

g h

Fig 6-34 Esthetic crown lengthening.

a An unattractive smile due to malposed teeth, short clinical crowns, and excessive gingival display.

b, c Adjunctive orthodontic therapy was performed to align the maxillary incisors.

d A flap was contoured and reflected, revealing thick marginal bone with an irregular crestal contour.

e Ostectomy and osteoplasty were performed to establish normal bone thickness and contour.

f Posttreatment correction of the esthetic problems.

g Following orthodontic treatment, the short clinical crowns detract from the orthodontic result.

h Following sugical treatment, normal tooth length, combined with proper tooth alignment, produces a beautiful smile.

Periodontist: Edward P. Allen, DDS, PhD

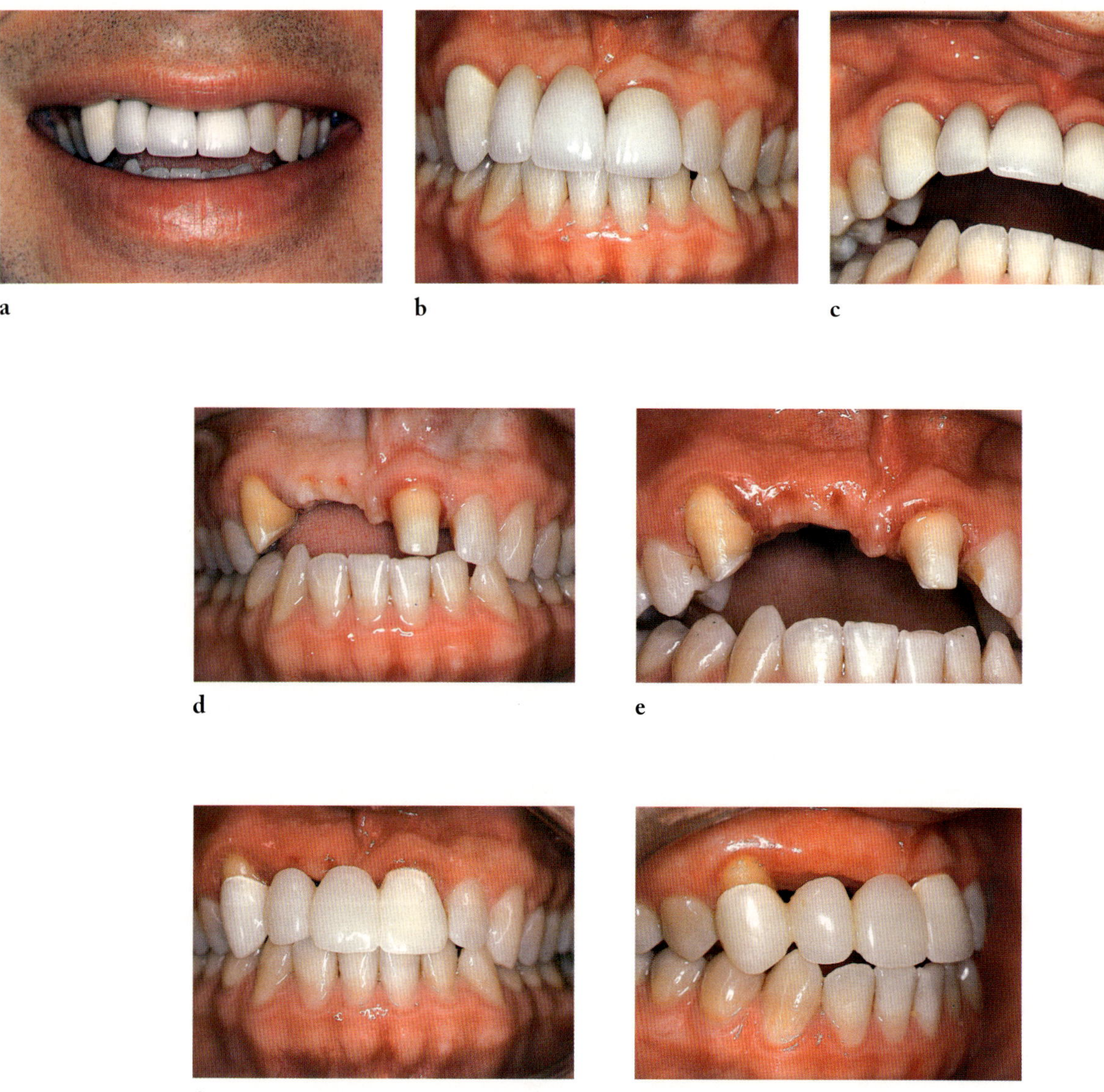

Fig 6-35 J.P. is a 35-year-old male who avulsed his maxillary right lateral and central incisors as an adolescent while playing football.

a, b, c Pretreatment smiling and intraoral views illustrating previously performed unidisciplinary compromised restorative therapy, with asymmetrical dental and gingival anatomy. Note extensive facial and buccal-lingual defect in alveolar ridge in the area of avulsed teeth 11 and 12. Also note gingival recession on tooth 13 and inflamed tissues around teeth 11 and 13, which were most likely caused iatrogenically by the overcontoured and overextended margins of the existing fixed partial denture.

d The fixed partial denture was removed and the abutment preparations examined. Knife-edge margins with minimal preparations were found.

e Abutment teeth 2 1 and 13 were reprepared for porcelain-shoulder restorations. The previous knife-edge margins were smoothed and polished, and the new margins were placed at the level of the gingival tissues on tooth 21 and 5 mm incisal to the previous restorative margin on tooth 13.

f, g Preparatory restorative-type III therapy was performed using a provisional fixed partial denture to illustrate the desired contours and ideal cervical extension position of the future definitive restoration. The provisional restoration was made to function as a template for the periodontist so that he could better visualize the desired result of the periodontal plastic procedures.

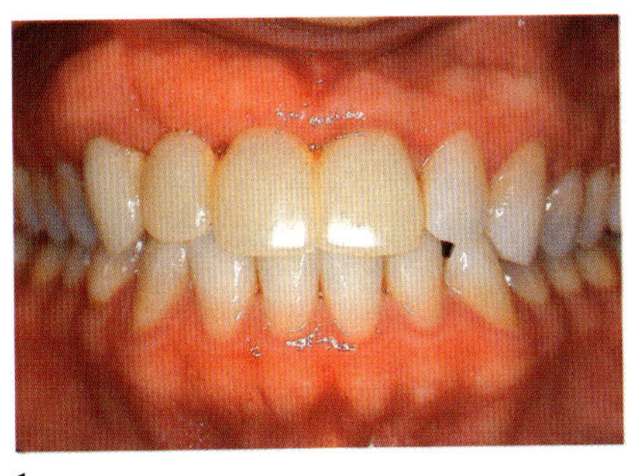
h

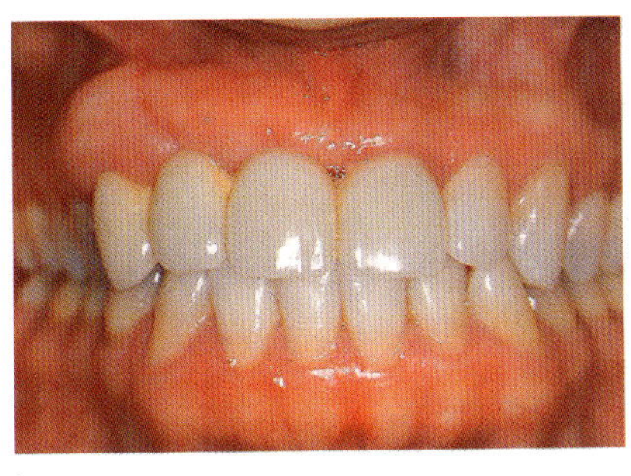
i

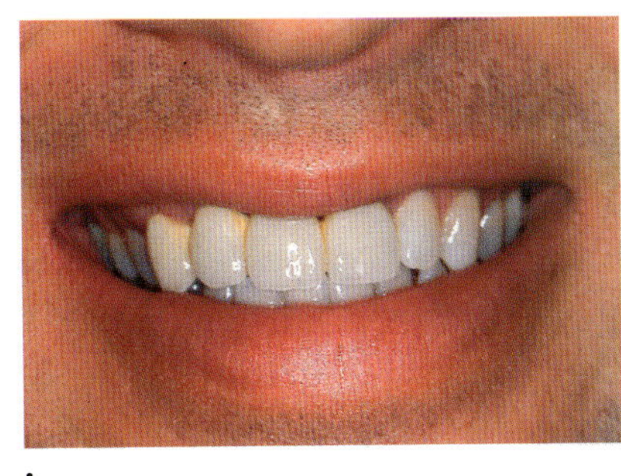
j

Fig 6-35 (continued)

h Postperiodontal view of the same provisional restoration after three different periodontal surgeries had been performed and the tissues allowed to heal for 3 months. The first surgery consisted of an initial soft tissue ridge augmentation. The second surgical procedure used a connective tissue graft to cover the exposed root surface of the canine and to further augment the alveolar ridge. In the third and final procedure, an onlay graft was placed to gain further ridge height in the area of the lateral incisor and a touch-up gingivoplasty was performed to finalize the periodontal contours in the previous surgical sites.

i, j Final intraoral and smiling views taken 2 months after placement of an all-ceramic fixed partial denture. Note the extent of the augmented tissues in relation to the initial photos and the enhanced symmetry in both the gingival and dental anatomy.

Periodontist: Edward P. Allen, DDS, PhD/*Restorative* Dentist: Richard D. Roblee, DDS, MS
Laboratory Technician: Jeffrey Singler, CDT

Occasionally, a partially edentulous ridge will be overcontoured and prevent placement of ideal restorations. In these instances, preparatory restorative-type III therapy can be performed using provisional restorations to illustrate the optimal incisal relationships of the future definitive pontic teeth of planned fixed partial dentures (Figs 5-25 i and 5-3j). The periodontist can then use this information to recontour the edentulous ridge to provide room for the correct size of pontic teeth (Fig 5-3k). Ridge recontouring can usually be accomplished by excising the appropriate amount of redundant soft tissue. In instances where there is a thin soft tissue coverage over the ridge, some osseous recontouring may also have to be performed. If moderate to severe recontouring of the ridge is needed, the provisional restorations should be extended into the recontoured area, which should then be allowed to heal and remodel before impressions are made for definitive restorations (Figs 5-31 and 5-3m). In cases where there is only a slightly overcontoured ridge, recontouring can be performed as part of the definitive restorative therapy after an ideally sized and shaped definitive pontic has been constructed (Figs 6-25j and 6-25m).

Preparatory Restorative-Type IV Therapy

Preparatory restorative-type IV therapy enables the prosthodontist or restorative dentist to provide valuable information to the implant surgeon to facilitate ideal implant placement. Little in interdisciplinary therapy is more frustrating and embarrassing to the entire team than when an implant has been improperly positioned and is unusable or unacceptable from a restorative, maintenance, and/or esthetic standpoint (Fig 2-4). The success of any implant system is highly dependent on the degree of cooperation between the implant surgeon and the restorative team member.[161,162] The restorative team member must be involved with the planning of the number and positions of implants, because it will be his or her responsibility to fabricate the implant prosthesis and maintain it over the life of the patient.[163]

When implants are going to be placed before or during definitive orthodontic and/or orthognathic surgical therapies, the orthodontic and/or orthognathic team members should also be consulted as to the ideal implant location to ensure that the implants do not interfere with their treatments and that the implant locations will still be appropriate when their therapies are completed. This is especially true when implants are going to be used for orthodontic or orthognathic anchorage (Fig 6-6).

The implant surgeon must also interact with other team members to make sure the information they provide will allow the implants to engage an adequate amount of bone and avoid vital contiguous structures, in addition to satisfying their therapy needs. Some of the contiguous structures to be avoided are nerves, arteries, maxillary sinuses, nasal floor, adjacent natural teeth, and other implants.

The number and approximate locations of the implants, as well as their prognosis, should have already been determined during treatment planning. This is accomplished by the diagnostic and treatment-planning process discussed in Chapters 4 and 5 and, when necessary, by the adjunctive diagnostic procedures of diagnostic waxup, tomograms (linear or multidirectional), and/or computed tomograms (CT scans). Often, preparatory restorative-type IV therapy is performed in conjunction with these adjunctive diagnostic procedures (Figs 6-36e and 5-5e).[164,165] Several aspects must be addressed to ideally position implants in all three dimensions: overall location, intra- and interarch spacing, parallelism, buccal-lingual relationship, and axial inclination. Errors in positioning as minimal as 2 mm or in angulation of just 10 degrees can render an implant unusable.[166] Other aspects that should be considered prior to implant placement are ease of future prosthetic procedures and the effectiveness, stability, esthetics, and maintenance of the prosthetic results.

Before surgery, the proposed implant positions should be simulated and radiographically evaluated[164,165] as to their relationship to contiguous structures (Figs 6-36 and 5-5e). Subsequent adjustment in implant placement should then be made as necessary to make the implants compatible with regional anatomy. The restorative team member usually conveys the final information to the implant surgeon by using implant surgical templates (guide stents) (Fig 6-37). There are many different methods for determining implant positions and constructing these templates,[167–173] and the various methods usually have different indications depending on the needs of each case. It is important that the template be constructed so that it can be used while the jaw is in the correct surgical position without interfering with the surgical techniques.[174] In order to ensure consistent optimal results, preparatory restorative-type IV therapy should be performed prior to any implant placement, no matter how limited.

Fig 6-36 Preparatory restorative-type IV therapy is often performed in conjunction with adjunctive diagnostic procedures to evaluate proposed implant positions. This computerized tomogram (CT scan) was taken after coating the patient's implant surgical template (guide stent) with radiopaque material. The outline of the stent can be seen in the upper right section of the image. This technique allows the implant team to more precisely plan implant placement, thereby improving the final result.

Periodontist and Implant Surgeon: Thomas G. Wilson, Jr, DDS/*Restorative Dentist:* John M. Kidwell, DDS
Laboratory Technician: Jeffrey Singler, CDT

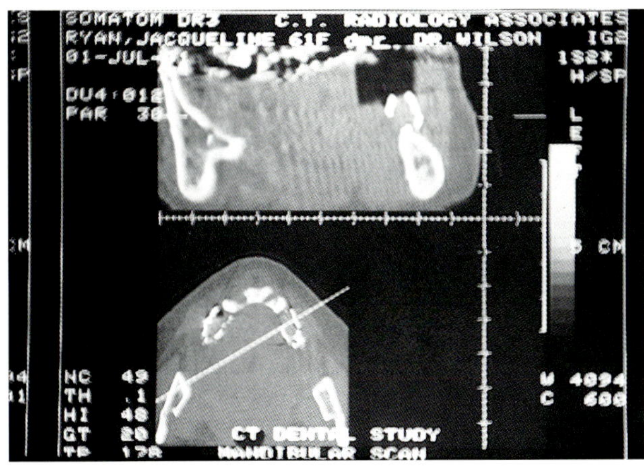

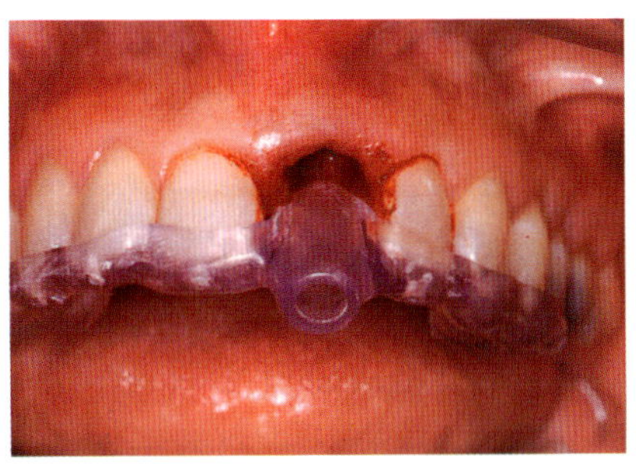

a

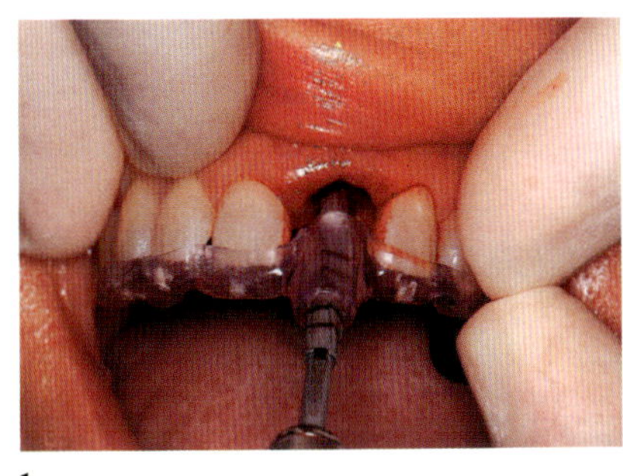

b

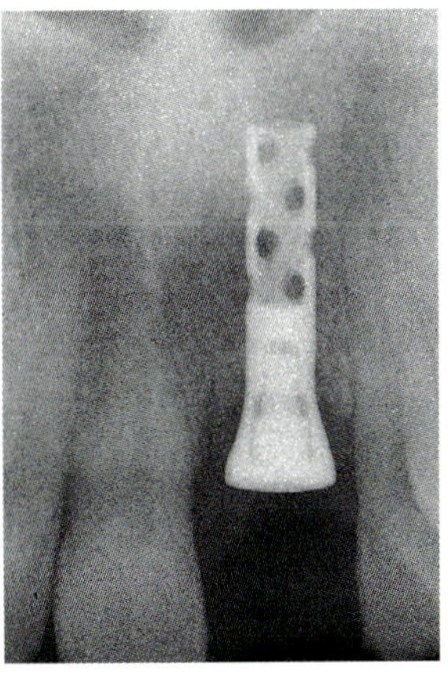

c

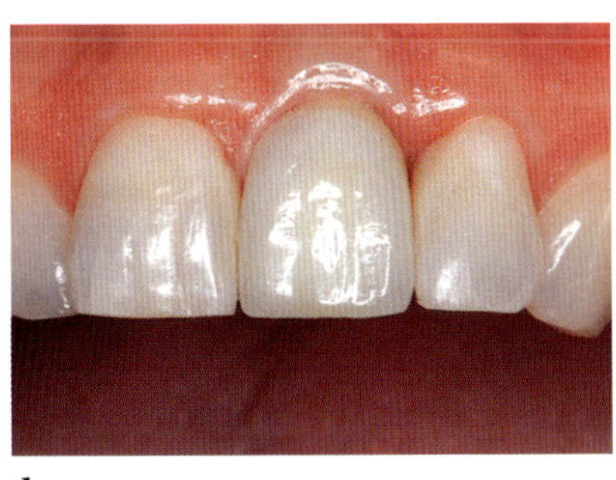

d

Fig 6-37 The information concerning optimal implant position acquired during preparatory restorative-type IV therapy is conveyed to the implant surgeon through the use of an implant surgical template (guide stents). There are many different methods for determining implant positions and constructing these templates.

a, b Implant surgical template in position and being used during implant placement.

c Radiograph of ideally positioned implant prior to restorative procedures.

d Final restoration with a natural, esthetic appearance due to proper planning of implant position.

Restorative Dentist: Frank Higginbottom, DDS/*Implant Surgeon:* Thomas G. Wilson, Jr, DDS
Laboratory Technician: Jeffrey Singler, CDT

Implant Surgical Therapy

Dental implants have become an increasingly viable treatment alternative for edentulous and partially edentulous patients (Fig 6-38). Dental implants can assist in restoring the form and function of the masticatory systems, and can also stabilize the process of residual ridge atrophy.[164,175] In addition, both retrospective and prospective studies show that dental implants can have a positive effect on a patient's well-being and quality of life.[176,177] Osseointegrated implants are being used for tooth replacement, to preserve and/or enhance formation of alveolar bone, for orthodontic anchorage,[68,69] for stability of orthognathic surgery,[178] and as sources of retention for extraoral prosthetic appliances.[179,180] These implants are particularly useful in restoring severe traumatic injuries with loss of normal anatomy[181] (Figs 6-39 and 6-26). There are many other exciting potential uses for osseointegrated implants.[182]

The commonly used types of implants can be categorized according to whether their attachment is through fibro-osseous integration or osseointegration. Fibro-osseous attachment is usually associated with blade and subperiosteal implants. This type of attachment is known to be the less stable of the two, and is known to have a reduced success rate due to tissue breakdown around the implant.[183]

Osseointegration of dental implants was first described by Brånemark.[184] He and others have shown that these implants have a high long-term success rate.[185,186] There are several osseointegrated dental implant systems currently available. All of them require a 3- to 8-month initial healing period, during which the implant must be protected from occlusal stress. Most osseointegrated systems require two surgical procedures.[184,185] The first surgery involves placement of the dental implant into bone, where it is left submerged beneath the mucosal tissues to protect it during healing and osseointegration. The second surgery uncovers the implant after the appropriate healing time has passed and prepares it for restoration. Some osseointegrated implant systems have a one-stage surgical technique in which the implant is placed and left unsubmerged. Recent studies have shown that the single-stage surgical procedure is also successful.[187,188]

The high predictability of osseointegrated implants and the many options they provide has added an exciting new dimension to interdisciplinary dentofacial therapy. This new dimension has also forced interdisciplinary treatment planning to be more creative, because the timing of implant placement must vary according to each patient's unique requirements. The placement should be done as early in therapy as possible to allow for an appropriate healing period with the shortest overall treatment time. In addition, dental implants should be placed and/or uncovered in conjunction with other surgical procedures whenever possible to minimize the number of surgeries. As previously mentioned, there are several indications for placing implants during preparatory therapy. In some situations, an implant can even be placed during initial periodontal therapy and uncovered during definitive periodontal surgery.[189]

Dental implants can be placed at various times in definitive therapy, depending on the circumstances of the case and the intended use or uses of the implants. They may be placed in extraction sites immediately following tooth removal, which results in shortened treatment time, as well as prevention of alveolar bone resorption.[190] In extraction sites with loss of a portion of the cortical plate or in alveolar ridges with inadequate buccal-lingual width, membranes may be used to promote bone growth around the implants.[191] As discussed in definitive periodontal therapy, the GTR technique has greatly expanded the use of implants in sites previously considered to have insufficient bone for successful placement of osseointegrated implants (Fig 6-40). The vertical dimension of maxillary bone can be significantly increased by using maxillary sinus lifts and onlay bone grafting during implant placement.[192,193] In the mandible, the amount of vertical bone available for implant placement can be increased through inferior alveolar nerve lateralization[194,195] and onlay bone grafting.[196,197] At implant uncovering, or after healing is complete with a single-stage implant system, soft tissue augmentation with connective tissue grafts can be used to enhance the soft tissue contours for construction of a prosthesis with a more natural form in harmony with the natural dentition.[198]

Implant techniques for replacing missing single teeth are becoming more favorable and predictable.[199] In areas of high esthetic concern, the implants can offer single-unit or multiple-unit restorations with a natural appearance (Fig 6-40).[200,201] Utilization of a single-tooth implant may prevent the need for preparation of healthy adjacent teeth for fixed partial denture abutments.

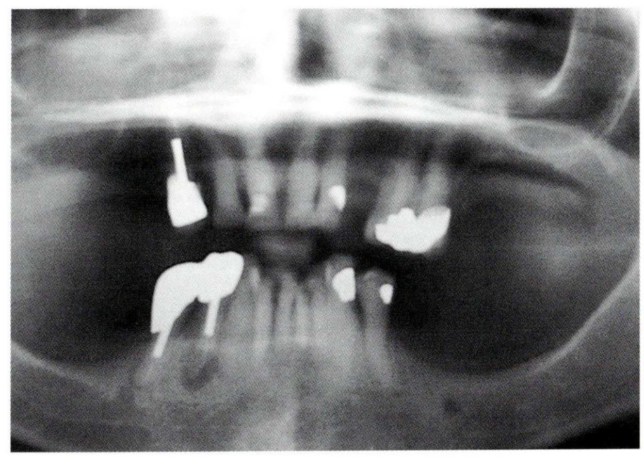

a

b c

d e

Fig 6-38 Transitional implant therapy.

a to d Initial radiograph and photographs and illustrating mutilated and failing dentition with bimaxillary dentoalveolar protrusion.

e The maxillary right canine and all remaining mandibular teeth except the canines were extracted. The mandibular canines were retained, even though they were given a hopeless prognosis, so that they could be used to maintain a provisional prosthesis during transitional implant therapy.

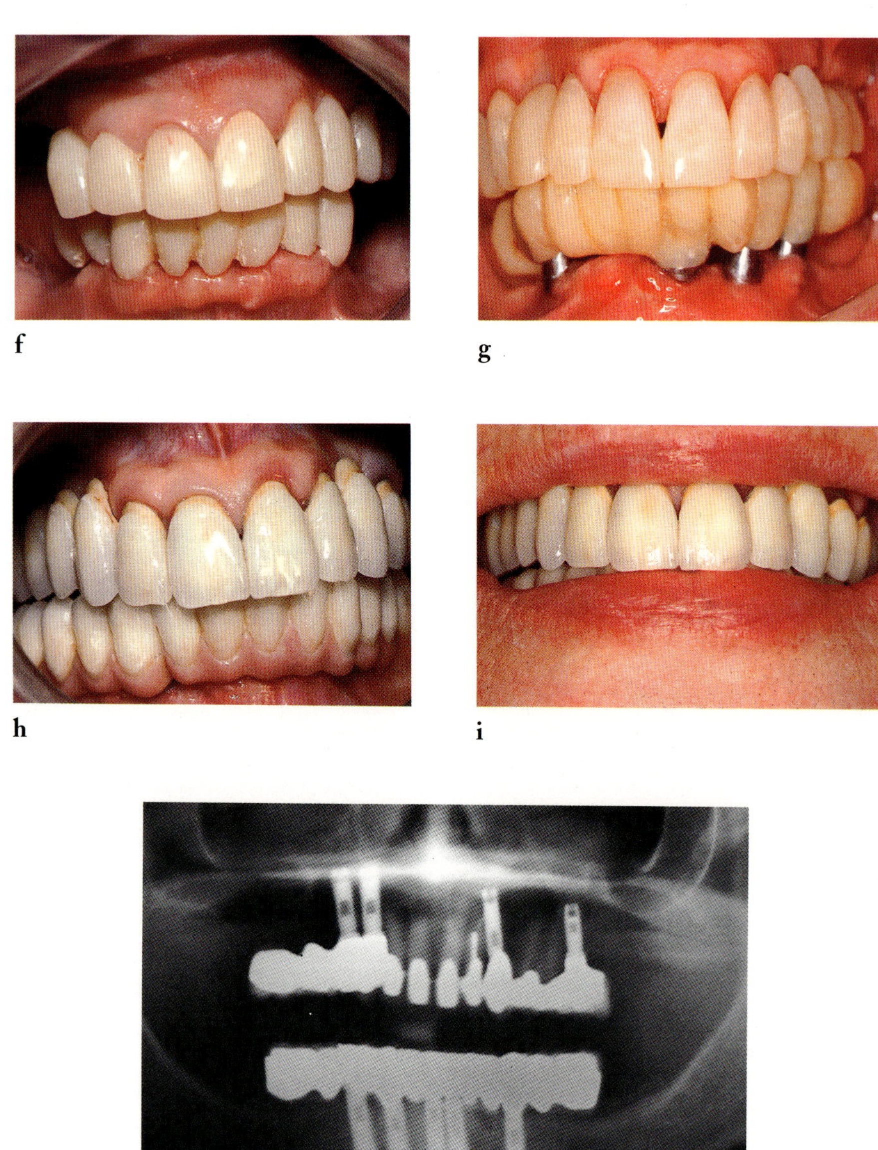

Fig 6-38 (continued)

f Full-mouth provisional restorations retained by remaining maxillary dentition and mandibular canines. The extraction sites were allowed to heal for approximately 45 days, at which time endosseous root-form dental implants were placed in both jaws. The provisional restorations were then reinserted and the dental implants were allowed to osseointegrate. After osseointegration, the implants were uncovered and put into function with new provisional restorations. At that time, the mandibular canines, whose usefulness was now exhausted, were removed and implants were immediately put into their place.

g After 3 months of healing, the mandibular canine implants were uncovered and put into function.

h to j Final intraoral, smile, and radiographic views of the definitive restorative therapy. This case clearly illustrates the tremendous impact implants have had on dentistry. It also illustrates the benefits, to patient and team, of proper planning and teamwork when restoring a failing natural dentition with transitional implant therapy. It is important not to extract hopeless teeth until a definitive treatment plan has been formulated. In this case, the failing mandibular canines played a key role in the transitional therapy, and without them the patient and the restorative dentist would have had a much more difficult time maintaining function while the first round of implants were osseointegrating.

Periodontist and Implant Surgeon: Thomas G. Wilson, Jr, DDS/*Restorative Dentist:* Frank L. Higginbottom, DDS
Laboratory Technician: Jeffrey Singler, CDT

Case Summary

Patient: S.B. is a 16-year-old female who was involved in a motor vehicle accident and sustained a severe fracture of her left zygomatic orbital complex and had a traumatic hemimaxillectomy of the left maxilla from the left lateral incisor through the third molar area.

Abbreviated Problem List

- Left maxillary continuity defect, secondary to trauma
- Left zygomatic orbital malunion
- Left enophthalmos
- Soft tissue deficiency in the left cheek area
- Missing maxillary left alveolus, palatal bone, and teeth from the lateral incisor through the third molar
- No bone around left central incisor except on mesial aspect
- Lack of stable prosthesis in left maxilla
- Impacted right maxillary and mandibular third molars

Treatment Plan

Interdisciplinary Dentofacial Therapy

- Surgery: Stage I
    - Cranial bone graft to reconstruct the left maxilla and create an alveolar ridge
    - Augmentation of left malar eminence and reconstruction of left orbital floor
    - Remove impacted right maxillary and mandibular third molars
    - Extract maxillary left central incisor
- Surgery: Stage II
    - Placement of osseointegrated implants into the bone graft in the left maxilla after proper maturation period
- Definitive Restorative Therapy
    - Prosthetic reconstruction after dental implants have osseointegrated

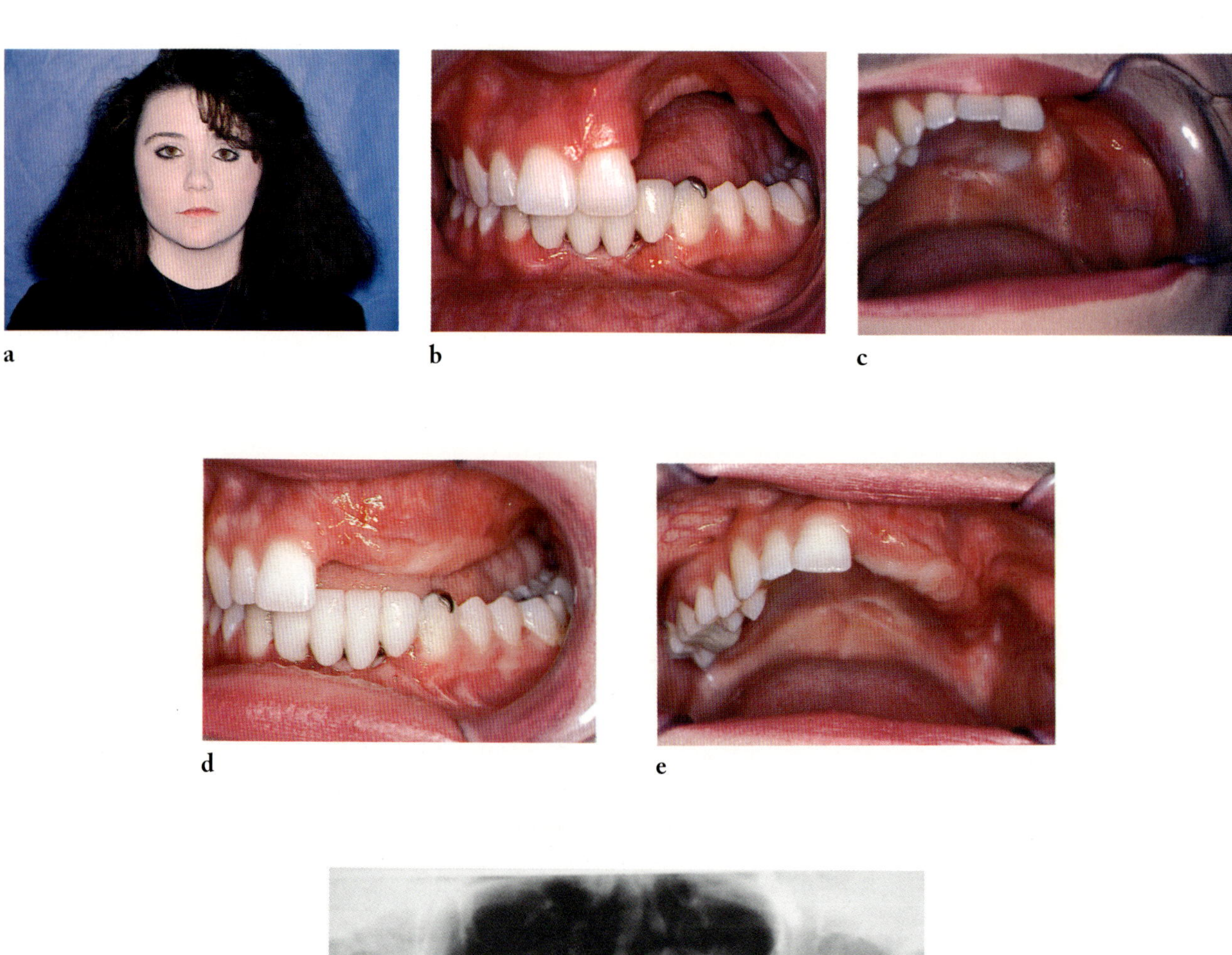

Fig 6-39

a to c This patient was involved in a motor vehicle accident, sustaining avulsion of her left maxilla, including the lateral incisor through the tuberosity and the associated palate. She also had left enophthalmus (sinking inward of the eye). Note the extent of the bony defect in the left maxilla.

d to f First-stage surgery was performed to reconstruct the avulsed alveolar ridge. Cranial bone grafts were used for the reconstruction. The left central incisor had to be removed at the time of surgery because there was no bone around three sides of it.

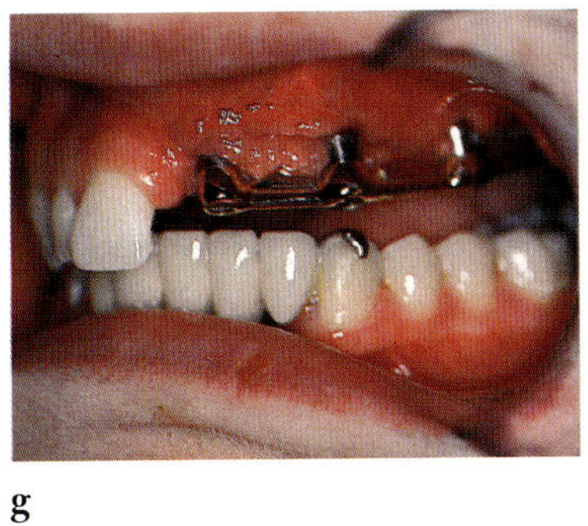
g

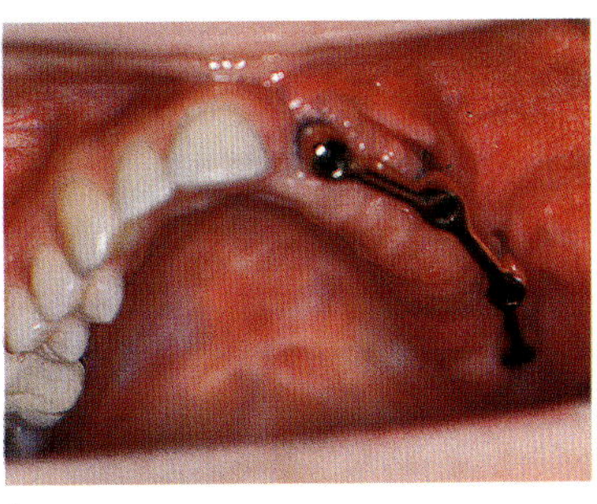
h

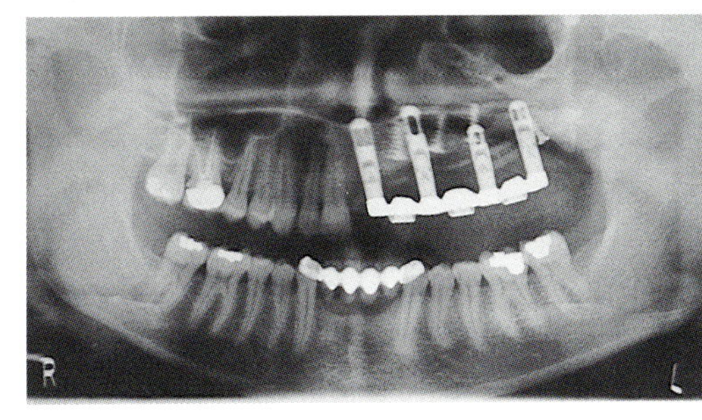

i

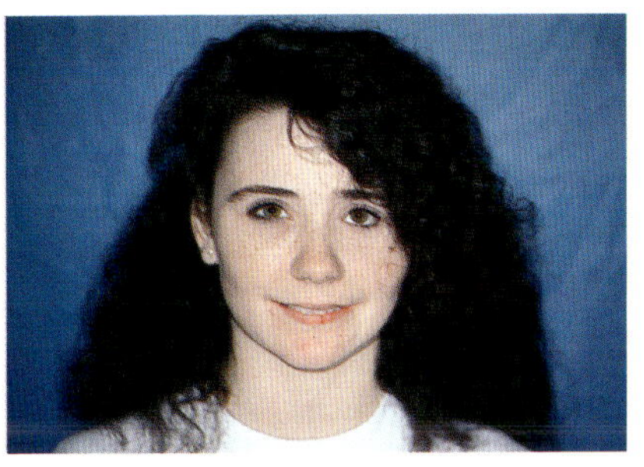
j

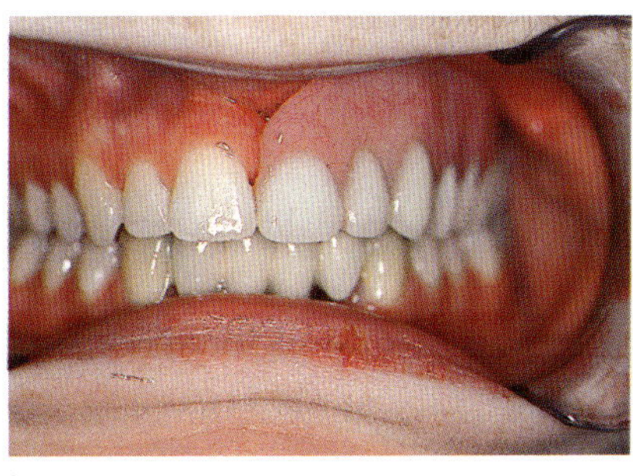
k

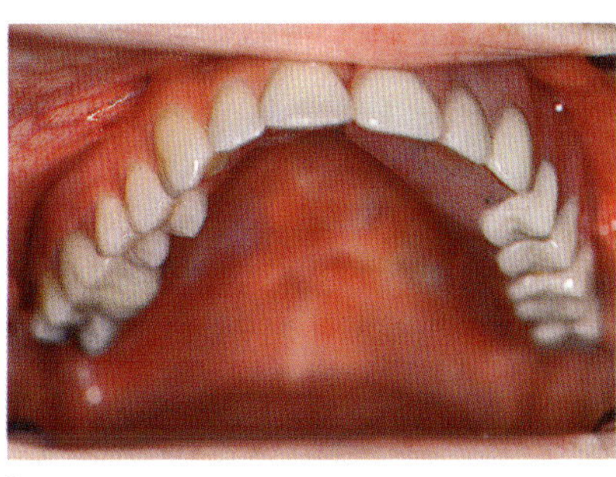
l

Fig 6-39

g to i Intraoral and panoramic views 6 months after implant placement into cranial bone grafts. A superstructure for prosthesis retention was constructed after the implants osseointegrated.

j to l The patient 2 years following injury, with correction of her left enophthalmus and reconstruction of her dentition.

Oral and Maxillofacial Surgeon (cranial bone reconstruction of the left maxilla and orbit): Larry M. Wolford, DDS
Oral and Maxillofacial Surgeon (implants): Colin Bell, DDS, MSD/*Restorative Dentist:* Donivan Ridgway, DDS

Discussion

Osseointegrated implants are especially useful in trauma cases with subsequent loss of normal anatomy. Due to the extent of the defect in this case, an extensive bone graft had to be performed in a separate surgery before the implants could be placed. In less extensive defects, the grafting and implant placement can frequently be performed during the same surgery.

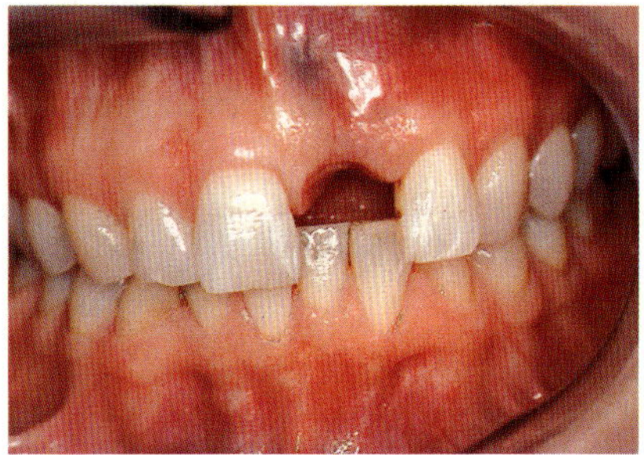

a

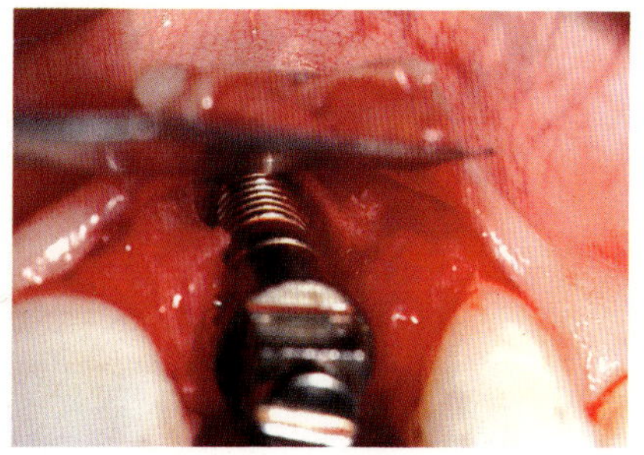

b

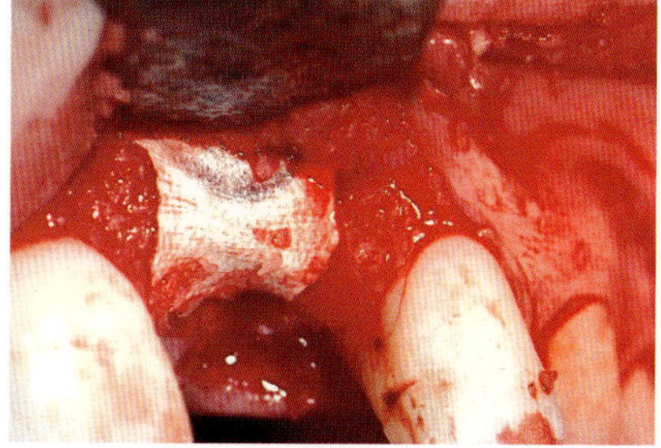

c

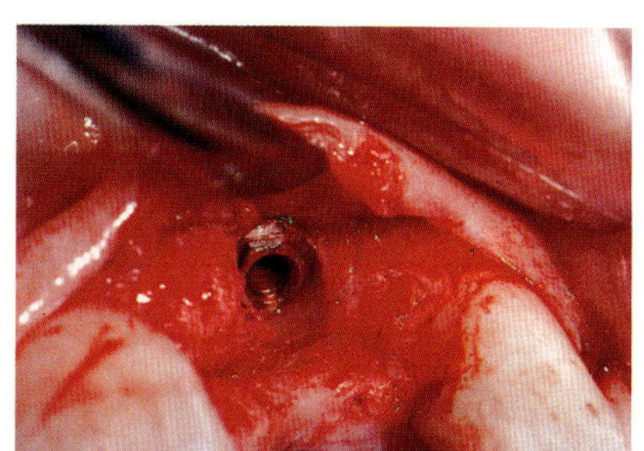

d

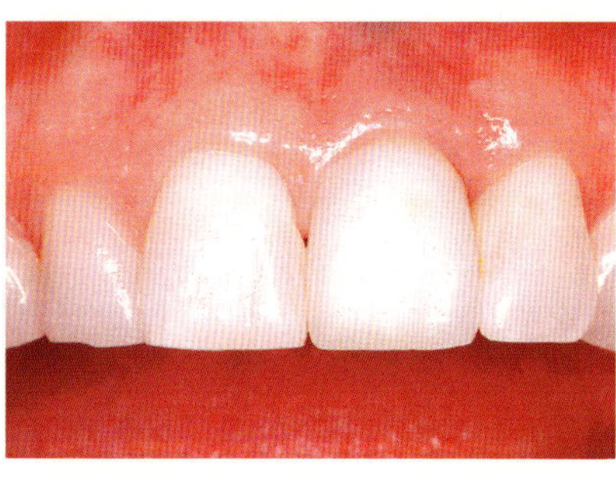

e

Fig 6-40

a Initial view of a patient who lost her maxillary left central incisor.

b An endosseous implant was optimally positioned in an area with bony and soft tissue deficiencies.

c Guided tissue regeneration using an expanded polytetraflouroethylene membrane was used to correct the deficiencies. Freeze-dried bone mixed with tetracycline was placed under the membrane to hold buccal space.

d Bone growth was evident 6 months later at reopening.

e This combined approach provided an increase in hard and soft tissues, which allowed construction of an esthetic replacement for the missing natural teeth.

Periodontist and Implant Surgeon: Thomas G. Wilson, Jr, DDS/*Restorative Dentist:* Frank L. Higginbottom, DDS
Laboratory Technician: Jeffrey Singler, CDT

Implants requiring two surgical procedures are usually uncovered just prior to definitive restorative therapy, but they may be uncovered earlier if they are to be used for another purpose, such as orthodontic or orthognathic anchorage. Implants should be placed by an appropriately-trained surgeon using surgical templates constructed by or in conjunction with the restorative team member (preparatory restorative-type IV therapy). Inappropriately positioned or failed dental implants resulting from poor surgical planning or techniques can be extremely frustrating and embarrassing to an interdisciplinary team (Fig 2-4). Dental implant systems are continuously improving and are sure to be of even greater value to the interdisciplinary dentofacial team in the future.

Definitive Restorative Therapy

Aspects of restorative therapy are discussed throughout this text. These discussions are necessary because optimal restorative results in IDT require proper planning and preparation by the entire team throughout the interdisciplinary process. Traditional multidisciplinary therapy, with its lack of team communication, frequently depends on definitive restorative procedures to compensate for inadequate planning and compromised results of previous therapies (Figs 2-3 and 2-4). This type of compensation frequently leads to iatrogenically induced problems in esthetics, function, stability, and periodontal health. These forced compromises, and their accompanying frustrations, might also explain why many restorative dentists and prosthodontists frequently hold a rather poor opinion of other specialists' ability to provide an optimal environment for definitive restorative procedures that are conducive to proper health and function. Interdisciplinary therapy, on the other hand, minimizes these problems.

There are many outstanding references on the broad and varied aspects of restorative therapy. Even a brief summary of these various aspects of restorative therapy is not practical in a text of this nature, so they are discussed in a generalized way, with important specifics given in relation to IDT, to enable the entire team to better use the knowledge and skills of the restorative team member. Definitive restorative therapies should be the last dental procedures performed in definitive therapy. At this point in interdisciplinary dentofacial therapy, the osseous, mucogingival, and dental/implant components should be optimally prepared to accept ideal definitive restorative procedures. This has been made possible through open-team communication during team conferencing and monitoring, and through the assistance and three-dimensional information provided by the restorative team member in preparatory restorative-type I, II, III, and IV therapies. Through the process of mutual or interdisciplinary compromise, difficult and complex problems can now be restored to the most satisfactory results possible. The restorative team member has the opportunity and responsibility to fine-tune and enhance the overall dentofacial results. To properly fulfill this role, the restorative dentist or prosthodontist must base his or her therapy on solid periodontal and occlusal principles to provide a result that will assist in the maintenance of the associated dentition, dental implants, periodontal, and temporomandibular complexes.

The restorative team member must, however, be very cautious about the overutilization of restorative procedures. Even ideal restorative therapy can increase the risk of periodontal disease.[202,203] All attempts should be made to maintain the natural tooth structures whenever possible (Fig 6-41), and when this is not possible, to place margins of restorations supragingivally.[204] Conservative restorative procedures such as bleaching (Fig 6-42), cosmetic recontouring (enameloplasty), composite resins (Fig 6-43), and all-ceramic restorations (Figs 6-44 and 6-45) can significantly enhance dental esthetics while helping maintain natural tooth structure and long-term periodontal health (Fig 6-41).

The restorative team member has many exciting materials and techniques in his or her restorative armamentarium. Many examples of the different kinds of restorations available today are presented throughout this text. These examples also illustrate how proper use of the restorative team member's knowledge and creativity throughout interdisciplinary dentofacial therapy can have a tremendous impact on overall results (Fig 2-5). The selection of the optimal type or types of restorative procedures depends on each patient's and each tooth's unique requirements. This selection should have been made in the treatment-planning phase so that all the

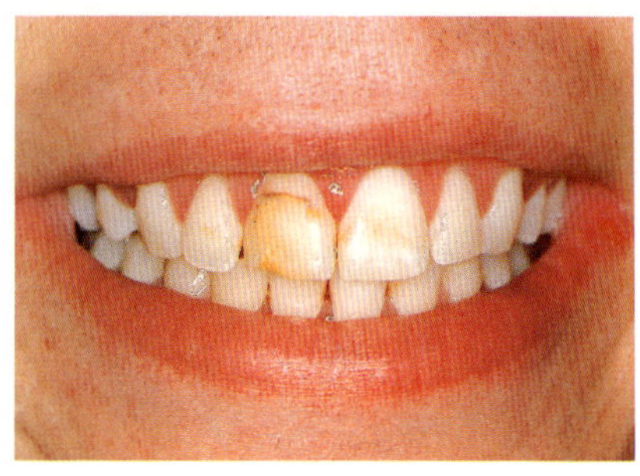

a

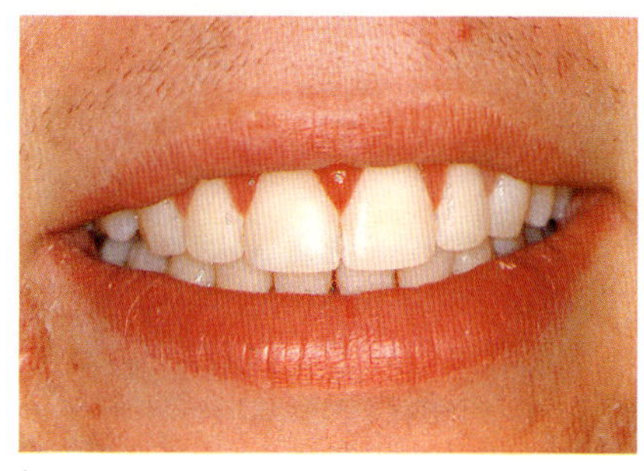

b

Fig 6-41

a Patient presented for restorative therapy after orthodontic therapy had been completed. Note unesthetic appearance of anterior dentition due to asymmetry of dental shapes, defective restoration on facial aspect of tooth 21, and yellow and white discoloration across remaining anterior teeth. Also note severe gingival inflammation due to poor oral hygiene.

b Final dental appearance after conservative restorative therapy was completed. This therapy consisted of esthetically recontouring the dentition, followed by chemical abrasion to remove discoloration on anterior teeth. A direct composite-resin labial veneer that matched the adjacent teeth was then placed on tooth 21. Without the chemical abrasion, it would have been difficult, if not impossible, to match the adjacent teeth with composite resin. All attempts should be made to maintain natural tooth structure whenever possible, especially when periodontal inflammation already exists. In this case, extensive restorative therapy (even conservative porcelain veneers) is contraindicated, due to the patient's inadequate maintenance of periodontal health. Instead, other conservative restorative procedures were used to dramatically improve the esthetic appearance of the dentition without exacerbating the periodontal problems.

preparatory and definitive therapies could be performed to prepare for the specific type of final restorations. Of course, each case must be reevaluated after those other therapies are completed to see if the planned restorative procedures are still optimal. Often, it is necessary to modify definitive restorative therapy when results of previous therapies are more or less satisfactory than originally expected.

The restorative dentist or prosthodontist should now optimally prepare the necessary teeth and use provisional restorations as outlined in preparatory restorative-type III therapy. If provisionals were used previously in preparatory restorative therapy-types I, II, or III and are still functionally, anatomically, and esthetically correct, they can often be relined to fit the final tooth preparation and thus prevent a total reconstruction of the provisional restorations.

If definitive periodontal therapy is performed, no restorative therapy should be performed for a minimum of 2 months[146] (preferably 3 months[189]) after periodontal surgery and 6 months after bone-grafting procedures to allow proper postoperative maturation of the periodontal tissues. Restorative procedures should be delayed for 3 to 6 months following periodontal surgical procedures in the anterior maxillary region to allow time for stabilization of the marginal gingival tissues.[151] After this time, an evaluation should be completed to make sure that the periodontal tissues have responded favorably and that no further periodontal procedures are indicated. The final restorative treatment plan should be reassessed and then carried through.

Definitive restorations or prostheses should permanently restore the proper function, periodontal relationships, phonetics, and esthetics acquired diagnostically through the provisional restorations or occlusal rim waxups. This use of provisional restorations minimizes the chances of unforeseen problems, both for the restorative dentist and the patient, and can greatly enhance the overall success and prognosis of the final restorations.

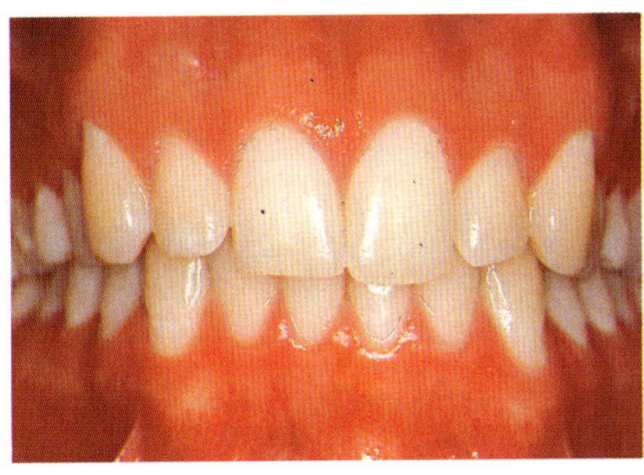
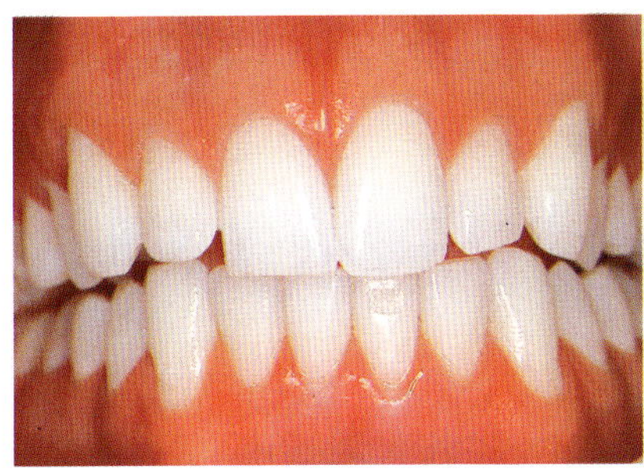

Fig 6-42 Before and after photographs of patient who was concerned about her dental appearance due to the generalized discoloration of her teeth. This problem was successfully treated using patient-administered vital bleaching. Conservative procedures such as these can not only enhance dental esthetics, but can also be used by dental professionals to motivate a patient to a higher level of dental health.

Restorative Dentist: Frank L. Higginbottom, DDS

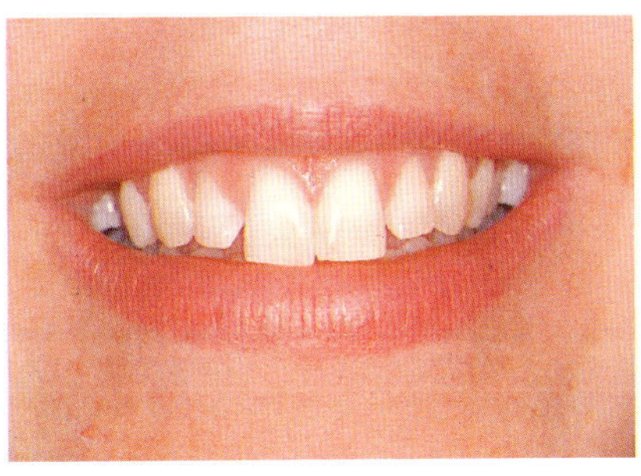
a

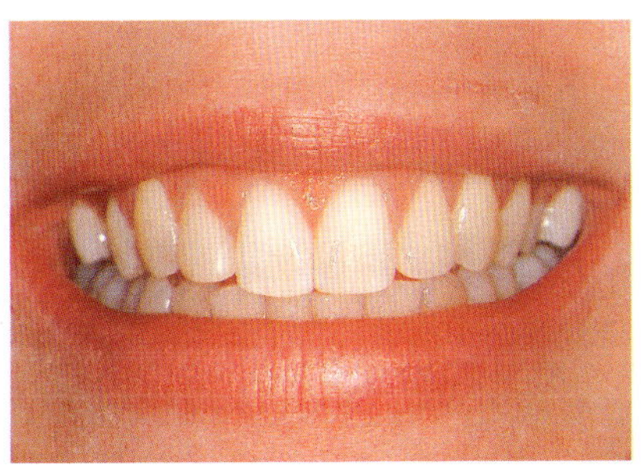
b

Fig 6-43 Conservative restorative procedures can be used in some circumstances to enhance a patient's dental appearance quickly without compromising oral health or long-term maintenance when functional and periodontal problems do not already exist.

a Female model presented because she was unhappy with her dental appearance. Note mild dental irregularities and unesthetic shape of the maxillary anterior dentition.

b Dental appearance after one short restorative appointment in which unesthetic and irregular teeth were reshaped and composite resin directly placed to mesial-incisal angles of lateral incisors. Note the tremendous esthetic enhancement of the patient's smile, accomplished with procedures that should not compromise future oral health or require excessive maintenance.

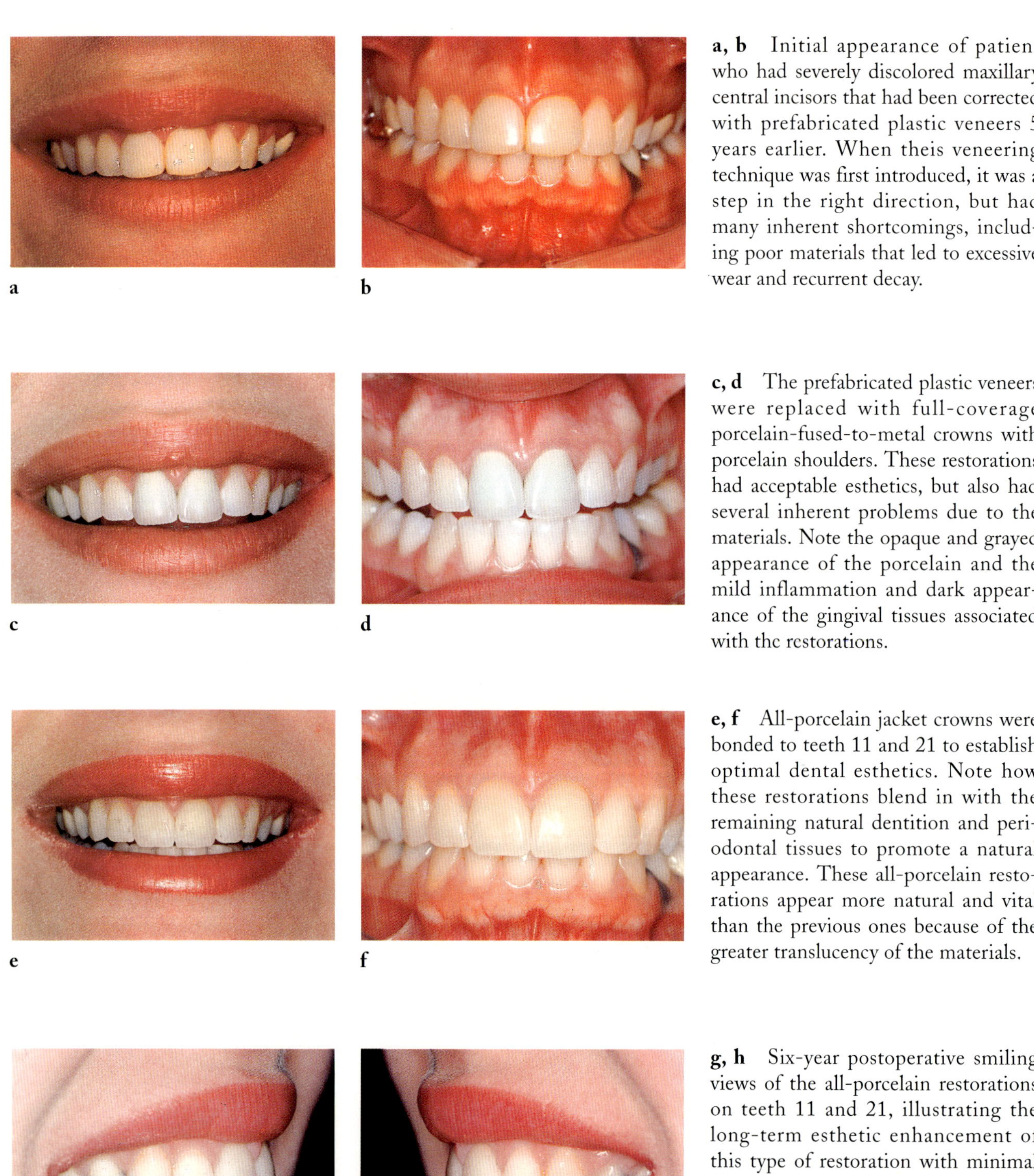

a, b Initial appearance of patient who had severely discolored maxillary central incisors that had been corrected with prefabricated plastic veneers 5 years earlier. When theis veneering technique was first introduced, it was a step in the right direction, but had many inherent shortcomings, including poor materials that led to excessive wear and recurrent decay.

c, d The prefabricated plastic veneers were replaced with full-coverage porcelain-fused-to-metal crowns with porcelain shoulders. These restorations had acceptable esthetics, but also had several inherent problems due to the materials. Note the opaque and grayed appearance of the porcelain and the mild inflammation and dark appearance of the gingival tissues associated with thc rcstorations.

e, f All-porcelain jacket crowns were bonded to teeth 11 and 21 to establish optimal dental esthetics. Note how these restorations blend in with the remaining natural dentition and periodontal tissues to promote a natural appearance. These all-porcelain restorations appear more natural and vital than the previous ones because of the greater translucency of the materials.

g, h Six-year postoperative smiling views of the all-porcelain restorations on teeth 11 and 21, illustrating the long-term esthetic enhancement of this type of restoration with minimal compromise to the periodontal health.

Fig 6-44 Restorative techniques and materials have changed dramatically over the last 15 years.

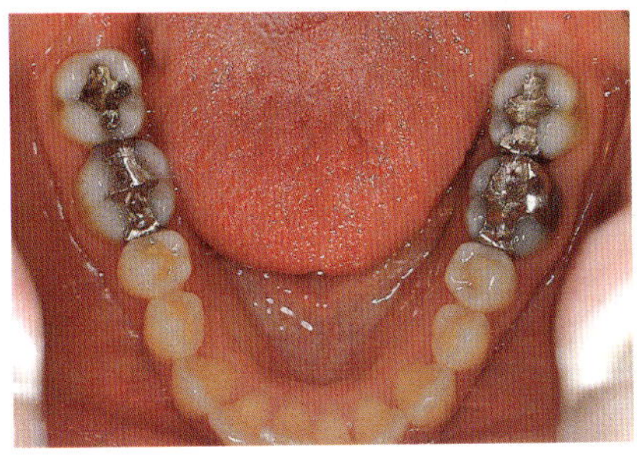

a

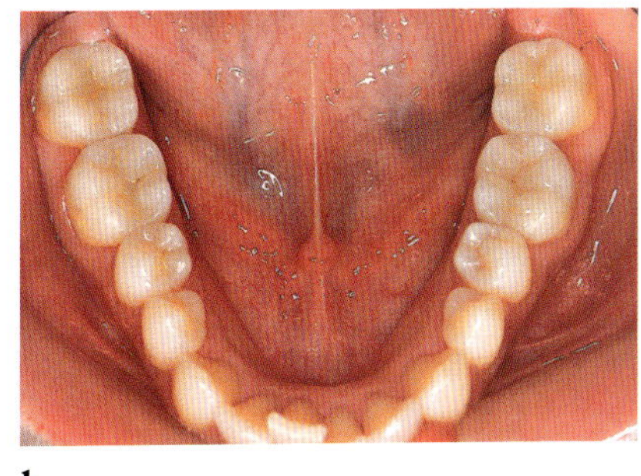

b

Fig 6-45 All-porcelain restorations can frequently be used in the posterior dentition to esthetically and conservatively restore and maintain dental health.

a Preoperative occlusal view of large amalgam restorations with numerous areas of recurrent decay.

b Occlusal view of final restorations 6 years after placement. Bonded porcelain onlays were placed on all four molars and a bonded porcelain inlay was placed on the right second premolar. Note the natural appearance of these restorations with no deleterious effects to the periodontal tissues.

Restorative Laboratory Procedures

The restorative team member has already played an integral role in several of the other therapies by providing valuable information concerning the final definitive restorations. Now is an important time for him or her to provide highly detailed information to another team member: the laboratory technician. Unfortunately, the laboratory technician is usually an improperly used member of an interdisciplinary team. A good laboratory technician who participates throughout the entire interdisciplinary dentofacial therapy process can frequently enhance overall function, periodontal condition, esthetics, and long-term prognosis of a complex dentofacial therapy. It behooves the rest of the team, especially the restorative dentist or prosthodontist, to use the laboratory technician to his or her full potential.

Problems can arise from the fact that laboratory technicians are rarely consulted during diagnostic or treatment-planning procedures. To make matters worse, they are often given less-than-adequate working casts with improper tooth preparations and virtually no diagnostic information except a standard tooth shade, and then asked to construct good-looking restorations. To attain optimal results in complex interdisciplinary dentofacial therapy, laboratory technicians often need information concerning facial form, lip support, incisor exposure, smile line, phonetics, function, detailed tooth coloration, age, sex, and various other pertinent information about the patient and his or her expectations. Without this information, a laboratory technician cannot be expected to sit behind a lab bench with a working cast and construct restorations that will optimally finalize dentofacial therapy.

The first and most important way to properly involve laboratory technicians is to include their expertise in the diagnostic and treatment planning phases of IDT. They can provide invaluable information concerning optimal prosthetic procedures so that the other team members can plan their therapies accordingly. The restorative dentist or prosthodontist must also provide laboratory technicians with all the pertinent diagnostic information needed to ideally construct the final restorations. This can be done in the following ways: *(1)* written and verbal communication, *(2)* diagnostic and working casts, *(3)* photographs, and *(4)* posttreatment feedback.

The written and verbal communication usually uses a shade diagram. This diagram should be highly detailed, especially if one is trying to match adjacent natural teeth (Fig 6-46). The laboratory technician needs the patient's age, gender, and various unique characteristics of the patient's dentition, such as base shades, translucency/opacity, presence of cracks, internal and external color characterizations, etc. If the restorative team member cannot adequately provide this information, then he or she needs to allow the technician to see the patient to acquire the information. All of these factors can influence the overall shape and characteristics of the restorations.

Dental casts can provide detailed information to the technician that cannot be adequately expressed otherwise. The most important casts are the working casts. They should be made with precision, and the working dies of tooth preparations should be trimmed by the restorative team member to help ensure the accurate location of the margins on the definitive restorations. For extensive restorative procedures, the casts should be mounted in a semiadjustable articulator in centric relation using an accurate technique.[205] It is also useful to send diagnostic casts of the pretreatment dentition and, most importantly, the provisional restorations. The pretreatment diagnostic casts can give the technician information about the natural shape and size of the dentition, as well as about surface texture and wear.

To construct optimal restorations, the technician needs to customize them to the unique dentofacial characteristics (facial form, lip support, smile line, etc) of the patient. The restorative dentist should have already developed these characteristics into the provisional restorations, along with critical functional relationships (Fig 2-5m). A diagnostic cast of these provisionals can precisely relay the necessary information to the technician and remove any guesswork associated with the shapes, sizes, positions, and functions of the teeth being restored (Fig 2-5n). In addition, a soft tissue cast using resilient material to represent gingival tissues can greatly assist the technician in producing contours in restorations that will achieve proper esthetics while maintaining healthy gingival relationships (Fig 6-47). These procedures again illustrate how the interdisciplinary team members can work together to greatly enhance their individual results by proper communication. It is also beneficial to properly mount the casts of the provisional restorations in centric relation to the opposing working casts (Fig 2-5n.2).

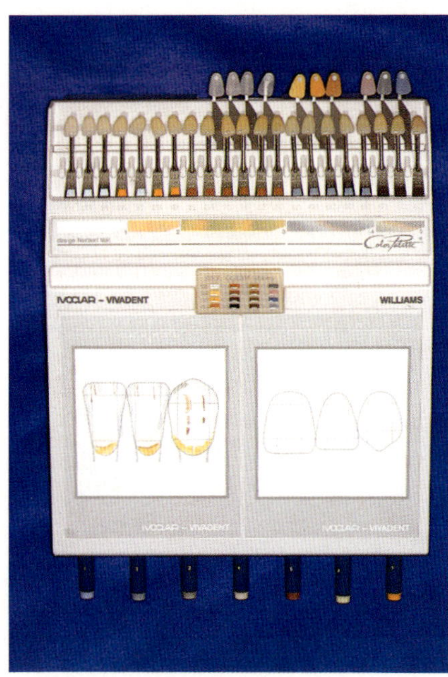

Fig 6-46 Shade diagrams should be highly detailed when matching adjacent teeth. Unique characteristics such as base shades, translucency/opacity, cracks, stains, and other characterizations should be illustrated. The restorative team member and the laboratory technician must develop a system that accurately communicates this information before successful matching of color characteristics can be consistently expected.
Prosthodontist: Conrad L. Cloetta, DDS

High-quality photographs or transparencies (slides) can provide additional information about the color characteristics of teeth that are to be matched in the final restorations (Fig 6-48). Shades cannot accurately be selected from photographs or transparencies, but areas of translucency, opacity, and color characteristics can easily be made from them.

One of the best ways to develop and maintain optimal laboratory results is through posttreatment feedback between the restorative team member and

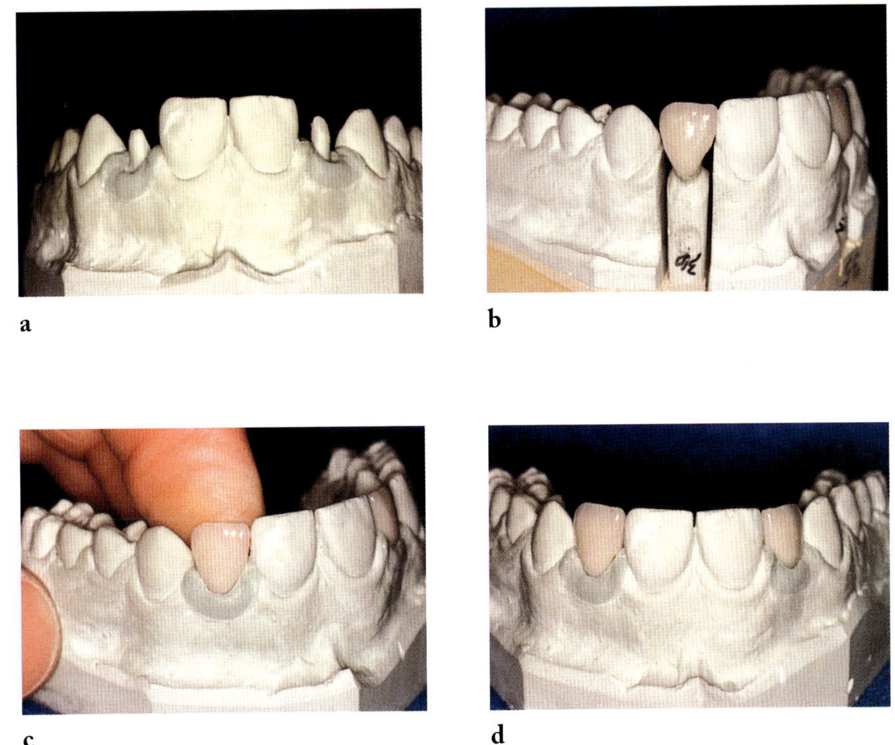

Fig 6-47

a A soft tissue model was constructed by removing stone replication of gingival margins around prepared peg laterals on the dental cast and then reinserting casts into the original impression to reform the gingival contours in resilient impression material.

b Margins of a restoration have to be made on an accurate trimmed die, but it is difficult to achieve optimal esthetic contours and healthy gingival relationships on this cast.

c A soft tissue model allows the technician to optimally contour the restoration for proper esthetic and gingival contours.

d Final restorations on soft tissue model. Without soft tissue replication, the laboratory technician must guess about gingival relationships to the restoration. This can lead to over- or undercontouring with subsequent results that have less-than-ideal esthetics and gingival health.

Prosthodontist and Laboratory Technician: Conrad L. Cloetta, DDS

the technician. The laboratory technicians are at a tremendous disadvantage compared to other interdisciplinary team members because they seldom have an opportunity to see their work clinically. For this reason, the restorative dentists and prosthodontists need to provide both positive and negative feedback to enable laboratory technicians to learn from their results and grow in their knowledge and skill. It is also important for laboratory technicians to have good working relationships with their restorative counterparts, so that they can give positive and negative feedback to restorative dentists or prosthodontists concerning their tooth preparation, impressions, and preparatory laboratory procedures. Through this mutual feedback process, both restorative team members and laboratory technicians can improve their skills needed to provide optimal restorative dentistry.

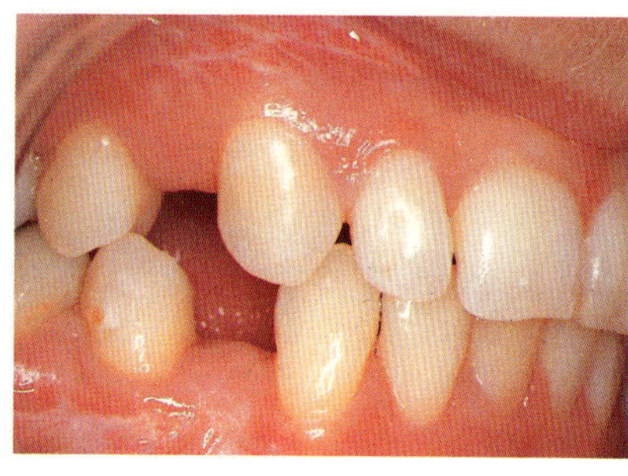

a

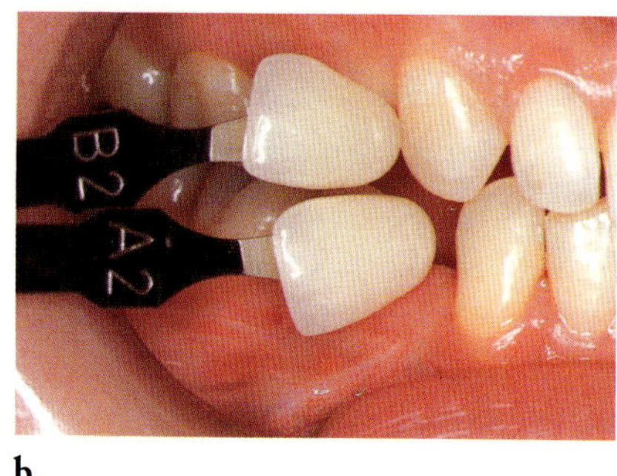

b

Fig 6-48

a High-quality photographs or slides can tremendously augment a shade diagram and communicate valuable information to the laboratory technician about the color characteristics of teeth that are to be matched in the final restorations.

b It is helpful to take a second picture with the appropriate shade tabs adjacent to the teeth to be matched. Shades cannot be selected accurately from photographs or slides, but information about translucency/opacity and other color characteristics can be interpreted from them.

Adjunctive Facial Cosmetic Surgery

Facial balance and harmony must be addressed throughout interdisciplinary therapy if optimal dentofacial results are to be obtained. *Adjunctive facial cosmetic surgery* is considered adjunctive because it is part of IDT, but it is not essential to dentofacial function. However, facial cosmetic surgery can make a significant contribution to the quality of life by improving the appearance of facial features and countering the effects of aging on the facial appearance.[206] Improved appearance will often enhance a person's self-image and change the way they are perceived by others. Qualified surgeons may use adjunctive facial cosmetic surgery to enhance or revise facial esthetics after the net dentofacial enhancements have been realized from the other definitive therapies, or they may use it for facial cosmetic changes without other dentofacial therapy. These cosmetic procedures may involve both hard and soft tissues in areas of the face, neck, chin, lips, nose, cheeks, eyelids, eyebrows, forehead, and scalp.

Success in facial cosmetic surgery depends on a thorough knowledge of facial and dental anatomy and physiology, as well as an artistic understanding of facial esthetics. This knowledge must be combined with sound surgical skills and training. Even though some guidelines have been presented for ideal facial proportions and esthetics,[207,208] they are often difficult to establish for each patient because factors such as sex, age, ethnic background, individual subjectivity, and others play an important role.[209] However, the continued increase in sophistication, scientific background, and patient acceptance of cosmetic facial surgery are making it a more predictable and accepted way to enhance the overall well-being of patients.

One must remember that the underlying bony skeleton and dentition play a key role in overall facial balance[210] and esthetics. Correction of irregularities in these underlying structures has been addressed in the discussion of orthognathic surgery and in discussion of other definitive therapies. The adjunctive facial cosmetic surgery treatment plan should usually not be completed until after all other dentofacial procedures have been finalized.[211,212] This is because the changes in facial features and esthetics associated with dentofacial therapy (especially in orthognathic surgery) are difficult to predict, due to the variability of soft tissue draping and bone and soft tissue remodeling.[112,124] However, certain cosmetic surgeries are occasionally performed simultaneously with orthognathic surgery during orthognathic surgical therapy. These cosmetic procedures frequently involve the nose,[213] chin,[214] and neck,[215,216] and they have various indications for being performed concurrently with the orthognathic procedures.

The different procedures in adjunctive facial cosmetic surgery can be used for *(1)* redefining facial features or *(2)* facial rejuvenation.[217] This section will describe cosmetic procedures in both categories that the IDT team may consider. These procedures can be performed separately or in combination, depending on the specific needs of each patient.

Redefining Facial Features

Irregularities and disproportions of the nose, ears, cheeks, chin, submental area, and neck may upset the balance of the face and affect overall facial appearance. This category of cosmetic surgery is designed to improve excesses or deficiencies in the above areas and bring them into balance with the rest of the face. Augmentation, reduction, or repositioning of the chin (genioplasty or mentoplasty) can be accomplished surgically,if needed, for facial harmony. These procedures do not alter the dental occlusion when performed alone, without orthognathic surgery. Ears can also be cosmetically recontoured or repositioned (otoplasty) if they protrude more than normal or are too large and out of proportion.

The neck and submental regions frequently host a number of cosmetic definition problems. These areas may accumulate excessive fat (lipomatosis) which may be surgically removed (lipoplasty) through direct lipectomy or liposection techniques. If platysmal dihisences or banding are evident, these may be surgically improved through platysmoplasty.

Probably the most challenging cosmetic surgical procedure is the correction of nasal deformities (rhinoplasty) (Fig 6-49).[218] Depending on the deformity, rhinoplasty may require reduction and/or augmentation of both the bony and cartilaginous components of the nose. This is frequently combined with septoplasty, which is the surgical correction of the internal nasal septum.

Facial Rejuvenation

Facial rejuvenation procedures were developed to create a more youthful appearance of the face. This is done by removing or reducing features such as wrinkling, sagging skin and muscles, fatty deposits, age spots, etc, that are associated with the aging process. Facial rejuvenation therapy may involve surgeries of

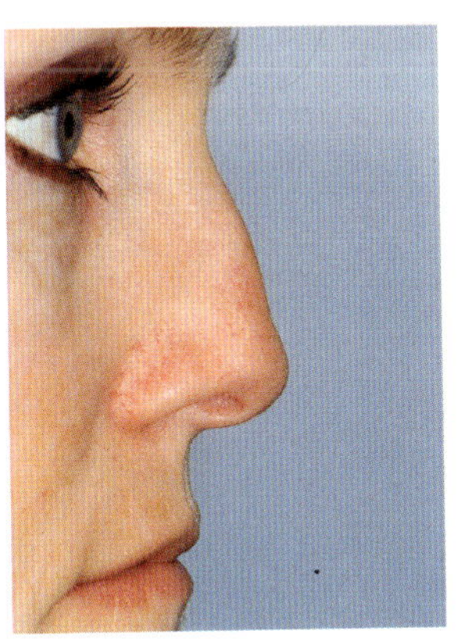
a

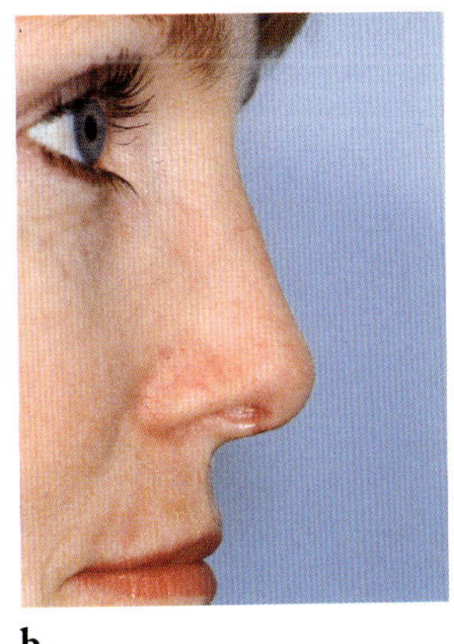
b

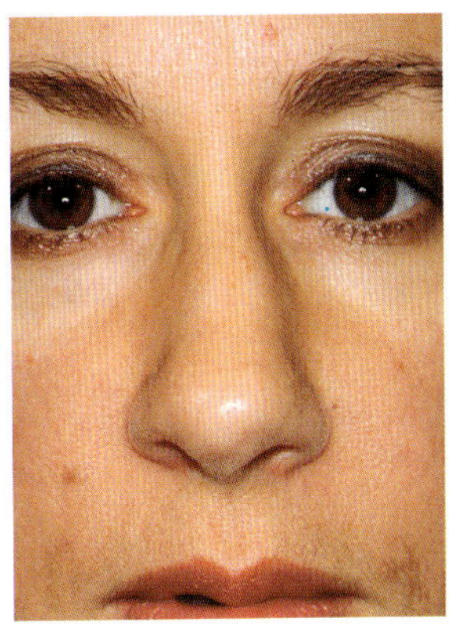
c

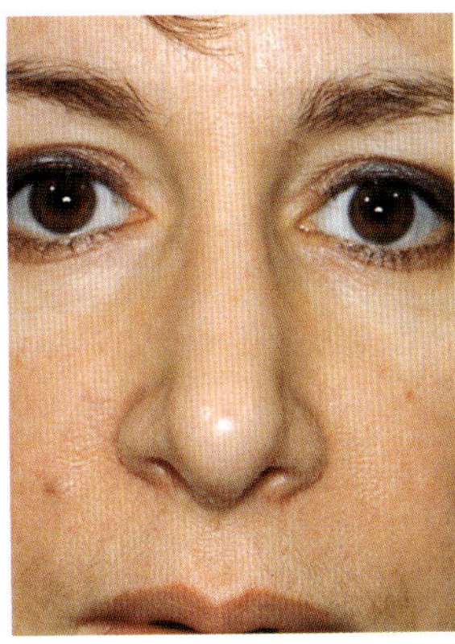
d

Fig 6-49 Surgical correction of nasal deformities (rhinoplasty).

a Preoperative lateral view of nose with large dorsal hump.

b The postoperative lateral view after open external rhinoplasty.

c Preoperative frontal view of nose with broad dorsum.

d Postoperative frontal view of nose after open external rhinoplasty.

Cosmetic Surgeon: Scott L. Bolding, DDS, MS

the face, neck, eyelids, forehead, and eyebrow areas, and procedures to reduce fine skin lines. Several of the surgeries for redefining facial features and orthognathic surgical procedures will also create a more youthful facial appearance.

A restorative, periodontal, and/or orthodontic team can also help counteract the dentofacial aging process by taking a worn, broken-down, or maligned dentition and establishing a more ideal dental and periodontal anatomy in proper relationship to the face. These procedures can add tremendously to the facial rejuvenation of a patient, Sometimes even without any orthgnathic or adjunctive facial cosmetic surgery (Figs 5-3 and 6-50.)

The rhytidectomy or face lift is a surgical procedure used to correct excess skin laxity and jowling of the face.[219] The forehead, eyebrows, and eyelids are also sites for wrinkling and sagging deformities that are generally secondary to aging characteristics.[219] These problems can cause a perpetual tired or sad look (Fig 6-51a). The forehead/brow lift and eyelid surgery (blepharoplasty) are used to remove excessive forehead and/or orbital skin and fat to give a more youthful appearance (Fig 6-51b). The rhytidectomy, forehead/brow lift, and eyelid surgeries are frequently performed simultaneously to rejuvenate the appearance of the entire face (Fig 6-52).

There are frequently fine lines and wrinkles around mouth, forehead, and cheek areas that are in the skin itself and may not be removed by surgically tightening the skin. These problems may usually be improved with procedures such as chemical peeling or dermabrasion.

Adjunctive facial cosmetic therapy can significantly enhance the esthetics of the overall dentofacial result. This adjunctive therapy should be used and suggested by the IDT team when indicated to finalize the definitive-therapy phase of IDT.

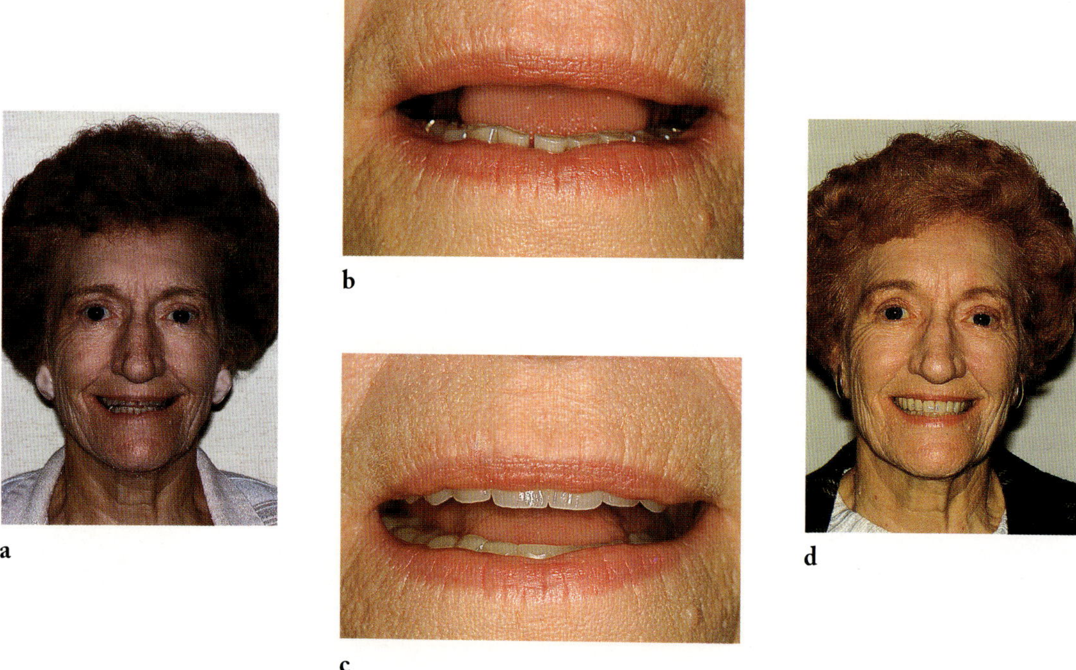

Fig 6-50 Facial rejuvenation with restorative dentistry performed from a dentofacial perspective.

a, b Preoperative facial smiling view and view with lips in repose, illustrating insufficient maxillary incisor exposure with an unesthetic worn dentition in poor dentofacial alignment. These problems can increase the apparent age of a patient.

c, d Postoperative view of lips in repose and facial smiling view after full-mouth dental reconstruction procedures were performed to restore proper length and anatomy to the anterior maxillary teeth in a more ideal dentofacial relationship. Note the profound influence on the overall facial appearance, with apparent facial rejuvenation.

Restorative Dentist: Richard D. Roblee, DDS, MS/*Laboratory Technician:* Jeffrey Singler, CDT

Fig 6-51

a Preoperative facial view illustrating wrinkling and sagging deformities of forehead, eyebrows, and eyelids that cause a perpetual tired or sad look.

b Postoperative facial view after forehead and eyebrow lift and eyelid surgery (blepharoplasty) to remove excess skin from forehead and excess skin and fat from orbital regions to give a more youthful and happier appearance.

Cosmetic Surgeon: Scott L. Bolding, DDS, MS

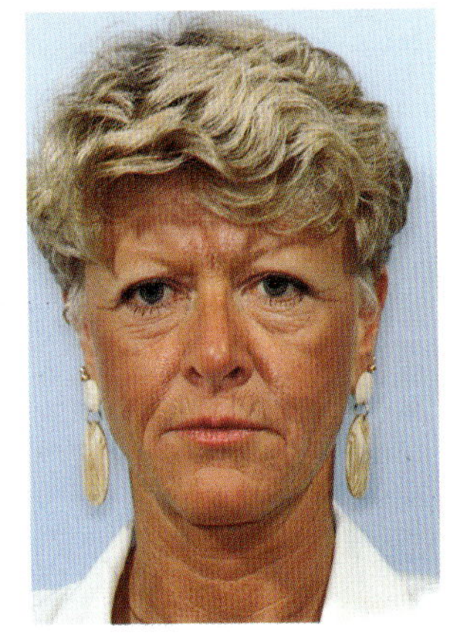

a

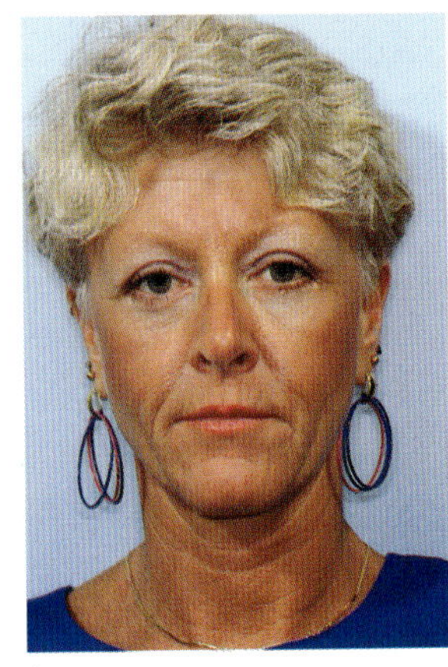

b

Fig 6-52

a, b Preoperative facial views illustrating excess skin laxity and wrinkling in all areas of face and neck.

c, d Postoperative facial views after forehead and eyebrow lift, upper and lower blepharoplasty, and cervicofacial rhytidectomy, with subsequent rejuvenated appearance of entire face.

Cosmetic Surgeon: Scott L. Bolding, DDS, MS

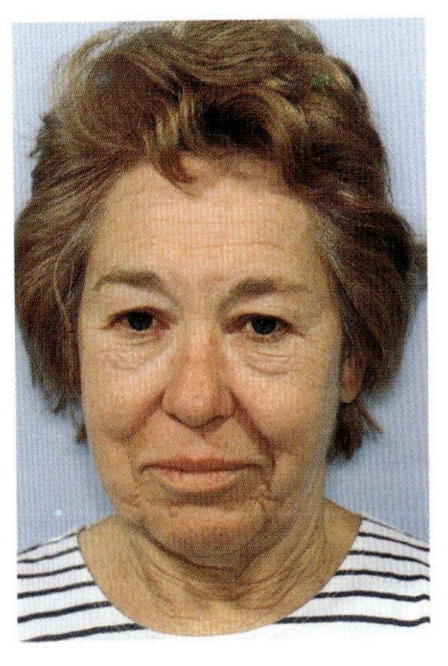

a

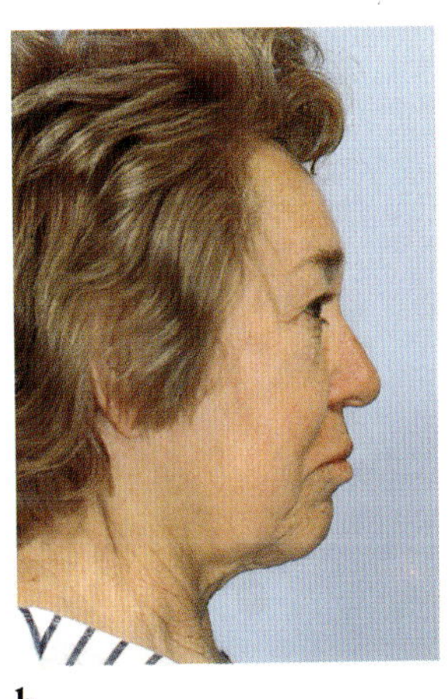

b

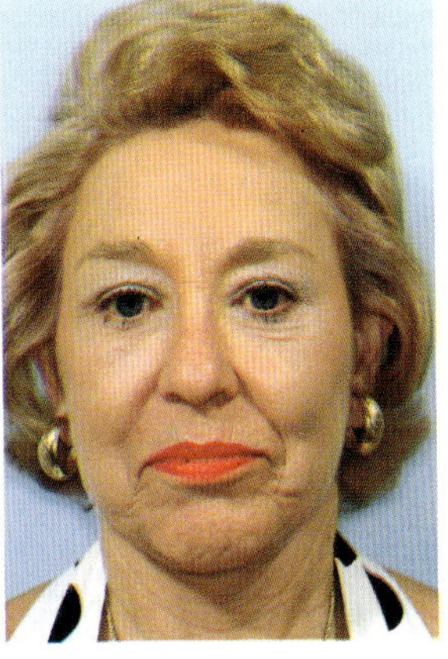

c

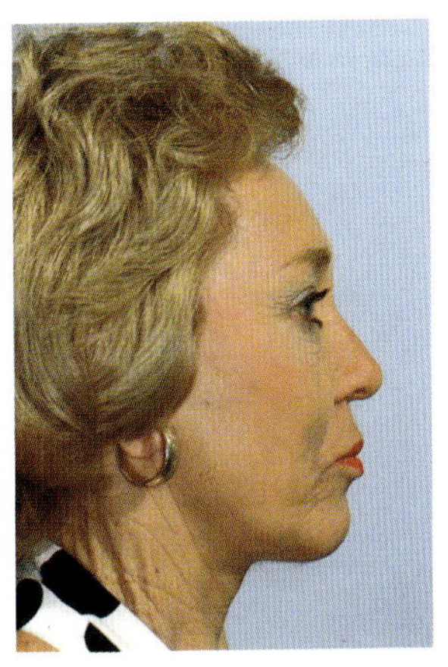

d

References

1. American Academy of Periodontology: Consensus report, supportive treatment [Proceedings of the World Workshop in Clinical Periodontics]. Chicago, American Academy of Periodontology, 1989: II-1 to IX-25.
2. Wilson TG. Supportive periodontal treatment for patients with inflammatory periodontal diseases. In: Wilson TG, Korman KS, Newman MG (eds). Advances in Periodontics. Chicago: Quintessence, 1992: 195–204.
3. Zachrisson BU, Alnags L. Periodontal condition in orthodontically treated and untreated individuals. Angle Orthod 1973;43:402–411.
4. Zachrisson BB. Cause and prevention of injuries to teeth and supporting structures during orthodontic treatment. Am J Orthod 1976;69:285–300.
5. Yeung SC, Howell S, Fahey P. Oral hygiene programs for orthodontic patients. Am J Orthod Dentofac Orthop 1989; 96:208–213.
6. Boyd RL, Murray P, Robertson PB. Effect of rotary electric toothbrush versus manual toothbrush on periodontal status during orthodontic treatment. Am J Orthod Dentofacial Orthop 1989;96:342–347.
7. Brightman LJ, Terezhalmy GT et al. The effects of a 0.12% chlorhexidine gluconate mouthrinse on orthodontic patients aged 11 through 17 with established gingivitis. Am J Orthod Dentofac Orthop 1991;100:324–329.
8. Geiger AM, Gorelick L et al. Reducing white spot lesions in orthodontic populations with fluoride rinsing. Am J Orthod Dentofac Orthop 1992;101:403–407.
9. Boyd RL. Comparison of three self-applied topical fluoride preparations for control of decalcification. Angle Orthod 1993;63:25–30.
10. Embler BF, Windchy AM, Zaino SW et al. The value of repetition and reinforcement in improving oral hygiene performance. J Periodontol 1990;51:228–234.
11. Chaves ES, Caffesse RG, Morrison EC, Stults DL. Diagnostic discrimination of bleeding on probing during maintenance periodontal therapy. Am J Dent 1990;3:167–170.
12. Wilson TG, Glover ME. Treatment sequencing. In: Wilson TG. Dental Maintenance for Patients with Periodontal Diseases. Chicago: Quintessence, 1989: 41–50.
13. Williams RC, Kaldahl WB, Kalkwarf KL. Periodontal disease activity. In: Wilson TG, Korman KS, Newman MG (eds). Advances in Periodontics. Chicago: Quintessence, 1992; 58–73.
14. Axelsson P, Lindhe J. Effect of controlled oral hygiene procedures on caries and periodontal disease in adults. J Clin Periodontol 1978;5:133–151.
15. Axelsson P, Lindhe J. Effect of controlled oral hygiene procedures on caries periodontal disease in adults. Results after 6 years. J Clin Periodontol 1981;8:239–248.
16. Mousques T, Listgarten MA, Phillips RW. Effect of sealing and root planing on the composition of human subgingival flora. J Periodont Rest 1991;15:144–151.
17. American Academy of Periodontology. Proceedings of the World Workshop in Clinical Periodontics. Chicago: American Academy of Periodontology, 1989, II-1 to II-20.
18. Marks MH. Management of the adult orthodontic patient. In: Marks MH, Corn H. Atlas of Adult Orthodontics: Functional and Esthetic Enhancement. Philadelphia: Lea and Febiger, 1989: 160–166.
19. Wilson TG. A typical maintenance visit. In: Wilson TG (ed). Dental Maintenance for Patients with Periodontal Diseases. Chicago: Quintessence, 1989:90–96.
20. Chivian N. Root resorption. In: Cohen S, Burns RC (eds). Pathways of the Pulp ed 5. St Louis: Mosby, 1991: 504–548.
21. Baumann MA, Ruppenthal T. A concept of restorative treatment during orthodontic therapy. Quintessence Intl 1992;23:695–700.
22. Buchanan LS: Cleaning and shaping the root canal system. In: Cohen S, Burns RC (eds). Pathways of the Pulp ed 5. St Louis: Mosby, 1991:166–193.
23. Nguyen NT. Obturation of the root canal system. In: Cohen S, Burns RC (eds). Pathways of the Pulp ed 5. St Louis: Mosby, 1991:193–283.
24. Radke RA, Eissman HF. Postendodontic restoration. In: Cohen S, Burns RC (eds). Pathways of the Pulp ed 5. St Louis:Mosby, 1991:640–682.
25. Hipp BR. The management of third molar teeth. Oral Maxillofac Surg Clin N Am 1993;5(1):77–86.
26. Verne D. A survey of indications for mandibular third molar surgery and complications using a distolingual approach. Oral Maxillofac Surg Clin N Am 1993;5(1): 87–94.
27. Lytle JJ. Etiology and indications for management of impacted teeth. Oral Maxillofac Surg Clin N Am 1993; 5(1):87–94.
28. Seibert JS. Treatment of moderate and localized alveolar ridge defects: Preventive and reconstructive concepts in therapy. Dent Clin N Am 1993;37:265–280.
29. Aren DE. Surgical endodontics. In: Cohen S, Burns RC (eds). Pathways of the Pulp ed 5. St Louis: Mosby, 1991: 574–611.
30. Carnevale GD, Febo G, Tonelli MP, Marvin D, Fuzzi M. A retrospective analysis of the periodontal-prosthetic treatment of molars with interradiculus lesions. Int J Peridont Restor Dent 1991; 11:189-205.
31. Newell DH. The role of the prosthodontist in restoring root–resected molars: a study of 70 molar root resections. J Prosthet Dent 1991;65:7–15.
32. Gutmann JL, Harrison JW. Surgical endodontics. Boston:Blackwell Scientific Publications, 1991.
33. Alling CC, Mills JC. Surgery for root canal therapy. Oral Maxillofac Surg Clin N Am 1993;5(1):145–157.
34. Bellizzi R, Loushine R. A Clinical Atlas of Endodontic Surgery. Chicago: Quintessence, 1991.
35. Fournier A, Turcotte J, Bernard C. Orthodontic considerations in the treatment of maxillary impacted canines. Am J Orthod 1982;81:236–239.
36. Zeitler DL. Management of impacted teeth other than third molars. Oral Maxillofac Surg Clin N Am 1993; 5(1):95–103.
37. Bishara SE. Impacted maxillary canines: A review. Am J Orthod Dentofac Orthop 1992;101:159–171.

38. Kokich VG, Matthews DP. Surgical management of impacted teeth. Dent Clin N Am 1993;37:181–204.
39. Brown IS. The effect of orthodontic therapy on certain types of periodontal defects. J Periodontol 1973;44:742.
40. Edwards JG. A surgical procedure to eliminate relapse. Am J Orthod 1970;57:35–46.
41. Crum RE, Anderson GF. The effect of gingival fiber surgery on the retention of rotated teeth. Am J Orthod 1974;65:626.
42. Kokich VC. Enhancing restorative, esthetic, and periodontal results with orthodontic treatment. In: Schluger S, Youdelis R, Page RC, Johnson RH (eds). Periodontal Diseases, ed 2. Philadelphia: Lea and Febiger, 1990: 433–460.
43. Ericsson I, Thilander B. Orthodontic forces and recurrence of periodontal disease. Am J Orthod 1978;71:41–50.
44. Ericsson I, Thilander B, Lindhe J, Okamoto H. The effect of orthodontic tilting movements in the periodontal tissue of infected and non-infected dentitions in dogs. J Clin Periodontol 1977;4:278–293.
45. Ericsson I, Thilander B, Lindhe J. Periodontal conditions after orthodontic tooth movements in the dog. Angle Orthod 1978;48:210–218.
46. Caffesse RG, Sweeney PL, Smith BA. Scaling and root planing with and without periodontal flap surgery. J Clin Periodontol 1986;13:205–210.
47. Kornman KS, Wilson TG. Treatment planning for patients with inflammatory periodontal diseases. In: Wilson TG, Kornman KS, Newman MG (eds). Advances in Periodontics. Chicago: Quintessence, 1992: 87–97.
48. Kalkwarf KL, Barrington EP, Loughlin. Moderate chronic adult periodontitis. In: Wilson TG, Kornman KS, Newman MG (eds). Advances in Periodontics. Chicago: Quintessence, 1992: 143–180.
49. Mellonig JT. Severe chronic adult periodontitis. In: Wilson TG, Kornman KS, Newman MG (eds). Advances in Periodontics. Chicago: Quintessence, 1992: 181–194.
50. Lindhe J, Svanberg G. Influence of trauma from occlusion on progression of experimental periodontitis in the beagle dog. J Clin Periodontol 1974;1:3.
51. Lang NP, Loe H. The relationship between the width of the attached gingiva and gingival health. J Periodontol 1972;43:623.
52. Shiloah J, Frey HR, Abrams MA, Binley LH, Taylor RF. Soft tissue fenestration and osseous dehiscence associated with orthodontic therapy. Int J Periodont Rest Dent 1987; 4:43–51.
53. Miller PD. Root coverage using a free soft tissue autograft following citric acid application. Part I. Technique. Int J Periodont Rest Dent 1982;2:65–70.
54. Holbrook T, Ochseubein C. Complete coverage of denuded root surfaces with a one-stage gingival graft. Int J Periodont Rest Dent 1983;3:9–27.
55. Langer B, Langer L. Subepithelial connective tissue graft technique for root coverage. J Periodontol 1985;56: 715–720.
56. Langer L, Langer B. The subepithelial connective tissue graft for treatment of gingival recession. Dent Clin N Am 1993;37:243–264.
57. Harvey PM. Surgical reconstruction of the gingiva. Part II. Procedures. NZ Dent J 1970;66:42–52.
58. Allen EP, Miller PD. Coronal positioning of existing gingiva: Short term results in treatment of shallow marginal tissue recession. J Periodontol 1989;60:316–319.
59. Maynard JG. Coronal positioning of a previously placed autogenous gingival graft. J Periodontol 1977;48:151.
60. Wagenberg BD. Periodontal preparation of the adult patient prior to orthodontics. Dent Clin N Am 1988; 32:457–481.
61. Vanarsdall RL. Anatomy and morphology of the periodontium. In: Schutz JP, Joho JP (eds). Minor surgery in orthodontics. Chicago: Quintessence, 1992: 91–104.
62. Edwards JG. Soft tissue surgery to alleviate orthodontic relapse. Dent Clin N Am 1993;37:205–226.
63. Edwards JG. The diastema, the frenum, the frenectomy: A clinical study. Am J Orth 1977;71:489–508.
64. Allen EP. Use of mucogingival surgical procedures to enhance esthetics. Dent Clin N Am 1988;32:307–30.
65. Allen EP. Surgical crown lengthening for function and esthetics. Dent Clin N Am 1993;163–180.
66. Atherton JD. The gingival response to orthodontic tooth movement. Am J Orthod 1970;58:179–186.
67. Edwards JG. The reduction of relapse in extraction cases. Am J Orthod 1971;60:128–141.
68. Shapiro PA, Kokich VG. Use of implants in orthodontics. Dent Clin N Am 1988;32:539–550.
69. Roberts WE, Garetto LP, Simmons KE. Endosseous implants for rigid orthodontic anchorage. In: Bell WH (ed). Modern Practice in Orthognathic and Reconstructive Surgery. Philadelphia: Saunders, 1992: 1230–1264.
70. Brånemark P-I, Zarb GA, Albrektsson T. Tissue-Integrated Prostheses: Osseointegration in Clinical Dentistry. Chicago: Quintessence, 1985.
71. Williams JA, Billington RW. Increase in compression strength of glass ionomer restorative materials with respect to time: A guide to their suitability for use in posterior primary dentition. J Oral Rehabil 1989;16:475–479.
72. McCaghren RA, Retief DH, Bradley EL, Denys FR. Shear bond strength of light-curved glass ionomer to enamel and dentin. J Dent Res 1990;69:40–45.
73. Forss H, Seppä L. Prevention of enamel demineralization adjacent to glass ionomer filling materials. Scand J Dent Res 1990;98:173–178.
74. Mount GJ. Polyacrylic cements in dentistry. Am J Dent 1990;3:79–84.
75. Pogrel MA (ed). Malignant tumors of the maxillofacial region. Oral and Maxillofac Surg Clin N Am 1993;3: 189–408.
76. Jacobsen L. Mouth breathing and gingivitis. J Periodont Res 1973;8:269–277.
77. Tiner BD, Waite PD. Surgical and non-surgical management of obstructive sleep apnea. In: Peterson GJ, Indresano AT, Marciani RD, Roser SM (eds). Principles of Oral and Maxillofacial Surgery, vol 3. Philadelphia: Lippincott, 1992: 1531–1548.

78. Waite PD, Wooten V, Lachner J, Guyette RF. Maxillomandibular advancement surgery in 23 patients with obstructive sleep apnea syndrome. J Oral Maxillofac Surg 1989;47:1256–1261.
79. Proffit WR, Fields HW. Orthodontic treatment planning: from problem list to final plan. In: Proffit WR. Contemporary Orthodontics. St Louis: Mosby, 1986: 168–197.
80. Jones ML. The Barry Project: A further assessment of occlusal treatment change in a consecutive sample: Crowding and arch dimensions. Br J Orthod 1990;17:269–285.
81. Ingber JS. Forced eruption: Part I. A method of treating isolated one and two wall infrabony osseous defects: Rationale and case report. J Periodontol 1974;45:199–206.
82. Kusy RP. Materials and appliances in orthodontics: Brackets, archwires and friction. Curr Opin Dent 1991;1: 634–644.
83. Birnie O. Ceramic brackets. Br J Orthod 1990;17:71–74.
84. McNamara JA, Brudon W. Orthodontic and Orthopedic Treatment in the Mixed Dentition. Ann Arbor: Needham Press, 1993.
85. Gianelly AA, Anderson CK, Boffa J. Longitudinal evaluation of condylar position in extraction and nonextraction treatment. Am J Orthod Dentofac Orthop 1991;100: 416–420.
86. Kundinger KK, Austin BP, Christensen LV, Donegan SJ, Ferguson DJ. An evaluation of temporomandibular joint and jaw muscles after orthodontic treatment involving premolar extractions. Am J Orthod Dentofac Orthop 1991; 100:110–115.
87. Bolton WA. Disharmony in tooth size and its relation to the analysis and treatment of malocclusion. Angle Orthod 1958;28:113–130.
88. Sheridan JJ. Air rotor stripping. J Clin Orthod 1985; 19:43–57.
89. Radlanski RJ, Jager A, Zimmer B. Morphology of interdentally stripped enamel one year after treatment. J Clin Orthod 1989;23:748–750.
90. Crain G, Sheridan JJ. Susceptibility to caries and periodontal disease after posterior air-rotor stripping. J Clin Orthod 1990;24:84–85.
91. Radlanski RJ, Jager A, Schwestka R, Bertzbach F. Plaque accumulation caused by interdental stripping. Am J Orthod Dentofac Orthop 1988;94:416–420.
92. Reitan K. Tissue behavior during orthodontic tooth movement. Am J Orthod 1960;46:881–900.
93. Polson, J Dent Research 1982 .
94. Zachrisson BU. Cause and prevention of injuries to teeth and supporting structures during orthodontic treatment. Am J Orthod 1976;69:285.
95. Richter WA, Ueno H. Relationship of crown margin placement to gingival inflammation. J Prosthet Dent 1973; 30:156–61.
96. Than A, Duguid R, McKendrick AJW. Relationship between restorations and the level of the periodontal attachment. J Clin Periodontol 1982;9:193–202.
97. Bjorn AL, Bjorn H, Grkovic B. Marginal fit of restorations and its relation to periodontal bone levels. Part II. Crowns. Odontol Rev 1970;21:337–346.
98. Boyd RL, Baumrind S. Periodontal considerations in the use of bonds or bands on molars in adolescents and adults. Angle Orthod 1992;62:117–126.
99. Roblee RD, Hugey S. Indirect Bonding-Clinical (videotape). Atlanta: Specialty Appliances Video Tape, 1992.
100. Roblee RD, Hugey S. Indirect Bonding-Laboratory (videotape). Atlanta: Specialty Appliances Video Tape, 1992.
101. Zachrisson BU, Brobakken BL. Clinical comparisons of direct verses indirect bonding with different bracket types and adhesives. Am J Orthod 1978;74:62–78.
102. Proffit WR, Ackerman JL. Diagnosis and treatment planning in orthodontics. In: Graber TM, Swain BF (eds). Orthodontics: Current Principles and Techniques. St Louis: Mosby, 1985:3–100.
103. Waters NE. Orthodontic products update: Super-elastic nickel-titanium wires. Br J Orthod 1992:19:319–322.
104. Hans S, Quick DC. Nickel-titanium spring properties in simulated oral environment. Angle Orthod 1993;63:67–72.
105. Reitan K. Tissue behavior during orthodontic tooth movement. Am J Orthod 1991;46:881–900.
106. Brown IS. The effect of orthodontic therapy on certain types of periodontal defects. Part I: Clinical Findings. J Periodontol 1973;44:742–756.
107. Vanarsdall RL. Correction of periodontal problems through orthodontic treatment. In: Hosl E, Zachrisson BU, Baldauf A (eds). Orthodontics and Periodontics. Chicago: Quintessence, 1985: 127–167.
108. Schmitt SM, Cronin RJ, Berg S. Anterior mandibular subapical osteotomy: A useful treatment for patients with severely worn anterior teeth. J Prosthet Dent 1992;67: 468–471.
109. Bell WH. Modern Practice in Orthognathic Reconstructive Surgery, vols 1, 2, 3. Philadelphia: Saunders, 1992.
110. Epker BN, Wolford LM. Dentofacial Deformities: Surgical-Orthodontic Correction. St Louis: Mosby, 1984.
111. Wolford LM, Hilliard FW. Correction of Dentofacial Deformities. In: Waite DE (ed). Textbook of Practical Oral and Maxillofacial Surgery ed 3. Philadelphia: Lea & Febiger, 1987:427–471.
112. Van Sickels JE, Flanary CM. Stability associated with mandibular advancement treated by rigid osseous fixation. J Oral Maxillofac Surg 1985;43:338–341.
113. Wolford LM. The use of porous block hydroxyapatite in orthognathic surgery. In: Bell WH (ed). Modern Practice in Orthognathic and Reconstructive Surgery. Philadelphia: Saunders, 1992: 854–871.
114. Wolford LM, Davis WM. The mandibular inferior border split: A modification in the sagittal split osteotomy. J Oral Maxillofac Surg 1990;48:92–94.
115. Wardrop RW, Wolford LM. Maxillary stability following downgraft and/or advancement procedures with stabilization using rigid fixation and porous block hydroxyapatite implants. J Oral Maxillofac Surg 1989;47:336–342.
116. Wolford LM, Bennett MA, Raffery CG. Modification of the mandibular ramus sagittal split osteotomy. Oral Surg Oral Med Oral Path 1987;64:146–155.

117. Bennett MA, Wolford LM. The maxillary step osteotomy modification and Steinmann pin stabilization. J Oral Maxillofac Surg 1985;43:307–311.
118. Satrom KD, Sinclair PM, Wolford LM. The stability of double jaw surgery: A comparison of rigid versus wire fixation. Am J Orthod Dentofac Orthop 1991;6:550–563.
119. Vallino LD. Speech, velopharynegeal function, and hearing before and after orthognathic surgery. J Oral Maxillofac Surg 1990;48:1272–1281.
120. Will LA. Mandibular advancement using the bilateral sagittal osteotomy: past, present and future. Oral Maxillofac Surg Clin N Am 1990;2:717–728.
121. Phillips C, Turvey TA, McMillian. Surgical orthodontic corrections of mandibular deficiency by sagittal osteotomy: Clinical and cephalometric analysis of 1-year data. Am Ortho Dentofac Orthop 1989;96:501–506.
122. Simmons KE, Turvey TA, Phillips C, Proffit WR. Surgical orthodontic correction of mandibular deficiency: Five-year follow-up. Int J Adult Orthod Orthognath Surg 1992; 7:67–79.
123. Schendel SA, Williamson LW. Muscle reorientation following superior repositioning of the maxilla. J Oral Maxillofac Surg 1983;41:235–240.
124. Schendel SA, Carlotti AE. Nasal considerations in orthognathic surgery. Am Orthod Dentofac Orthop 1991;100: 197–208.
125. Moenning JE, Bussard DA, Lapp TH, Garrison BT. A comparison of relapse in bilateral sagittal split osteotomies for mandibular advancement: Rigid internal fixation (screws) versus inferior border wiring with anterior skeletal fixation. Int J Adult Orthod Orthognath Surg 1990; 5:175–182.
126. Moenning JE, Garrison BT, Lapp TH, Bussard DA. Early screw removal for correction of occlusal discrepancies following rigid internal fixation in orthognathic surgery. Int J Adult Orthod Orthognath Surg 1990;5:225–232.
127. Nanda R, Burstone CJ. Retention and Stability in Orthodontics. Philadelphia: Saunders, 1993.
128. Joondeph DR, Riedel RA. Retention. In: Graber TM, Swain BF (eds). Orthodontics: Current Principles and Techniques. St Louis: Mosby, 1985:857–898.
129. Proffit WR, Fields HW. Retention. In: Proffit WR. Contemporary Orthodontics. St Louis: Mosby, 1986;455–470.
130. Lamberth RE. Maintenance for the adult in fixed appliances. In: Wilson TG. Dental Maintenance for Patients with Periodontal Diseases. Chicago: Quintessence, 1989; 142–147.
131. Little RM. Stability and relapse of dental arch alignment. Br J Orthod 1990;17:235–241.
132. Hawley CA. A removable retainer. Int J Orthod 1919; 5:291–305.
133. Edwards JG. A study of the periodontium during orthodontic rotation of teeth. Am J Orthod 1968;54:441–461.
134. Shulman J. A technique for biteplane constructions. J Prosthet Dent 1973;29:334–339.
135. Ramfjord SP, Ash MM. Occlusion ed 3. Philadelphia: Saunders, 1983.
136. Youdelis RA, Weaver JD, Sapkos S. Facial and lingual contours of artificial complete crown restorations and their effects on the periodontium. J Prosthet Dent 1973;29:61.
137. Donaldson D. Gingival recession associated with temporary crowns. J Periodont 1973;44:691.
138. Ferencz JL. Maintaining and enhancing gingival architecture in fixed prosthodontics. J Prosthet Dent, 1991;65(5): 650–657.
139. Higginbottom FL. Maintenance of fixed prosthetics. In: Wilson TG: Dental Maintenance for Patients with Periodontal Diseases. Chicago: Quintessence, 1989:117–133.
140. Edwards JG. A surgical procedure to eliminate relapse. Am J Orthod 1970;57:35–46.
141. Campbell PM, Moore JW, Matthews JL. Orthodontically corrected midline diastemas: The histologic study and surgical procedure. Am J Orthod 1975;67:139–158.
142. Vanarsdall RL, Musich DR. Adult orthodontics: diagnosis and treatment. In: Graber TM, Swain BF (eds). Orthodontics: Current Principles and Techniques. St Louis: Mosby, 1985: 791–856.
143. Kokich VC. Enhancing restorative, esthetic, and periodontal results with orthodontic treatment. In: Schluger S, Youdelis R, Page RC, Johnson RH (eds). Periodontal Diseases ed 2. Philadelphia: Lea and Febiger, 1990: 433–460.
144. Wilson TG. Treatment sequencing. In: Wilson TG: Dental Maintenance for Patients with Periodontal Diseases. Chicago: Quintessence, 1989: 41–50.
145. Ingber JS, Rose LF, Coslet JG. The "Biologic Width"—a concept in periodontic and restorative dentistry. Alpha Omegan 1977;10:62–65.
146. Nevins M, Skurow HM. The intraceviation restorative margin, the biologic width and the maintenance of the gingival margin. Int J Periodont Rest Dent 1981;4:43–47.
147. Gottlow J, Nyman S, Karring T. Maintenance of new attachment gained through guided tissue regeneration. J Clin Periodontol 1992;19:315–317.
148. Mellonig JT, Triplett RG. Guided tissue regeneration and endosseous dental implants. Int J Periodont Rest Dent 1993;13:109–120.
149. Wilson TG. Guided tissue regeneration around dental implants in immediate and recent extraction sites: Initial observations. Int J Periodont Rest Dent 1992;12:185–194.
150. Werbitt MJ, Goldbert PV. The immediate implant: Bone preservation and bone regenerations. Int J Periodont and Rest Dent 1992;12:207–217.
151. Brägger U, Lauchenauer D, Lang NP. Surgical lengthening of the clinical crown. J Clin Periodontol 1992;19:58–63.
152. Abrams H, Kopczyk RA, Kaplan AL. Incidence of anterior ridge deformities in partially edentulous patients. J Prosthet Dent 1987;57:191–194.
153. Langer B, Calagna L. The subepithelial connective tissue graft: a new approach to the enhancement of anterior cosmetics. J Prosthet Dent 1980;44:363–367.
154. Langer B, Calagna L. The subepithelial connective tissue graft: a new approach to the enhancement of anterior cosmetics. J Periodont Rest Dent 1982;2:23–33.

155. Abrams L. Augmentation of the deformed residual edentulous ridge for fixed prosthesis. Compend Contin Educ Dent 1980;1:205–214.
156. Seibert JS. Reconstruction of deformed, partially edentulous ridges, using full thickness onlay grafts. Part II. Prosthetic/periodontal interrelationships. Compend Contin Educ Dent 1983;4:549–562.
157. Seibert JS. Reconstruction of deformed, partially edentulous ridges, using full thickness onlay grafts. Part I. Technique and wound healing. Compend Contin Educ Dent 1983;4:437–453.
158. Seibert JS, Nyman S. Localized ridge augmentation in dogs: A pilot study using membranes and Hydroxylapatite. J Periodontol 1992;61(3):157–165.
159. Buser D, Dula K, Belser U, Hirt H-P, Berthold H. Localized ridge augmentation using guided bone regeneration. Part I. Surgical procedure in the maxilla. Int J Periodont Rest Dent 1993;13:29–45.
160. Nevins M, Mellonig JT. Enhancement of the damaged edentulous ridge to receive the dental implant: A combination of allograft and the Gore-Tex membrane. Int J Periodont Rest Dent 1992;12:97–111.
161. Langer B, Sullivan D. Osseointegration: Its impact on the interrelationship of periodontics and restorative dentistry. Part 1. Int J Periodont Rest Dent 1989;9:85–105.
162. Langer B, Sullivan D. Osseointegration: Its impact on the interrelationship of periodontics and restorative dentistry. Part II. Int J Periodont Rest Dent 1989;9:165–183.
163. Barnett BC, Krump JL. Implant dentistry: The significance of a team approach. J Prosthet Dent 1987;58:69–73.
164. Mecall RA, Rosenfeld AL. The influence of residual ridge resorption patterns on implant fixture placement and tooth position. Part 1. Int J Periodont Rest Dent 1991;11:9–23.
165. Israelson J, Plemons JM. Barium-coated surgical stents and computer-assisted tomography in the preoperative assessment of dental implant patients. Int J Periodont Rest Dent 1992;12:53–61.
166. Watson RM, Davis DM, Forman GH, Coward T. Considerations in design and fabrication of maxillary implant-supported prosthesis. Int J Prosthodont 1991;4:232–239.
167. Neidlinger J, Lilien BA, Kalant DC. Surgical implant stent: A design modification and simplified fabrication technique. J Prosthet Dent 1993;69:70–72.
168. Lima Verde MAR, Morgano SM. A dual-purpose stent for the implant-supported prosthesis. J Prosthet Dent 1993;69:276–280.
169. Render RJ, Fondak JT. A surgical guide for implant placement. J Prosthet Dent 1992;67:831–832.
170. Blustein R, Jackson R, Rotskoff K, Coy RE, Godar D. Use of splint material in the placement of implants. Int J Oral Maxillofac Implants 1986;1:47–49.
171. Murrell GA, Davis WH. Presurgical prosthodontics. J Prosthet Dent 1988;59:447–452.
172. Engelman MJ, Sorensen JA, Moy P. Optimum placement of osseointegrated implants. J Prosthet Dent 1988;59: 467–473.
173. Zinner ID, Small SA, Panno FV. Presurgical prosthetics and surgical templates. Dent Clin N Am 1989;33:619–633.
174. Adrian ED, Ivanhoe JR, Krantz WA. Trajectory surgical guide stent for implant placement. J Prosthet Dent 1992; 67:687–691.
175. Chaytor DV, Zarb GA, Schmitt A, Lewis, DW: The longitudinal effectiveness of osseointegrated dental implants—The Toronto study: Bone level changes. Int J Periodont Rest Dent 1991;11:113–125.
176. Kent GK. Effects of osseointegrated implants on psychological and social well-being: A literature review. J Prosthet Dent 1992;68:515–518.
177. Grogono AL, Lancaster DM, Finger IM. Dental implants: A survey of patients' attitudes. J Prosthet Dent 1989; 62:573–576.
178. Eckhart JE, Davis WH, Marshall MW, Hochwald DA. The use of osseointegration to stabilize a surgical elongation of the maxilla: A case report. Int J Adult Orthod Orthognath Surg 1992;7:235–243.
179. McCartney JW. Osseointegrated implant-supported and magnetically retained ear prosthesis: A clinical report. J Prosthet Dent 1991;66:6–9.
180. Tjellström A, Jacobsson M. The bone-anchored maxillofacial prosthesis. In: Albrektsson T, Zarb G (eds). The Brånemark Osseointegrated Implant. Chicago: Quintessence, 1989: 235–244.
181. Wein JP. The use of osseointegrated implants in the treatment of patients with trauma. J Prosthet Dent 1992;67: 670–678.
182. Fenton A. The role of dental implants in the future. J Am Dent Assoc 1992;123:37–42.
183. Smithloff M, Fritz ME. The use of blade implants in a selected population of partially edentulous adults: A ten-year report. J Periodontol 1982;53:413–418.
184. Brånemark P-I, Breine U, Adell R, Hansson BO, Lindstrom J, Ohlsson A. Intra-osseous anchorage of dental prosthesis. Scand J Plast Reconstr Surg 1969;3:81–100.
185. Brånemark P-I, Hansson BO, Adell R, Breine U, Lindstrom J, Hallen O et al. Osseointegrated implants in the treatment of the edentulous jaw. Experience from a 10-year period. Scand J Plast Reconst Surg 1977;16 (suppl):1–132.
186. Adell R, Lekholm U, Rockler B, Brånemark P-I. A 15-year study of osseointegrated implants in the treatment of the edentulous jaw. Int J Oral Surg 1981;10:387–416.
187. Gotfredsen K, Hansen EH, Jorgensen EB. Clinical and radiographic evaluation of submerged and nonsubmerged implants in monkeys. Int J Prosthodont 1990;3:463–469.
188. Buser D, Weber HP, Donath K, Fiorellini JP, Paquette DW, Williams RC. Soft tissue reactions to non-submerged unloaded titanium implants in beagle dogs. J Periodontol 1992;63:226–236.
189. Wilson TG, Glover ME. Treatment sequencing. In: Wilson TG. Dental Maintenance for Patients with Periodontal Diseases. Chicago: Quintessence, 1989: 41–50.
190. Lazzara R. Implant placement into extraction sites: Surgical and restorative advantages. Int J Periodont Rest Dent 1989;9(5):332–343.

191. Becker W, Lynch SE, Lekholm U, Becker BE, Caffesse R, Konath K et al. A comparison of ePTFE membranes alone or in combination with platelet-derived growth factors and insulin-like growth factor-I or demineralized freeze-dried bone in promoting bone formation around immediate extraction socket implants. J Periodontol 1992;63:929–940.
192. Triplet RG, Bolding SL: Management of the Atrophic Maxilla. In: Controversies in Oral and Maxillofacial Surgery. Philadelphia: Saunders, in press.
193. Tidwell JK, Blijdorp PA, Steolinga PJ, Brouns JB, Hinderks F. Composite grafting of the maxillary sinus for placement of endosteal implants: A preliminary report of 48 patients. Int J Oral Maxillofac Surg 1992;21:204–209.
194. Smiler DG. Repositioning the inferior alveolar nerve for placement of endosseous implants: Technical note. Int J Oral Maxillofac Implants 1993;8:145–150.
195. Friberg B, Ivanoff CJ, Lekholm U. Inferior alveolar nerve transposition in combination with Brånemark implant treatment. Int J Periodont Rest Dent 1992;12:447–450.
196. Astrand P. Onlay bone grafts to the mandible. In: Worthington P, Brånemark P-I (eds). Advanced Osseointegration Surgery: Applications in the Maxillofacial Region. Chicago: Quintessence, 1992: 123–128.
197. Ohrnell LD, Palmquist J, Brånemark P-I. Single tooth placement. In: Worthington P, Brånemark P-I (eds). Advanced Osseointegration Surgery: Applications in the Maxillofacial Region. Chicago: Quintessence, 1992: 129–144.
198. Langer B. Dental implants used for periodontal patients. J Am Dent Assoc 1990;121(4):505–508.
199. Ohrnell LD, Palmquist J, Brånemark P-I: Single tooth placement. In: Worthington P, Brånemark P-I (eds). Advanced Osseointegration Surgery: Applications in the Maxillofacial Region. Chicago: Quintessence, 1992: 221–232.
200. Spitzer D, Kastenbaum F, Wagenberg B. Achieving ideal esthetics in osseointegrated prosthetics. Part II: The single unit. Int J Periodont Rest Dent 1992;12:501–507.
201. Kastenbaum F. Achieving ideal esthetics in osseointegrated prostheses. Part I: Multiple units. Int J Periodont Rest Dent 1992;12:153–159.
202. Silness J. Fixed prosthodontics and periodontal health. Dent Clin N Am 1980;24:317–329.
203. Reeves WG. Restorative margin placement and periodontal health. J Prosthet Dent 1991;66:733–736.
204. Bader JD, Rozier RG, McFall WT, Ramsey DL. Effect of crown margins on periodontal conditions on regularly attending patients. J Prosthet Dent 1991;65:75–79.
205. Roblee RD. The determination of the accuracy and reproducibility of six maxillomandibular relation techniques [master's thesis]. Dallas, Baylor College of Dentistry, 1989.
206. Kiyak HA. Aging, appearance and surgical interventions. In: Bell WH (ed). Modern Practices in Orthognathic and Reconstructive Surgery. Philadelphia: Saunders, 1992: 1438–1446.
207. Powell N, Humphreys B. Proportions of the Aesthetic Face. New York: Thieme-Stratton, 1984.
208. McCarthy JG. Introduction to plastic surgery. In: McCarthy JG. Plastic Surgery, vol I. Philadelphia: Saunders, 1990: 1–68.
209. Kolar JC. Anthropologic guidelines for aesthetic craniofacial surgery. In: Oosterhout OK (ed). Aesthetic Contouring of the Craniofacial Skeleton. Boston: Little, Brown, 1991: 15–30.
210. Sarver DM, Matukas VJ, Weissman SM. Incorporation of facial plastic surgery in the planning and treatment of orthognathic surgical cases. Int J Adult Orthod Orthognath Surg, 1991;6:227–239.
211. Hupp JR. Early delayed rhinoplasty after orthognathic surgery using external approach. Oral Maxillofac Surg Clin N Am 1990;2:327–338.
212. Muller-Schelken H. Esthetic correction in cases of orthognathic surgery. Int J Adult Orthod Orthognath Surg 1989; 4:47–55.
213. Waite PD. Simultaneous orthognathic surgery and rhinoplasty. Oral Maxillofac Surg Clin N Am 1990;2:339–350.
214. Bell WH. Genioplasty strategies. In: Bell WH (ed). Surgical Correction of Dentofacial Deformities—New Concepts. Philadelphia: Saunders, 1985: 57–64.
215. Epker BN, Stella JP. Simultaneous orthognathic and cosmetic neck surgery. Oral Maxillofac Surg Clin N Am. Philadelphia: Saunders, 1990: 259–272.
216. Bach DE, Newhouse RF, Boice GW. Simultaneous orthognathic surgery and cervicomental liposuction. Oral Surg Oral Med Oral Pathol 1991;71:262–266.
217. Guide to Aesthetic Plastic Surgery. Long Beach, California: American Society for Aesthetic Plastic Surgery, Inc, 1991.
218. McCollough EG. Rhinoplasty. J Oral Maxillofac Surg 1989;47:1132–1141.
219. Alexander RW, Kinnebrew MC. Soft-tissue aesthetic surgery of the maxillofacial region. In: Peterson LJ, Indressano A, Marciani RD, Roser SM (eds). Principles of Oral and Maxillofacial Surgery, vol 3. Philadelphia: Lippincott, 1992:1665–1771.

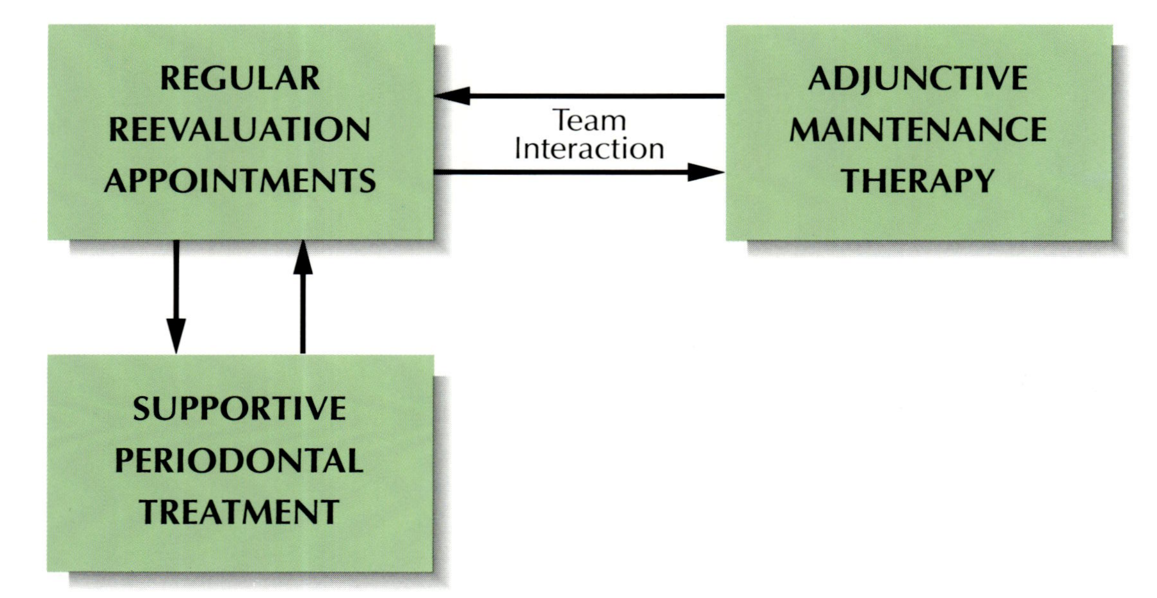

MAINTENANCE: IDT PHASE IV

7

Maintenance

Phase IV of IDT

The definitive therapy phase is now completed and the results of dentofacial therapy can be evaluated. This marks the beginning of the maintenance phase of therapy, which will maintain the results of the previous phases. All too frequently, this phase of dentofacial therapy is overlooked, but it is very important, because without proper maintenance, even the most sophisticated treatment results may be short-lived and destined to fail.[1]

There are three major areas in which the maintenance phase helps the patient sustain the results achieved through interdisciplinary dentofacial therapy. The first aspect is regular supportive periodontal treatment (SPT) to maintain optimal periodontal health throughout the patient's life. The second aspect is to perform regular reevaluation appointments for early detection of problems associated with previously performed dentofacial therapies or the occurrence of new dentofacial problems. Lastly, this phase promotes proper team interaction of detected problems so that proper adjunctive maintenance therapy can be performed to resolve the problems optimally.

The other benefits from the maintenance phase of IDT, besides the ones which benefit the patient undergoing the therapy, are realized by scientifically evaluating the final results and continuing a reevaluation process throughout the life of the patient. From this information, the interdisciplinary team can learn from each case and carry that knowledge forward to refine and improve the treatment of future patients. By sharing the knowledge with others, the profession will also continue to grow and ultimately provide even more advanced services for its patients.

Supportive Periodontal Treatment (SPT)

Overall maintenance of a dentofacial result usually centers on periodontal maintenance, or *supportive periodontal treatment* (SPT). Of all the different disciplines associated with interdisciplinary dentofacial therapy, the periodontal (including dental implants) and restorative aspects are usually the only ones in which long-term maintenance must be addressed on a relatively frequent basis. Most other areas (such as orthodontics, endodontics, and orthognathic surgery) rarely schedule maintenance appointments after the first year of posttreatment maintenance. In fact, maintenance can be considered the most important phase of periodontal therapy, and should be continued throughout the patient's life.

The frequency of the SPT depends upon the disease type, the form of previous periodontal therapy, and the level of oral hygiene attained by the patient. The average periodontal case should generally be seen for SPT every 3 months.[1,2] For a nonperiodontally involved patient, a 6-month maintenance interval is usually adequate. These maintenance intervals should be adjusted for the level of patient compliance with oral hygiene and for the amount of disease activity.[3]

Wilson has described typical maintenance visits for inflammatory periodontal disease[3,4] and for dental implants[5–7]. The guidelines he established for these visits should be individualized for each patient. Special attention should be given to cleaning implants so that their surfaces are not altered, increasing plaque accumulation.[8] Metal scalers should be avoided when cleaning titanium or hydroxyapatite implants because their use can impair cell attachment to treated surfaces relative to untreated control surfaces.[9] SPT is usually performed by a dental hygienist and should include monitoring with the appropriate periodontal disease indicators[7,10] in addition to treating areas of active disease. Peri-implant disease must also be monitored, because early detection and treatment is crucial to the long-term success of implants.[11] It is also of utmost importance that the patient's oral hygiene is monitored, documented, and discussed with the patient at these appointments. Positive reinforcement for good oral hygiene should always be given to patients, and it is also important to give positive feedback and further instructions to patients with less-than-adequate oral hygiene.

Patients with little or no periodontal problems are usually seen for maintenance in the office of the restorative dentist. Patients with moderate periodontal problems are usually best handled by alternating the SPT with visits to the periodontal specialist and the restorative dentist. When patients have severe periodontal problems, they should be maintained by the periodontist and have periodic monitoring by the restorative dentist or prosthodontist.[4,12] With this alternating schedule, periodontal maintenance and dentofacial reevaluation can be regularly provided from different dentofacial perspectives to help ensure that no problems are overlooked.

Regular Reevaluation Appointments

Much has been written about orthodontic and orthognathic surgical relapse. Posttreatment problems are also associated with restorative, endodontic, and periodontal therapies. These problems must be detected and treated as early as possible in order to maintain the results initially attained. The detection of these problems is usually accomplished through regular reevaluation appointments.

One of the most important tools needed for proper reevaluation is a thorough set of posttreatment records. These records should be an update of the records initially made by the interdisciplinary team leader during the generalized evaluation. These updated records will be used as a baseline from which changes can be monitored throughout the patient's life. For the average orthodontist and oral and maxillofacial surgeon, regular reevaluation appointments are frequently not scheduled for more than 1 year after active therapy is completed. Because of this, it is frequently the responsibility of the periodontal and/or restorative team members to reevaluate the dentofacial status of patients during SPT appointments. This can be accomplished by performing a brief update of the information gathered at the time of the posttreatment records.

Team Interaction

Any pertinent information gained through the supportive periodontal treatment and regular reevaluation appointments should be passed on to the rest of the interdisciplinary team at the regular team meetings, through other verbal communication, or through correspondence. This information should include any problems found, as well as positive information regarding successful treatment. The team members will obviously learn from their mistakes, but they also need positive feedback in order to follow those therapies which have been successful, and observe the length of time of the success. In this way, the team members will continue to grow in their expertise and be able to provide higher levels of interdisciplinary dentofacial therapy.

Posttreatment problems should undergo the process of team interaction. The team must repeat the relevant aspects of the diagnostics and treatment-planning phases of therapy to generate a problem list and then formulate the optimal treatment plan to correct the problems. The scope of this team interaction will vary according to the magnitude of the problem.

For example, if the problem is an isolated event, such as a porcelain fracture on an anterior crown, then little or no team interaction is necessary before the restorative team member repairs or replaces the restoration. However, if the problem is more extensive, such as relapse of the orthognathic surgical result, then the entire diagnostics and treatment-planning phases of therapy may have to be repeated to develop an appropriate strategy.

Regular reevaluation appointments with all the different team members are highly impractical. However, through proper team interaction, all the team members can stay abreast of the status of their posttreatment patients.

Adjunctive Maintenance Therapy

Adjunctive maintenance therapy consists of any procedures that are needed, in addition to SPT, to maintain or reestablish the dentofacial health in the patient. These procedures should typically be planned through proper team interaction. Then the plan must be presented to the patient in a patient conference similar to the one held during the original treatment-planning phase. Only in this way can optimal definitive treatment plans be made consistently for necessary adjunctive maintenance therapy.

References

1. Ramfjord SP, Morrison PC, Burget FG, Nissle RR, Schick RA, Zann GJ et al. Oral hygiene and maintenance of periodontal support. J Periodontol 1982;3:26–30.
2. American Academy of Periodontology: Consensus report, supportive treatment [Proceedings of the World Workshop in Clinical Periodontics]. Chicago, American Academy of Periodontology, 1989: II-1 to IX-25.
3. Wilson TG. Supportive periodontal treatment for patients with inflammatory periodontal diseases. In: Wilson TG, Korman KS, Newman MG (eds). Advances in Periodontics. Chicago: Quintessence, 1992: 195–204.
4. Wilson TG. A typical maintenance visit. In: Wilson TG (ed). Dental Maintenance for Patients with Periodontal Diseases. Chicago: Quintessence, 1989:90–96.
5. Wilson TG, Higginbottom FL. Diagnosis and management for dental implants. In: Wilson TG (ed). Dental Maintenance for Patients with Periodontal Diseases. Chicago: Quintessence, 1989: 191–196.
6. Orton GS, Steele DL, Wolinsky LE. The dental professional's role in monitoring and maintenance of tissue integrated prostheses. Int J Oral Maxillofac Implants 1989; 4:305–310.
7. Lang NP, Wilson TG. Choice of implant systems and clinical management. In: Wilson TG, Korman KS, Newman MG (eds). Advances in Periodontics. Chicago:Quintessence, 1992:346–376.
8. McCollum J, O'Neal RB, Brennan WA, Van Dyke TE, Horner JA. The effect of titanium implant abutment surface irregularities on plaque accumulation in vivo. J Periodontol 1992;63:802–805.
9. Dmytryk JJ, Fox SC, Moriarty JD. The effects of scaling titanium implant surfaces with metal and plastic instruments on cell attachment. J Periodontol 1990;61:491–496.
10. Williams RC, Kaldahl WB, Kalkwarf KL. Periodontal disease activity. In: Wilson TG, Korman KS, Newman MG (eds). Advances in Periodontics. Chicago: Quintessence, 1992; 58–73.
11. Rapley JW, Mills MP, Wylam J. Soft tissue management during implant maintenance. Int J Periodont Rest Dent 1992;12:373–381.
12. American Academy of Periodontology. Proceedings of the World Workshop in Clinical Periodontics. Chicago: American Academy of Periodontology, 1989, II-1 to II-20.

8

Coordinating an Interdisciplinary Team

IDT Communications

Most dental and medical providers will agree that an interdisciplinary dentofacial approach is the most efficient and consistent way to achieve optimal dentofacial results. Very few providers, however, practice interdisciplinary care because of the complexity and difficulty in developing and maintaining an interdisciplinary team. This chapter will deal with these problems and give the philosophy and methodology necessary to help establish and manage an interdisciplinary team approach to dentofacial therapy. All the figures for this chapter appear at the end, and they are arranged in the order they would be used in IDT.

Hallmarks of IDT

Successful interdisciplinary teams can be established in virtually any type of solo or group practice; in private, hospital, or university settings; and in urban, rural, or long-distance treatment situations. It is not the demographics of a group of providers that determines the level of care; instead, it is the underlying principles on which the team practices. These underlying principles can be summarized by the three hallmarks of IDT: *(1)* common philosophy, objectives, and knowledge; *(2)* regimental sequencing of diagnostic, treatment planning and therapeutic procedures; and *(3)* extensive communication between team members.

Common Philosophy, Objectives, and Knowledge

To become a successful interdisciplinary team, a group of providers must have a common philosophy of treatment with common objectives for their results. In addition, individual team members must have common knowledge about IDT methodology and all the possible treatment options the various disciplines offer so that they will know how and when to best utilize the other team members. The common philosophy, objectives, and knowledge are discussed throughout this book, which can be utilized as a team reference. A team can greatly expand upon this common information, and stay current with advancements at the same time, by properly performing IDT and through interdisciplinary team or study group meetings as outlined in this chapter.

Regimental Sequencing of Diagnostic, Treatment Planning and Therapeutic Procedures

To obtain consistent, high-quality results, dental and dentofacial problems must be analyzed and treatment must be planned in a highly ordered fashion to ensure that all necessary expertise has been included at the most appropriate time and that no problems or potential solutions have been overlooked. It is also critical to regimentally sequence all aspects of therapy to help maximize the team's individual and overall results; and to help minimize the possibility of one or more members having to make unplanned compromises in their therapy because another team member performed improper therapy and/or therapy out of the proper order. The interdisciplinary dentofacial therapy flowcharts were developed to regimentally sequence the actions of an interdisciplinary team and to assist them in providing consistent optimal results. These flowcharts (Fig 8-8) are discussed in detail in chapters 3, 4, 5, 6, and 7, and should be closely followed by the team.

Extensive Communication Between Team Members

The first two hallmarks of IDT lay down the foundation of the team and give it direction. Extensive communication, however, fuels the team, sustains its proper function, and promotes its growth. This hallmark is frequently the most difficult to maintain, and its absence or ineffectiveness is commonly the source of breakdown in interdisciplinary therapy and in the relationship of team members. IDT communications will be the primary focus of this chapter and the information previously presented throughout this text will serve as the foundation from which it is practiced.

Setting up an Interdisciplinary Team

The first step in performing IDT is setting up a new team or properly organizing a team that has already been established. As mentioned previously, team demographics are not as important as the underlying principles on which the team practices. If a group of providers is already working together as a team, it is fairly easy to implement the interdisciplinary philosophy and objectives by using this text as a reference. It is much more difficult, however, to initiate IDT when a core team has not already been established. In these cases, an effective approach to establishing or developing an interdisciplinary team involves formation of an interdisciplinary study group.

IDT Study Group

An interdisciplinary (IDT) study group may consist of a core group of providers who routinely work with one another, or it may consist of a larger group of providers that brings together several core groups to further their overall level of patient care. A brochure outlining the objectives of an established and successful interdisciplinary study group is presented in Fig 8-1.

Like an interdisciplinary team, an interdisciplinary study group should be founded on solid principles to help ensure its success and longevity. The most successful study groups have their principles spelled out in sound bylaws, including strict attendance policies and mandatory active participation by all members. Attendance and participation are critical to the longevity and success of the study group, because without them, a few members will usually end up doing most of the work, eventually becoming "burned out." Team meetings should follow a regular schedule, with a fixed monthly day and time, to encourage regular attendance.

The main focus of the meetings should be case study and continuing education, not social activities. Experience has shown that the most effective meetings are scheduled in the afternoon and do not revolve around refreshments. Night meetings are frequently ineffective, because the individual members are usually tired and strict attendance policies are not enforceable due to family and other personal time conflicts. Potential team members should be assured that the practice time lost for these meetings will be more than compensated for by the resulting increased effectiveness and productivity in their therapy. IDT study groups should strive to have representatives from all the major dental disciplines. Competition within each discipline should be overcome, and multiple representatives from each discipline, especially restorative dentistry, should be welcomed and encouraged.

To initiate an IDT study group, an organizational meeting should be set up to present IDT principles and objectives to all interested practitioners. Figure 8-2 shows a sample letter promoting this meeting, to be sent to all dental practitioners in the community. It is paramount that the strict attendance and participation policies are maintained after the interdisciplinary study group and/or team is established. At first, there will be professionals who join just to see what the group is about and who do not want to be left out. Those group members not committed to providing the best possible dentofacial care and furthering themselves in their own professional roles will eventually drop out of the group because of the rigid policies. The group that remains will be even more effective and committed to excellence.

The format for a typical interdisciplinary meeting should focus on group diagnosis, problem solving, and treatment planning of actual interdisciplinary dentofacial cases. This problem-based learning is an excellent medium for developing and enhancing an interdisciplinary team. To be most effective, these cases should be presented in a structured, consistent fashion. A suggested checklist for IDT case presentations is shown in Fig 8-3. A comprehensive case presentation is critical for the attainment of optimal group treatment planning. Furthermore, the discussion surrounding a well-presented case is an excellent means of problem-based learning, especially when the discussion includes experts from all the various disciplines. As the group matures, the meetings should include monitoring the progress of current IDT patients and critical analysis of completed cases. This will allow members to make adjustments in treatment plans and to learn from their previous therapy.

In addition to case presentation and study, there are several other aspects of team meetings that can further a team's common knowledge. At each meeting, one or more members should be scheduled to make presentations on topics including updates on advances in their area of expertise, summaries of recent dental meetings that they have attended, literature review, and "clinical pearls." Guest lecturers can occasionally be planned and participation by medical colleagues should be encouraged whenever possible. Additional meetings of core interdisciplinary teams should be scheduled as necessary to meet the demands of their IDT caseloads.

Shared IDT Resources

An IDT team or study group can pool the resources of individual providers to establish an interdisciplinary library (for textbooks, journals, audiotapes, videotapes, etc) and to sponsor presentations by national and international speakers on topics of team interest. These shared IDT resources can advance the common knowledge of a team, reduce continuing education expenses for each team member, and provide greater access to references and expertise than if providers functioned individually.

IDT Communications

Extensive communication between team members is crucial to the success of IDT. As mentioned previously, lack of communication or improper communication between team members is frequently the most common source of breakdown of therapy and of the team. Nowhere in interdisciplinary therapy are the first two hallmarks more important than in IDT communications.

Ineffective communications can result when various team members have differing philosophies and objectives in their patient care. The resulting verbal or written communication is usually difficult to utilize effectively. Often in multidisciplinary therapy, two or more team members from different disciplines will independently construct their own problem list and treatment plan for the same patient. Due to varied philosophies, objectives, and knowledge, the formats, terminologies, and scopes of these communications will be vastly different, making it difficult, if not impossible, to combine them into a useful interdisciplinary problem list and treatment plan. That is why common philosophy, objectives, and knowledge are so important during communications. The various team members must have a common purpose with the same objectives, as well as common knowledge that allows them to communicate intelligently and effectively with one another. Some highly successful interdisciplinary teams utilize common forms for questionnaires, histories (Figs 8-5 and 8-18), diagnostic procedures (Fig 8-6), treatment-planning procedures (Figs 8-9 to 8-11) and common formats for correspondence (Figs 8-13 and 8-15).

The total lack of communication or improper coordination of communication stems from a disjointed team without a proper philosophical and therapeutic format. This is where regimental sequencing of diagnostic, treatment-planning, and therapeutic procedures becomes extremely valuable. Timing of correspondence is an integral part of the philosophy, and regimental sequencing defines for the various team members both when and what type of communications are needed. Through this regimental sequencing with the same format and the same terminology of various treatment aspects, all providers can communicate more precisely about the different phases and types of therapy. The IDT flowcharts (Fig 8-8) are a valuable reference, and should be included whenever possible in correspondence and records so that team members can properly sequence all procedures related to interdisciplinary therapy.

Types of IDT Communications

The philosophy of IDT communications should be the same for all teams; however, due to differing team demographics, sophistication, and maturity, the methods of communication between team members may vary. There are four basic types of interdisciplinary communications: *(1)* team conferencing; *(2)* correspondence; *(3)* visual communication, and *(4)* electronic communication. Different teams need to combine these to effectively fulfill the requirements for their specific needs and demographics. As a team matures and becomes more sophisticated, communication between team members will change.

Team Conferencing

The first type of IDT communication is team conferencing. This occurs when two or more members of a team confer directly (perhaps at a team meeting) or by telephone. Team conferencing is an integral and extremely important part of the IDT concept and should be utilized throughout the four phases of IDT. Team conferencing is most beneficial for a new team that has not yet established common therapeutic knowledge. Team conferencing is one of the most valuable tools for establishing this common understanding, and extensive use of this format should be made whenever feasible. Team conferencing is the underlying concept for IDT study groups and interdisciplinary team meetings. As a team matures and members become more efficient in their understanding and performance of IDT and of each other's therapies, face-to-face or telephone interaction will become less and less necessary. Eventually an interdisciplinary team can function extremely well with minimal team conferencing or detailed problem-solving, relying on the IDT record and associated correspondence outlined in this chapter. When the team reaches that level, the interdisciplinary process will become highly efficient at providing optimal care and will require considerably less of each provider's time.

Correspondence

Correspondence entails any written communication between team members. Correspondence is invaluable to team success, not only for communication, but also because it serves to outline and ultimately to document the diagnostic findings and different stages of treatment. Thus, correspondence serves as a road map for future treatment as well as a historical perspective of the therapy already performed. Correspondence needs to be thorough yet concise to be effective. Correspondence between team members should be use similar formats with a common philosophy, so that it can be used as efficiently as possible by all team members.

Correspondence in medicine and dentistry has become considerably easier to perform in recent years. In the past, handwritten and typed correspondence was the norm. The introduction of dictation recorders made medical correspondence easier and more efficient. With the advent of electronic word processing, correspondence has become even easier. Commonly used sentences, paragraphs, and letters can be saved and modified as needed, greatly reducing provider and clerical time, as well as making the content of the correspondence more consistent. Intelligent use of electronic word processing can ensure the use of correct terminology, grammar, and meaning. Electronic communication methods will be discussed in more detail later in this chapter.

Visual Communication

Visual communication can be a highly useful tool for communicating and supporting complex information about IDT cases. The most common visual communications are diagnostic records. Photographs, radiographs, study casts, and other visual records are invaluable to the various team members, especially during the diagnostic and treatment-planning phases of therapy. Visual communications are also used during preparatory restorative therapy-types II, III, and IV (Figs 6-7, 6-23, 6-35, and 6-37), in which team members convey three-dimensional information to each other to facilitate treatment. In addition, orthodontists and restorative dentists frequently use visual communications for communicating complex information to laboratory technicians (Figs 6-46, 6-47, and 6-48) to help ensure a better and more consistent laboratory result.

Electronic Communication

The most recent and exciting advance in interdisciplinary communication is electronic communication. Electronic communication provides an extremely efficient, versatile modality for IDT communication. There are many types of electronic communication methods, including faxes, voice mail, electronic record storage and transfer, computer imaging, computer modems, and electronic mail. This is a new and exciting area for IDT and will be discussed in more detail later in this chapter.

The four types of IDT communication (team conferencing, correspondence, visual communication, and electronic communication) are utilized in various combinations by different teams. The particular type of combination depend on the demographics, as well as the maturity and sophistication of the team. A versatile and highly effective vehicle for coordinating IDT communications and actual therapy is through the use of an IDT diagnostic and treatment-planning record.

IDT Diagnostic and Treatment Record (IDT Record)

One of the most common sources of breakdown in therapy involving two or more providers is the fractionalization of records and associated treatment information among the various team members. Because of this fractionalization, it is often difficult for team members to know what records (initial and progress) have been made and what procedures have been or should be performed. This can cause confusion between providers, which frequently leads to needless repetition of diagnostic records or performance of other inappropriate procedures. This is frustrating to the providers and often results in the patient losing confidence in the team.

Individual team members maintaining their own specific diagnostic records and associated information, without coordinating and sharing them with other team members, is both highly inefficient and confusing to the team. With this fractionalization, the individual providers do not know what records have been made, where they are located, or at what point a patient's therapy is in the IDT flowcharts. The different phases of IDT run much more efficiently when all diagnostic and treatment records and associated information (past, present, and planned) are stored as one concise formatted reference. The *IDT diagnostic and treatment record,* or *IDT record,* was developed for this purpose. The IDT record is the main reference for IDT communication and therapy, and is used by the entire team during all phases of therapy.

The IDT record will be circulated to the different providers as needed for evaluation and therapy appointments and then immediately returned between appointments for storage either in the team leader's office or in one central location, called *IDT headquarters.* The IDT headquarters is typically in a team member's office, which may also house an IDT library and/or other centers (diagnostic, voice mail, and electronic network) that will be discussed later in this chapter. Central storage in an IDT headquarters is effective and efficient, as it may serve a single team or an entire dental community.

Contents of the IDT Record

The contents of the IDT record vary according to the phase of IDT; some materials are present in all phases (Fig 8-7). The IDT record usually consists of a binder that contains all of the IDT diagnostic records, including the general evaluation records (photographs, radiographs, dental and periodontal charting, etc) (Fig 4-1), any completed specialized records (eg, cephalometric analyses), and all progress records to date. The original records, or at the very least high-quality duplications, should be used. The diagnostic study casts, along with the articulator in which the casts were centrically mounted, should accompany this binder. It is most helpful if an interdisciplinary team selects (and each member purchases, possibly at a group discount) a high-quality interchangeable articulator system that can be periodically calibrated to ensure accurate interchangeability. This will permit study casts to be transferred easily among the various team members.

In addition to diagnostic records and treatment records, the IDT record should include an instruction page, an IDT progress notes page, and the IDT flowcharts. The instruction page (Fig 8-18) is necessary to make sure that the proper protocol is followed with the IDT record. These instructions will become less necessary as the team matures. The IDT progress notes page (Fig 8-16) assists the team in documenting therapeutic progress and helps guide members through future IDT procedures. This notes page is used both to document all procedures completed and to list the procedures that are planned next according to the preliminary or definitive treatment plan. This helps to ensure a smooth transition of the IDT record between providers. The progress notes page should be signed by the team member making the notation after all other appropriate documentation has been completed. The IDT flowcharts (Fig 8-8) are included in the IDT record as references for the team members and their auxiliaries to follow for proper sequencing and terminology.

Any relevant IDT correspondence between team members should also be included in the IDT record. This usually includes the preliminary or interdisciplinary problem list and preliminary or definitive treatment plan (depending on the stage of therapy), along with any associated correspondence referring to changes or additions to the problem lists or treatment plans. IDT record correspondence will be discussed in more detail later in this chapter.

The IDT record can only be as effective as its level of use by the team. The entire team must strive to properly employ the IDT record, because if any one member fails to fulfill their role, the actual process and results of IDT may suffer. However, one team member must oversee each IDT case to ensure the highest level of therapy.

IDT Team Leader

The IDT team leader is responsible for team coordination, data collection, treatment planning, and eventual therapy. The team leader also organizes and maintains the IDT record and associated correspondence. The team leader, commonly referred to as the "team quarterback," is an important position around which the interdisciplinary therapy will revolve.

A newly established team frequently has only one or two team members that can properly fulfill the team leader role. These team members are usually one of the specialists who, due to their training and the nature of their specialty, have enough interdisciplinary common knowledge to perform the general evaluation and formulate both the preliminary problem list and preliminary treatment plan. Due to the nature of their practices, these specialists may initially be the most capable of producing the extensive correspondence necessary for proper IDT communication. It should be the goal of a mature team to enable any team member to function as the team leader, because the burden of that position needs to be shared. This can be accomplished through interdisciplinary study groups, team meetings, and/or correspondence to enhance the team's overall common knowledge. It is also helpful for the to team have a common format for correspondence, including common database and word-processing programs, so that the team leader's correspondence can easily be accomplished by all members.

The general practitioner or restorative team member is the most logical first choice for team leader for several reasons. First, the general practitioner is usually the team member who first sees the interdisciplinary problems, and has usually already established a solid rapport with the patient. This positions the general practitioner ideally to initiate the interdisciplinary process and to relay the IDT procedures and communications between the team and the patient. Second, the definitive restorative procedures are usually the last dental procedures to be performed in IDT; accordingly, the restorative team member should coordinate the entire process, because his or her therapy will be affected by all other previous therapies. Third, the general practitioner is usually the team member who will eventually be responsible for overseeing the long-term maintenance of the interdisciplinary results, so supervision of the entire interdisciplinary process would be most beneficial to him or her.

The IDT record and associated correspondence should play a major role in helping the team leader orchestrate an optimal progression of IDT. These aspects will be discussed in greater detail later in this chapter.

IDT Coordinators and Managers

To further facilitate interdisciplinary communication and optimal utilization of the IDT record, it is helpful for each team member to assign one of his or her staff members as an *IDT coordinator*. IDT coordinators can relieve the practitioner of many of the burdens of maintaining continuity in IDT protocol and serve as contacts for the IDT coordinators of other team members, as well as for the patient. The IDT coordinators should also be in charge of transferring the IDT record to the various offices as needed.

In teams that have an IDT headquarters for central record storage, the IDT coordinator in that office is called the *IDT manager*. The IDT manager is in charge of organizing, tracking, distributing and storing all IDT records. Central storage with an IDT manager is the most effective arrangement, because IDT records are quickly accessible to the team (for tracking, requesting, updating, etc) and there is less chance of records being misplaced or lost in a team member's office. An IDT manager can be even more beneficial when he or she also functions as the IDT transcriptionist for the team, and oversees the IDT library or other various IDT centers (diagnostic, voice mail, and electronic network) that a team may have established.

In situations where there is not an IDT headquarters, the IDT coordinator from the team leader's office of each case should assume the role of IDT manager and be in charge of tracking and storing that specific IDT record. In some communities, a dental laboratory or dental supply company may volunteer the use of their shuttle service for transferring IDT records between team members. The IDT coordinator and/or manager should work closely with this shuttle service to coordinate the timely pickup and delivery of the records.

IDT Communication in the Four Phases of IDT

The role of the team leader and the use of the IDT record and IDT communications changes throughout the various phases of therapy. More specific information on the team leaders responsibility and the utilization of the IDT record and associated correspondence for each of the different phases of therapy is outlined in the remainder of this chapter.

Diagnostic Phase

After the patient has elected to enter into the interdisciplinary diagnostic and treatment-planning process from the preliminary therapy stage of IDT (Chapter 3), the team leader must accumulate the general diagnostic information needed to effectively initiate the team approach. The first step in this is to complete the general evaluation and records as outlined in Fig 4-1. The team leader of each case will make the diagnostic records. An IDT diagnostic center can also be established in a team member's office to standardize these records and ensure consistent quality. The team leader, however, must always perform the evaluation and analyze the records for the case.

To assist the team leader in performing a thorough and consistent generalized evaluation, a standardized *IDT general evaluation and initial therapy form* has been developed (Fig 8-6). The team leader completes this general diagnostic database and devises the preliminary problem list from it (Chapter 4). Problem lists can be most efficiently and effectively utilized by the interdisciplinary team when they are consistently arranged. For this reason, the problem list should be divided into standard categories (see page 72); a *problem list worksheet* (Figure 8-9) can be very useful in this process.

After the preliminary problem list is completed, the team leader will attempt to solve the problems by formulating one or more preliminary treatment plans. This problem-solving and treatment-planning process should be performed with the philosophy outlined in Chapter 5, except that it is usually accomplished solely by the team leader, without any team conferencing. The preliminary problem list and treatment plan are thus not as comprehensive as the final interdisciplinary problem list and definitive treatment plan established by the efforts of the entire team. The preliminary problem list and treatment plan serve only to initiate the interdisciplinary diagnostic and treatment-planning process. They will typically change significantly during the specialized evaluations and team-conferencing session.

The preliminary treatment plans, as well as the tentative and definitive treatment plans, can be divided into three sections: *(1)* diagnostic and treatment planning, *(2)* definitive therapy, and *(3)* maintenance. A *treatment plan worksheet* (Figure 8-10) helps establish the proper format and sequence of this plan. More specific treatment-planning information can be outlined for each individual tooth on the IDT dental treatment planning worksheet (Fig 8-11). The process of synthesizing the database into a discrete list of problems and formulating preliminary treatment plans will suggest what expertise among the different disciplines will be needed to optimally diagnose, plan treatment, and treat the patient's unique dentofacial problems. With this information, the team can be selected and organized.

The team leader's role then switches to counseling and the preliminary patient conference. At this appointment, the team leader will present and discuss the patient's general dentofacial problems and preliminary treatment options. During this dentofacial counseling (Chapters 3 and 4), the patient should determine whether to pursue the IDT diagnostic and treatment-planning phases of therapy. If the patient elects to proceed, the team leader then refers the patient to the appropriate team members for specialized evaluations (the team leader's IDT coordinator should schedule and track these appointments), assembles the IDT record, and sends the appropriate correspondence.

An *IDT diagnostic and treatment-planning summary* should now be made, which will include the patient's name, current date, list of team members, and the *preliminary problem list* and *preliminary treatment plan* (Fig 8-12). The preliminary treatment plan should list all the completed diagnostic procedures to date, including the records made to help prevent procedures from being repeated. This summary page is an integral part of the IDT record during the diagnostic and treatment-planning phases of therapy and will also be incorporated into the initial correspondence referring the patient to the various team members. Problem lists and treatment plans should be properly numbered (Fig 8-12) so the interdisciplinary team can easily refer to a specific part during team conferencing. The team leader must list all specialized evaluations on the preliminary treatment plan, along with the appropriate dates, so the preliminary treatment plan can guide the proper and timely distribution of the IDT record to the appropriate practitioners.

Figures 8-13 and 8-15 show examples of initial correspondence to the interdisciplinary team and the patient. The preliminary problem list and preliminary treatment plans are easily inserted into the bodies of these standard letters, so that the patient and team members will have copies for their office files. Copies of the completed *IDT patient information and history forms* (Figs 8-4 and 8-5) should also be included in the IDT record, and copies mailed with the initial correspondence to all team members, so the patient (or IDT manager, when applicable) will not have to fill out new forms at each office.

The team leader, or his or her IDT coordinator (or IDT manager, when applicable), should oversee the delivery of the IDT record to the appropriate team member at least one day (when possible) before their specialized evaluation. This will give each provider a chance to review the general evaluation records, the preliminary problem list, and the preliminary treatment plan before seeing the patient. After team members perform their specialized evaluations, they should include any specialized records in the IDT record and fill out a *specialized evaluation summary* (Fig 8-19). The specialized evaluation summary is a very efficient communication tool. It simplifies each provider's correspondence by requiring them to write only the information needed to add to or change the preliminary problem list and preliminary treatment plan according to their specialized findings. In this process, the unidisciplinary databases described in Chapter 4 can be immediately arranged into an interdisciplinary problem list format. This summary can easily and quickly be filled out by the provider and the information can be reviewed by the other team members before their specialized evaluation. The various team members may also initiate any appropriate initial therapy as described in Chapter 4, and include any associated information on the specialized evaluation summary. The team or team leader (depending on the maturity of the team) will eventually incorporate the information on these summaries into the interdisciplinary problem list and tentative treatment plan(s). The specialized evaluation summaries relieve each team member from having to dictate long letters, which are often very difficult to combine into one workable problem list and treatment plan. This simplified system of correspondence saves a tremendous amount of time for all team members. Specialized evaluation forms have been developed for the various disciplines to expand on a specific area of information from the IDT general evaluation and initial therapy form (Fig 8-6). An example of an *IDT dental and periodontal specialized evaluation form* is illustrated in Fig 8-18; when completed, specialized evaluation forms, or copies of them, are also included in the IDT record.

After all of the specialized evaluations and forms, along with the appropriate initial therapy, have been completed, the team should have all the necessary diagnostic information to properly formulate treatment plans. It is at this stage when the case is usually presented at a team or study group meeting for group problem solving and treatment planning (Fig 8-3). Presenting IDT cases before the diagnostic phase has been completed is inefficient, because the team conferencing may have to be repeated if all the pertinent information is not yet available. The IDT problem list, treatment planning, and dental treatment planning worksheets (Figs 8-9 to 8-11) are very helpful for efficiently documenting and organizing the information developed during team conferencing.

Treatment-Planning Phase

The interdisciplinary problem list was developed in the diagnostic phase from all the information gathered during the general and specialized evaluations, and is used as a reference during all the team conferencing (ie, team problem-solving) needed to properly formulate the tentative treatment plan(s). Even though team conferencing is an extremely useful tool during the treatment-planning phase of therapy, it is not always necessary for a well-organized and experienced team. A mature team frequently does not have to perform team conferencing in order to arrive at an optimal treatment plan. By properly utilizing the communication outlined in this chapter, an experienced team whose members understand the common IDT information can often "conference indirectly." This will frequently enable the team leader to combine all the information from the specialized evaluation summaries, with the preliminary problem list and treatment plan(s), directly into an interdisciplinary problem list and tentative treatment plan(s). This streamlined format is particularly useful in long-distance situations or in situations where there are tremendous time constraints on the various providers.

The result of interdisciplinary treatment planning is one or more tentative treatment plan(s). These treatment plans are tentative because they are suggested by the team as a trial. They will undergo the scrutiny of adjunctive diagnostic procedures (Fig 5-5) and the patient before the definitive treatment is selected. The team leader continues the dentofacial counseling process at the definitive patient conference, and presents the tentative treatment plan(s) to the patient to help them determine the best overall treatment option.

Definitive-Therapy Phase

The definitive treatment plan was finalized by the team and patient in the treatment-planning phase. The team leader now combines all the pertinent information in preparation for the definitive therapy phase and develops the *IDT summary*. The IDT summary (Fig 8-14) is the updated version of the IDT diagnostic and treatment-planning summary (Fig 8-12), and includes the patient's name, date, list of team members, the interdisciplinary problem list, and definitive treatment plan. It also has space for team members to list any additional diagnostic records (progress, presurgical, etc) they make during therapy. A letter outlining the definitive treatment plan is sent along with the IDT summary to all the team members to ensure that everyone fully agrees on the final treatment plan (Fig 8-13). This gives them one last chance to make any alterations before definitive treatment is initiated. Subsequent changes are made in the definitive treatment plan as necessary, then the IDT summary is included into the IDT record. The final IDT summary is sent to the patient and all the team members to serve as a road map for the definitive therapy phase of IDT.

It is the team leader's role to oversee definitive therapy to help ensure a smooth therapeutic progression. The IDT record, now containing the IDT summary, should be distributed to each provider as they are performing their therapies. Proper documentation, as outlined on the *IDT record instructions* (Fig 8-17), is important, as are team monitoring and conferencing, which should be performed as necessary and as dictated by the IDT philosophy (Chapter 6). Changes are made in the definitive treatment plan as necessary during the team monitoring aspects of treatment; they should be reflected in the IDT summary.

Maintenance Phase

After definitive treatment is completed, the team leader should make final records, using the same protocol as the general evaluation records (Fig 4-1), and include them in the IDT record. These records will be used in the maintenance phase to monitor any changes and/or relapse in the final result. Any significant dentofacial problems found by the team leader or other team members during the maintenance phase should be subjected to the interdisciplinary process as needed for proper treatment (Chapter 7). The final records are also useful for the interdisciplinary team and individual providers to critically evaluate their treatment. The resulting information can be used to further IDT common knowledge and improve future interdisciplinary therapy.

The IDT communication protocol utilizing the IDT record is very useful and should be followed by interdisciplinary teams to maximize their results and minimize the problems typically associated with a team approach. IDT communications and the IDT records can be even more efficient and effective when performed through IDT electronic communications.

IDT Electronic Communications

Electronic communication is the newest of the four types of IDT communications. Its versatility continues to increase as the pace of technological advance increases. It may be only partially used by an IDT team, or it can be expanded to provide a comprehensive platform on which the three other forms of communication (team conferencing, correspondence, and visual communication) can be performed. The more completely and effectively an IDT team can use electronic communications, the more efficient it will be in optimally performing all aspects of IDT, especially the diagnostic and treatment-planning procedures. The following are some specific examples of electronic communication, some or all of which may be utilized by the IDT team or the individual members.

Personal Computer

Personal computers are the main vehicles of electronic communications. They are central to data processing (accounting, practice management, scheduling, etc) in most modern dental and medical offices. They are used to prepare, store, manipulate, and communicate large amounts of information.

The versatility and speed of high-quality personal computers gives IDT teams and individual members great latitude to choose and tailor specific applications to their particular needs. There are computer programs, also called applications or software, available to perform extensive IDT communications, as well as interdisciplinary diagnostic and treatment-planning procedures. Most computer programs suitable for IDT fall into one of the following categories.

Word Processing

Word processing applications use the computer to help create, edit, proofread, format, and print documents. It is by far the most popular computer application. Word processing makes the creation and alteration of text much easier than on traditional typewriters, which require large amounts of retyping. Using a word processing application, one can easily correct, insert, delete, or rearrange words as necessary, without retyping the entire document. It is also possible to store and retrieve frequently used documents or portions of documents, such as letters, questionnaires, problems for problem lists, procedures for treatment plans, and other correspondence, altering them as necessary to fit a particular situation. This saves provider and staff clerical time during the initial creation of documents. Most word processing software also contains grammar, punctuation, and spelling correction, which greatly reduces revision time. The IDT correspondence in shown in the figures for this chapter were created and stored with word processing applications, and customized with information directly from the patient record. In the highly detailed correspondence in Figs 8-13 to 8-16 only about 10% of the documents needed to be written or dictated by the provider.

Word processing programs are now available that contain IDT databases, allowing highly customized documents to be easily created. This can be done by the doctor or treatment assistant while the patient is being evaluated in the office or during a private or group treatment-planning session. This IDT word processing application can be highly specialized for specific disciplines, yet will include information common to all disciplines, along with standardized IDT document terminology and formatting. This allows all team members to easily undertake the role of team leader, and enables detailed and highly specific correspondence from different team members (especially problem lists and treatment plans) to be easily consolidated into a single comprehensive document.

Patient Record Storage

One of the most useful computer applications is the database, which is a collection of related information about a subject organized into a useful manner that provides a foundation for other procedures. A computer database can be used to store highly organized patient records that can be easily retrieved and utilized. These patient records can include all written and visual patient information, as well as voice messages. The patient's personal, medical, and dental histories can be stored in a format that matches an interdisciplinary team's standard history and diagnostic forms (Figs 8-4 to 8-6 and 8-18) and coordinates with their practice-management software. Diagnostic and treatment information can also be stored to match the IDT philosophy and standardized forms.

Patient images, including facial and dental photographs and radiographs, can also be easily and quickly recorded, stored and retrieved. Photographic-quality images can now be produced and stored digitally, and can be altered and printed in many ways, making duplication of records easy and economical. Images can also be made of completed diagnostic forms, such as periodontal probing charts. In some dental software programs, these charts are completed electronically.

Voice notations and messages attached to a patient file are also possible with some applications. Other computer applications can even recognize voice commands and eliminate using a keyboard or mouse for certain functions. This "hands off" use of the computer can be very useful for procedures such as computer charting and image capturing (especially when maintaining asepsis). The use of voice technology in computers is a rapidly growing area and is sure to be increasingly important.

Patient databases significantly enhance the use of the IDT diagnostic and treatment-planning record, facilitating formulation of problem lists and treatment plans, team conferences, and dentofacial counseling with patients. Computer databases permit organized, centralized storage of patient records that can be accessed and printed quickly for all team members. The stored information, including images, can also be integrated into word-processing applications to produce customized documents for patients, insurance companies, and team members.

Image Manipulation

Computer-based imaging has made enhancement and alteration of pictures easier and faster. Patient pictures can be quickly adjusted to ensure the esthetics of the final image. Images can also be altered to realistically simulate dental and dentofacial changes expected during IDT, enabling visualization of the completed procedures. Cephalometric images can also be analyzed and manipulated to assist in diagnosis and treatment planning. Both cephalometric and image manipulation can be valuable to the interdisciplinary team as adjective diagnostic procedures. Image manipulation can also serve as a powerful educational tool during patient consultations and patient dentofacial counseling (Fig 5-6).

Networks

Computer databases and applications can be maximized through the use of networks. A network is a data exchange system created by physically connecting two or more computers. There are two basic types of computer networks.

The first, smaller type is the *local area network* (LAN), which is usually found within a single team member's office. A LAN connects a few computers so that they can share databases, applications, and expensive peripheral equipment, such as laser printers. LANs link computers together within a limited area by high-performance cables; desktop computers (in networks, often known as workstations) can then run application programs and access shared network resources. In more complex LANs, central computers (file servers) are used to enable other users (workstations) to communicate with each other interactively. This allows users to communicate via electronic mail and to share multiuser programs, databases and expensive peripherals. They can also draw on resources of massive secondary storage units. A LAN system could be a tremendous asset for an IDT team member because it allows patient databases to be shared between imaging, word-processing, diagnostic, treatment-planning, and consultation systems and personnel.

The second type of network, the *wide area network* (WAN), is much larger. A WAN employs telephone lines to connect individual computers or LANs over large distances. It operates like a LAN, but enables the user to access information from libraries, medical and dental schools, and other practitioners worldwide.

Telecommunications

IDT information can be transmitted between team members as voice or computer signals by using telephone and data communications, or telecommunications. Telecommunications can be a highly effective and efficient means of interdisciplinary communication and may be performed through several modalities depending on the needs of the team and the equipment available. Some examples of these modalities are as follows.

Fax

Fax (short for "facsimile") is the transmission of a printed page between two locations connected by telecommunications. The fax machine scans a sheet of paper and convert its image into a coded form that can be transmitted via telephone system. The fax machine on the other end receives and translates the code, and prints a replica of the original page. This technology can allow team members to transmit IDT correspondence to one another virtually instantaneously. This not only saves time but also can save expenses when performed within a local telephone area. In addition to sending correspondence, black and white images and other graphics can also be sent via fax.

Voice Mail

With voice mail, voice messages can be sent, over telephone lines, to a communication system where they are transformed into digital form and stored on a computer hard drive. This digitally stored voice message can then be retrieved at any time by the person to whom it was directed. Voice mail has opened up an entirely new avenue for efficiency in IDT communications.

Team conferencing via telephone is a commonly necessary during IDT diagnostic, treatment-planning, and therapeutic procedures. Simple voice communication, however, is often inefficient, as many busy practitioners have limited time for telephone conversations, which, because they are not written down, may be misinterpreted or misremembered, causing communication problems.

To counteract these problems and enhance telephone team conferencing, an IDT voice mail network can be set up. Each team member thus has a voice mailbox that confidentially stores messages from other team members. Messages can be sent to multiple team members or to the entire team at once. Voice mail reduces telephone-call interruptions and allows more efficient and convenient communication. Team members can review messages at convenient times, playing the message as many times as needed for the best understanding. Voice mail messages are highly efficient because they are usually short, concise, and contain little "small talk." On advanced voice mail systems, the reply to a message can be stored immediately in the original sender's voice mailbox.

Voice mail messages may be transferred to printed form by transcription to create correspondence or electronic messages via word processing. A voice mail center can even be used as a transcription service so that one transcriptionist can produce the interdisciplinary correspondence for all team members in the same format. Voice mail technology is sure to become an important vehicle for providing effective IDT communications.

All of the above electronic communications applications can be used either alone or in any combination, depending on the sophistication of the interdisciplinary team. Fig 8-20 shows several ways correspondence may be produced and transmitted by electronic means, sometimes in combination with non-electronic means. By far the most effective and exciting form of electronic communications though, is through the coordination of the various applications in an IDT electronic network.

IDT Electronic Network

The IDT record is an invaluable tool for organizing and storing patient records and for coordinating IDT communication in therapy. It should be used by all interdisciplinary teams to optimize therapy and reduce confusion between team members. But having all patient records in a single file has its shortcomings; the file may be misplaced or in the wrong office at the wrong time. IDT team conferencing can also be very challenging to coordinate efficiently due to providers' time constraints. The *IDT electronic network* is designed to minimize these problems, and can take a team to the highest level of sophistication in IDT.

A new team should initially use the IDT record in a non-electronic form, because the members need to determine their specific interdisciplinary needs according to their demographics. The standard IDT communication process, especially team conferencing, should also be used at first, because it strengthens the common philosophy, objectives, and knowledge of the team. But as a team matures and becomes more sophisticated in the understanding of and approach to IDT, the IDT electronic network can decrease the effects of time constraints and tremendously increase the efficiency and effectiveness of communications among team members and patients.

An IDT electronic network combines some or all of the personal computer and telecommunication modalities described previously. Its configuration is extremely flexible and can be customized to meet the needs of a particular team. The ideal network configuration presented in Fig 8-21 shows how an IDT team might use many of the tools now available.

After a document has been completed in the computer, the information can be transferred to the various team members through several different avenues. The most common are outputting the documents to a printer to make a hard copy. This hard copy can then either be hand delivered, mailed via the postal service, or faxed to the appropriate team members and the patient. In more advanced settings, a paperless communication medium can be used, sending a document from one computer to another via a fax/modem; telecommunications systems thus transfer the information to the various team members. The receiver can either output the electronic document to a printer, storing it in the computer for use and for paperless correspondence.

Network Configuration

The IDT electronic network (Fig 8-21) can best be described in two major parts. The IDT network center houses the main computer on which all the IDT patient records and information are stored. The IDT network periphery consists of the team members' electronic communications equipment connected to the network center via telecommunications.

IDT Network Center. The heart of an IDT network is the network center, which consists of a network server or file server and several workstations. The server, usually located in a team member's office or an IDT records center, is typically a powerful computer, dedicated to network record storage and data-processing. The server stores all the patient databases and interfaces with team members through telecommunications, especially high-speed computer fax/modems. Large-volume storage, such as optical disks, is necessary to facilitate storage and transmission of high-quality digital images. An imaging workstation should be included for processing diagnostic, progress, and final images of IDT cases, along with hardware for scanning documents, photographs, radiographs, and other materials into digital form. High-quality printers are necessary to create hard copies of correspondence and diagnostic records. Other workstations are typically connected at the server's location in a LAN; these are used for IDT word processing, patient dentofacial counseling, and IDT communications. A voice mail center can also be connected to the network via telecommunications, although it may be in a different, separate location than the IDT network center.

IDT Network Periphery. The IDT network periphery consists of the team members' electronic communication equipment connected to the network center via telecommunications (Fig 8-21). Individual team members' electronic communications equipment can vary considerably, depending on level of participation in interdisciplinary therapy and financial constraints. Electronic equipment can be as basic as a telephone with or without a fax, or as extensive as a complete LAN with the same capabilities as the IDT network center. The minimum suggested equipment is a high-power personal computer with software to view IDT patient records (including images), that are received via telecommunications or floppy disks, as well as IDT word-processing capabilities so that each team member can update information on the network server. But a provider can be part of the team without this minimum equipment. Using voice mail and the IDT transcriptionist, a team member can update the main patient file. In addition, the flexibility of the main LAN system allows all records to be printed for any member who wants a hard copy of patient records.

IDT Electronic Record

The *IDT electronic record* is an IDT diagnostic and treatment record (IDT record) that is stored and managed electronically. The IDT record is the fundamental tool in the interdisciplinary team process. Electronic processing of the IDT record makes it more efficient and effective. Electronic communications in IDT will surely grow in importance with new technological developments. The IDT electronic network described above can provide a number of functions and advantages through the IDT electronic record. The configuration and the complexity of a team's IDT electronic network will determine the functions available to team members.

Central Storage and Management of IDT Record and Correspondence. Electronically storing and managing patient records in a central location allows instantaneous access by team members. They can thus review a patient's IDT electronic record at any time and know exactly where the patient is in the interdisciplinary process. Team members can also immediately update the records with specialized evaluation findings and therapies they have performed. Updating can be performed either directly, via computer modem and telecommunications, or through the telephone or voice mail system, using a transcriptionist at the IDT network center who updates the IDT electronic record.

Word processing on an IDT electronic network allows highly formatted and compatible correspondence between team members. The contents of correspondence can easily be consolidated in the central IDT electronic record, further reducing team-leader and team-conferencing time. Specialized IDT record processing and storage software is now available for IDT team members. This software creates detailed problem lists and treatment plans quickly and easily.

Record Duplication. Centrally storing and managing patient records and images is a tremendous asset, but it is still very useful for each team member to have a personal set of records. Electronic communications allows inexpensive, high-quality record duplication to provide each member with a set of patient diagnostic and treatment records to store in their standard patient filing system in their office.

Variable Levels of Electronic Communication. The flexibility of electronic communication technology permits different team members to participate at various levels in an IDT electronic network depending on sophistication of their equipment. This allows any provider to participate, at least at some level, in an IDT electronic network without having to spend large amounts of money for a comprehensive system.

Patient Confidentiality. A common concern with central electronic storage and accessibility of patient files is that patient confidentiality may be lost. This can be prevented by using security codes and identification numbers for both patient files and team members. These allow providers to access only IDT electronic records for IDT cases in which they are participating. A team or team leader can also determine the level of access to patient files by different team members. For example, some members may only permitted to view files, whereas others may be able to alter or copy them. All network systems have these security capabilities.

Electronic Tracking and Priority List. IDT can be electronically tracked to assist the team in following the status of each patient. Necessary tasks can listed and prioritized on the system, as well as sent to the appropriate team member(s) via electronic mail. Each team member can be updated daily as to which tasks must be completed and their order of priority.

Electronic Mail. Electronic mail is similar to voice mail, but messages are sent as electronic text files. IDT correspondence and patient records can thus be electronically mailed to one or more IDT team members. The recipient can examine the documents and reply when time is available. This is particularly useful when team conferencing is required. Electronic mail can also be prioritized so that more pressing messages can be dealt with first.

Team Leader Flexibility. The IDT electronic record enables different team members to be able to act as team leader whenever needed. Any team member who has access to the central electronic patient files can optimally perform the team leaders' responsibilities. This permits sharing of the team leader's burden, even when all the patient files are centrally stored at a different location.

Telecommuting. In a busy practice, it is often difficult for a provider to find the time or privacy needed to properly diagnose, treatment-plan, and monitor IDT cases, as well as formulate associated correspondence. Often, providers must bring patient records home to do this, which may jeopardize the safety of the records. The IDT electronic network enables team members to perform IDT tasks at home without taking records from the office. In telecommuting a provider links a home computer to the IDT network, or their office, by means of telecommunications. Telecommuting is now possible anywhere with portable computers. Correspondence can be electronically produced and then retrieved and processed at the central network location or in the team member's office.

Electronic Team Conferencing. Two or more team members with IDT network workstations can undergo electronic team conferencing via telecommunications. They can simultaneously view cases and interact electronically while conversing over the telephone, either from their offices or their homes (or, with portable computers, from any location). No longer must team members meet in one place; electronic team conferencing performs the same function, usually faster.

Advantages of IDT Electronic Records

IDT electronic records save enormous amounts of time for providers and their staffs. Daily practice tasks are less frequently interrupted, and IDT team roles can be more easily and efficiently fulfilled. Electronic communication can minimize the "paper chase" and "phone tag" typically associated with normal comprehensive care. Even though the technology for electronic communication is expensive, it more than pays for itself in increased productivity.

Electronic communication in conjunction with the IDT electronic record can be more effective than traditional communication. Patient information and records are more highly structured, communicated messages are typically more focused, and receivers have more flexibility in reviewing and replying to the information. Computerized records in themselves are tremendous assets, and can improve communication process better than common records. During team conferencing and patient dentofacial counseling, both team members and patients can better visualize dentofacial problems and potential solutions when records can be shared with them via electronic communications.

Electronic communications can be a tremendous asset to an interdisciplinary team, but it is important to point out that, with or without electronic communications technology, the team must practice interdisciplinary dentofacial therapy according to its fundamental principles.

Summary

This text presents a comprehensive philosophy and methodology for interdisciplinary management of dentofacial problems. The attainment of consistent and optimal treatment results often requires the expertise of several different disciplines. The most effective utilization of these different disciplines is through an organized interdisciplinary team which is coordinated to promote open communication through rigidly structured phases in therapy. The overall goal for an interdisciplinary team is to provide an unbiased diagnosis, formulate an optimal treatment plan that properly weighs and addresses all relevant factors, and produce and maintain an optimal dentofacial result that enhances the overall physical and psychological well-being of the patient.

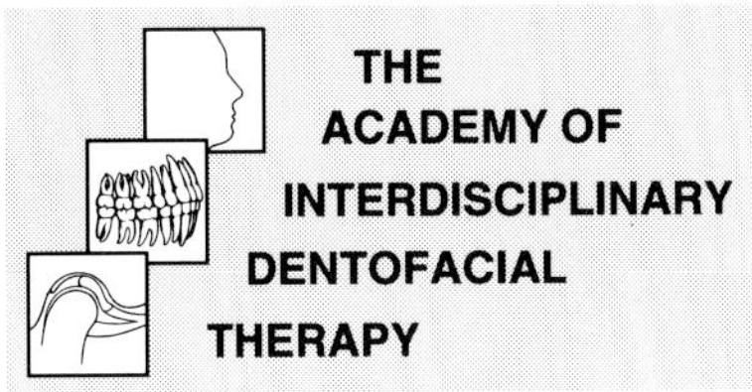

The Academy of Interdisciplinary Dentofacial Therapy

The Academy of Interdisciplinary Dentofacial Therapy was organized to advance its members professionally in the Art and Science of Dentistry and to promote good fellowship between members of the Academy and other members of the profession. It is the purpose of the Academy to present quality continuing education to augment the abilities of dental professionals in the delivery of optimal dentofacial care for their patients. The Academy provides a vehicle for exchange of expertise, literature review, and continuing dental education.

Study Groups

The Academy encourages the formation of affiliated local chapters where dental groups are committed to the delivery of excellent and comprehensive dental care to patients through an interdisciplinary perspective. Individual Study Groups meet monthly for group diagnosis, treatment planning and follow-up of Interdisciplinary Dentofacial Therapy. Study groups allow for intensive hands-on study in small groups and stimulate professional interaction and camaraderie through participatory problem-based learning and interdisciplinary therapy.

Lectures

The Academy pools the resources of the affiliated local chapters to bring in national and international speakers to share their expertise with the Academy's members and their guests.

Membership

Membership in the Academy and participation in its activities demonstrate an outstanding dedication to the practice of dentistry. Membership consists of dentists and other professionals in related areas who are interested in providing optimal dentofacial care for their patients. Active members fully participate in a local chapter study group and the large lectures. Associate memberships with the Academy allows participation in large lectures only at a discounted yearly rate.

Continuing Education Credit

The Academy is fully approved by the Academy of General Dentistry and the Arkansas State Board of Dental Examiners for continuing education credit.

The Academy of Interdisciplinary Dentofacial Therapy
is a nonprofit organization

1915 Green Acres Road, Fayetteville, AR 72703

Fig 8-1 Brochure outlining objectives from a successful IDT study group.

RICHARD D. ROBLEE, D.D.S, M.S.
ORTHODONTICS

1915 GREEN ACRES ROAD
FAYETTEVILLE, ARKANSAS 72703
(501) 521-6060
FAX (501) 521-4161

DATE

PREFIX FIRSTNAME LASTNAMESUFFIX
ADDRESS1
ADDRESS2
CITY, STATE ZIP

Dear SALUTATION:

There has been an overwhelming amount of interest from area dentists to organize a dental study group in (location). This organization is now in the process of being formed and you are invited to become a charter member in (name of group). The group's focus will revolve around the study of dental and periodontal health, dental occlusion, interdisciplinary therapy and dentofacial esthetics.

Regular meetings will be held monthly on the (first, last, etc.)(weekday) at 2:00 p.m. to minimize the chance of conflicts with nightly events. The typical meeting format will center around group diagnosis and treatment planning of actual interdisciplinary dentofacial cases as well as the continuous monitoring of cases in progress. Also at each meeting, one or more members will be scheduled to make presentations on topics such as (1) updates or advances in their area of expertise, (2) clinical pearls, (3) summaries of recent dental meetings they attended, or (4) literature reviews of dental journals/texts. Guest speakers will be included whenever possible.

In order for this group to have long-term success, I feel that we need to keep it scientifically based and nonsocial. We are currently filing for both AGD and state continuing education credit as well as nonprofit organization status. This group will have sound by-laws which will include an initiation fee plus annual dues, a strict attendance policy, and mandatory active participation by all members.

The first meeting for the (location) Interdisciplinary Dentofacial Study Group will be held on (date and time), at the (meeting place). I will have all the information about the study group at the meeting, and have also prepared a short presentation to introduce the philosophy. Please contact (name and phone number) to let us know whether or not you will be able to attend the meeting.

It will be the goal of this group to maintain a model dental community in (location) which provides optimal dentofacial care to their patients through the use of the most advanced techniques, technology and materials. I hope you will seriously consider joining us on (meeting date) if you are interested in this concept. Please do not hesitate to contact me if you have any questions, comments or suggestions.

Sincerely,

Richard D. Roblee, D.D.S, M.S.

Fig 8-2 Sample letter for initiating an IDT study group.

IDT Case Presentation Checklist

- Extraoral photographs
  - 1 anterior facial nonsmiling
  - 1 anterior facial smiling
  - 1 lateral facial relaxed

  Optional
  - 1 lips in repose
  - 1 lips during smiling
- Intraoral photographs
  - 1 anterior closed
  - 1 anterior slightly open
  - 1 lateral interincisal
  - 2 lateral occlusion
  - 2 occlusal
- Full-mouth radiographic survey
- Panoramic radiograph
- Diagnostic study casts mounted in centric relation in a semiadjustable articulator
- Specialized evaluations completed with appropriate specialized records
- Preliminary problem list completed
- Preliminary treatment plan completed
- Documented status of needed initial therapy

Fig 8-3 This suggested checklist for IDT case presentation helps ensure structure and completeness for cases presented at team meetings and study groups. With this information, proper group diagnosis, treatment planning, and problem-

Interdisciplinary Dentofacial Diagnostic Systems

Richard D. Roblee, DDS, MS

ORTHODONTICS

Chart Number: ______

Date: ______

PATIENT'S INFORMATION (please completely fill out first and second pages)

Patient's Full Name: ______ (First, Middle, Last) Name you like to be called by: ______

Patient's Address: ______ (Street, Apt. No., City, State, Zip) Soc. Sec. #: ______

Home Phone: (____) ______ Date of Birth: __/__/__ Marital Status: ❑ Single ❑ Married ❑ Divorced ❑ Separated ❑ Widowed

Place of Employment or School and Grade: ______ Phone: (____) ______

Person to contact in case of emergency: ______ Relationship: ______ Phone: (____) ______

Contact's Address: ______

Whom May We Thank for Referring You? ______ Names and Ages of Children or Siblings: ______

PERSON RESPONSIBLE FOR ACCOUNT

Full Name: ______ (First, Middle, Last) Relation to Patient: ______

Full Home Address: ______ (Street, Apt. No., City, State, Zip) Home Phone: (____) ______

If Less than 3 Years at above, Previous Address: ______ Date of Birth: __/__/__

Marital Status: ❑ Single ❑ Married ❑ Divorced ❑ Separated ❑ Widowed Occupation: ______

Driver's License No.: ______ Social Security No.: ______ Employer: ______

Work Phone: (____) ______ Years at Employer: ______ Employer's Address: ______

Name of ❑ Spouse ❑ Other Parent or ❑ Secondary Responsible Person: ______ (First, Middle, Last) Full Address: ______

Date of Birth: ______ Social Security No.: ______ Home Phone: (____) ______ Work Phone: (____) ______

Employer: ______ Occupation (type of business): ______ Years at Employer: ______

INSURANCE INFORMATION

If you have insurance, this section must be completed

Dental Insurance Company (name and address): ______
Name of Subscriber/Policy Holder: ______ Relationship to Patient: ______
Group #: ______ Identification #: ______ Other Number(s) ______

Secondary Dental Insurance Company (name and address): ______
Name of Subscriber/Policy Holder: ______ Relationship to Patient: ______
Group #: ______ Identification #: ______ Other Number(s) ______

Medical Insurance Company (name and address): ______
Name of Subscriber/Policy Holder: ______ Relationship to Patient: ______
Group #: ______ Identification #: ______ Other Number(s) ______

Secondary Medical Insurance Company (name and address): ______
Name of Subscriber/Policy Holder: ______ Relationship to Patient: ______
Group #: ______ Identification #: ______ Other Number(s) ______

RELEASE

I authorize the doctor or other dentists or health-care professionals (interdisciplinary team members) to perform diagnostic procedures and treatment as may be necessary for proper dentofacial care.

I authorize release of any information concerning my (or my child's) health care for advice and treatment provided for the purpose of evaluation and administering claims for insurance benefits.

I authorize release of any information concerning my (or my child's) health care for advice and treatment to interdisciplinary team members.

I consent to the release of credit reports and information regarding my credit history to the doctor(s).

I authorize the taking of photographs, radiographs and other diagnostic records before, during and after treatment, and to the use of the same by the doctor or interdisciplinary team members in scientific presentations or scientific literature.

Date: ______ **Patient or Guardian's Signature:** ______

Updated: ______ Patient or Guardian's ______

Fig 8-4 Example of standardized patient information form used by an interdisciplinary team.

Interdisciplinary Dentofacial Diagnostic Systems

MEDICAL AND DENTAL HISTORY (to be completed by patient)

Patient's Full Name: ______ ❑ Male ❑ Female
Date of Birth: ______ Age: (years)______ (months)______ Weight: ______ Height: ______
Patient's ❑ Current ❑ Previous Dentist(s): ______ Date of Last Dental Cleaning: ______
Patient's ❑ Current ❑ Previous Physician(s): ______ Date of Last Physical Exam: ______

All past medical and dental history may be important for your optimal care. Please take time to be as accurate and thorough as possible in answering the following questions (use bottom of page if necessary). THANK YOU.

A Please list your chief concerns for treatment: (# in order of priority): ______
B What or who motivated you to seek treatment and what do you expect? ______
C Describe anything that bothers you about the appearance of your teeth, smile or face: ______
D Describe any injuries or blows to your face, jaw, mouth or teeth: ______
E List all current medications including non-perscriptions: ______
F List all drug allergies: ______
G List all previous surgeries or hospitalizations: ______

Please ✓ if "yes" to every question appropriate, and thoroughly describe (use space at bottom of page if necessary)

MEDICAL

1 High Blood Pressure ❑
2 Chest pains or heart attack ❑
3 Stroke ❑
4 Rheumatic Fever ❑
5 Shortness of breath or swollen ankles ❑
6 Any heart trouble, murmur, or mitral valve prolapse ❑
7 Prosthetic devices (heart, valve, hip, etc.) ❑
8 Any lung disease (T.B., emphysema, etc.) ❑
9 Asthma ❑
10 Allergies or hay fever ❑
11 Sinus problems ❑
12 Mouthbreathing or excessive snoring ❑
13 Ulcers or stomach problems ❑
14 Diabetes ❑
15 Hepatitis or liver disease ❑
16 Kidney or bladder disease ❑
17 Thyroid trouble ❑
18 Connective tissue disease ❑
19 Sexually transmitted disease ❑
20 Arthritis or rheumatism ❑
21 Cancer (type, date) ❑
22 Serious illnesses not listed (list-type, date) ❑
23 Subject to prolonged bleeding or bruise easily ❑
24 A contact lens user ❑
25 Glaucoma ❑
26 Epilepsy, convulsions or seizures ❑
27 Psychiatric therapy or emotional problems ❑
28 Do you have HIV (AIDS)? ❑
29 Have you been exposed to HIV? ❑
30 Have you been tested for HIV? ❑
31 Pregnant or possible pregnant ❑
32 Taking birth control pills ❑
33 Drink coffee (cups per day) ❑
34 Use tobacco (types/how much) ❑
35 Consume alcoholic beverages ❑
36 Pain, popping, catching or locking in jaw joints ❑
37 Clench or grind your teeth ❑
38 Wake up with sore jaws ❑
39 Frequent headaches (How many per week?____) ❑
40 Dizziness, ringing or pain in ears ❑
41 Tenderness or stiffness in the jaw, neck or back ❑
42 History of TMJ (jaw joint) problems or therapy ❑

DENTAL

50 Treated for or told you have gum disease ❑
51 Treated or consulted for orthodontic therapy ❑
52 Had any oral surgery ❑
53 Dental x-rays taken in the last year ❑
54 Excessive fear of dental treatment ❑
55 Brush your teeth (how often) ❑
56 Floss your teeth (how often) ❑
57 Bad breath or unpleasant tastes in your mouth ❑
58 Bleeding gums ❑
59 Sore teeth ❑
60 Tooth sensitivity (hot, cold, sweets) ❑
61 Fever blisters or mouth ulcers ❑
62 Suck your thumb, finger or lip (now or in the past?) ❑
63 Tongue thrusting habit ❑
64 Gag easily ❑
65 Place a high priority on keeping your natural teeth ❑

Please expand on the above information (refer to letter or number) or add anything you feel is important: ______

The above information is accurate and complete to the best of my knowledge:

Date: ______ **Patient or Guardian's Signature:** ______ **Doctor's Signature:** ______
Updated:______ P or G's Initials:______ Doctor's Initials:______; ______, ______, ______; ______, ______,

Fig 8-5 Example of standardized patient history form used by an interdisciplinary team.

IDT General Evaluation and Initial Therapy **Dates:** Initial Exam:______ Diagnostic Records:______ Reevaluation:______ TMD:______ Perio:______

GENERAL TEMPOROMANDIBULAR AND OCCLUSAL EXAMINATION

Date	Initial						Reeval	
PALPATION	R	L	R	L	R	L	R	L
Lateral Capsule								
Posterior Capsule								
Masseter								
Inf. Border Mandible								
SCM								
Trapezius								
Temporalis								
EAM (ear canal)								
Medial Pterygoid								
Lateral Pterygoid								
LOADING w/o dep.								
(N,D,P) with dep.								
AUSCULTATION								
Opening (Click 1-5)								
Closing								
Right Lateral								
Left Lateral								
Protrusive								
Crepitation (1-3)								

Range of Motion (m.m.), (P)ain, (D)iscomfort or (N)egative

Date	Initial			Reeval
Opening				
Right Lateral				
Left Lateral				
Protrusive				

Mandibular Deviation (O)pen, (C)losing

date: Initial | date:____ | date:____ | date: Reeval

Radiographic Eval.: Date:________ RIGHT LEFT ❑Pan ❑Tomo ❑Trans ❑MRI

	RIGHT	LEFT
Condyle		
Fossa		
Jt. Space		
Meniscus		
R of M		

TM Trauma History:

TM Scale (0-10 worst): date Initial level_____; ____ ____; ____ ____; ____ ____; Reeval ____

Mand. Manip.: date Initial, E M D; ______, E M D; ______, E M D; ______, E M D

Dental Relationships: 6R 3 | 3 L6 ; CI ______ , Crossbite R 87654321 | 12345678 / 87654321 | 12345678

Centric Contact: R 87654321 | 12345678 / 87654321 | 12345678 ; CR to CO ____mm A,P,R,L ; Anterior Overlap: Vert._____mm, Horz._____mm

Functional Interferences: Right Lateral R 87654321 | 12345678 / 87654321 | 12345678 Left Lateral R 87654321 | 12345678 / 87654321 | 12345678 Protrusive R 87654321 | 12345678 / 87654321 | 12345678

Comments:

GENERAL DENTAL & PERIODONTAL EXAMINATION

FACIAL ANALYSIS:

Eyes: ___

Nose: ___

Dentition: ___

Chin: ___

Facial Profile __________

Lip Support __________

Misc. __________

Incisor Exp.: Rest ____mm Smile ____%

Cancer Screening: ✓for negative ❑ Face ❑ Lips ❑ Floor of Mouth ❑ Palate ❑ Tongue ❑ Neck & Lymph Nodes

X-rays taken: ❑ FMX ❑ BWX x_____ ❑ PA's x____ ❑ Pan ❑ Other______

Initial/Reeval Periodontal Exam:
(N)ormal (L)imited (M)oderate (S)evere

Date:	Init.			Reeval
Gingival inflam.:				
Soft plaque buildup:				
Hard calc. buildup:				
Bleed after probing:				
Home care effect.:				
X-ray bone loss:				

Periodontal Screening & Recording:
Date:____ Date:____ Date:____

Pathology
Existing Restorations
Date:______ Reeval Probing
Date:______ Initial Probing
Recession I/R

Periodontal Probing:
circle=bleeding
underline=supportation

Pathology:
A=Abscess
C=Thermal Cold
CM=Congen.Missing Perm.
CT=Cracked Tooth Syndrome
D=Decay
E+F=Erupted & Functioning
EX=Extracted
F=Fractured Tooth
FR=Fractured Restoration
H=Thermal Hot
I=Impacted
IF=Incomplete Fracture
NE=Non Erupted Perm.
OM-Open Margin
OC=Over-Contoured Margin
PER=Percussion
PL=Peg Lateral
RL/O=Radiolucent/Opaque Lesion
RP=Retained Primary
S=Space
SN=Supernumerary
T=Tipped into extraction site
U+E=Unopposed & Extruded

Restorations or Therapy:
A1, A2, A3=Amalgam
C1, C2, C3=Composite
CA=Cervical Abrasion/Abfraction
CC=Cast Crown
CI/O=Cast Inlay/Onlay
E=Enamelplasty
EQ=Equilibration
FB=Fixed Bridge
IM=Implant
M1, M2, M3=Mobility
P=All Porcelain Crowns
P+C=Post & Core
PI/O=Porcelain Inlay/Onlay
PM=Porcelain Fused to Metal
RB=Resin Retained Bridge
RC=Root Canal
SSC=Stainless Steel Crown
TB/C/F=Temp. Bridge/Crown/Filling
VC/P=Veneer Composite/Porcelain

P / E / RP / IP / R

[1] 1 (8) 2 (7) 3 (6) 4 (5) 5 (4) 6 (3) 7 (2) 8 (1) 9 (1) 10 (2) 11 (3) 12 (4) 13 (5) 14 (6) 15 (7) 16 (8) [2]

[5] A(5) B(4) C(3) D(2) E(1) F(1) G(2) H(3) I(4) J(5) [6]

R L

IR IP RP | IR IP RP

RP IP IR | RP IP IR

R L

[8] T(5) S(4) R(3) Q(2) P(1) O(1) N(2) M(3) L(4) K(5) [7]

[4] 32 (8) 31 (7) 30 (6) 4 (5) 5 (4) 6 (3) 7 (2) 8 (1) 9 (1) 10 (2) 11 (3) 12 (4) 13 (5) 14 (6) 15 (7) 16 (8) [3]

Recession I/R
Initial Probing
Reeval Probing
Existing Restorations
Pathology

R / IP / RP / E / P

Comments:

Fig 8-6 Example of standardized general evaluation and initial therapy form used by all team members.

Contents of the IDT Record

- **All Phases of IDT**
  - Instruction page
  - IDT progress notes page
  - IDT flowcharts
  - IDT personal, dental and medical forms
  - All diagnostic records
    - general evaluation
    - specialized evaluation(s)
    - adjunctive diagnostic(s)
    - progress
- **Diagnostic and Treatment-Planning Phase**
  - IDT diagnostic and treatment-planning summary
  - Specialized evaluations summary
- **Definitive-Therapy Phase**
  - IDT summary
- **Maintenance Phase**
  - Final records

Fig 8-7 The specific contents of IDT records varies during different phases of IDT, due to the changing needs of the team. Note that all diagnostic records become permanent parts of the record as soon as they are made.

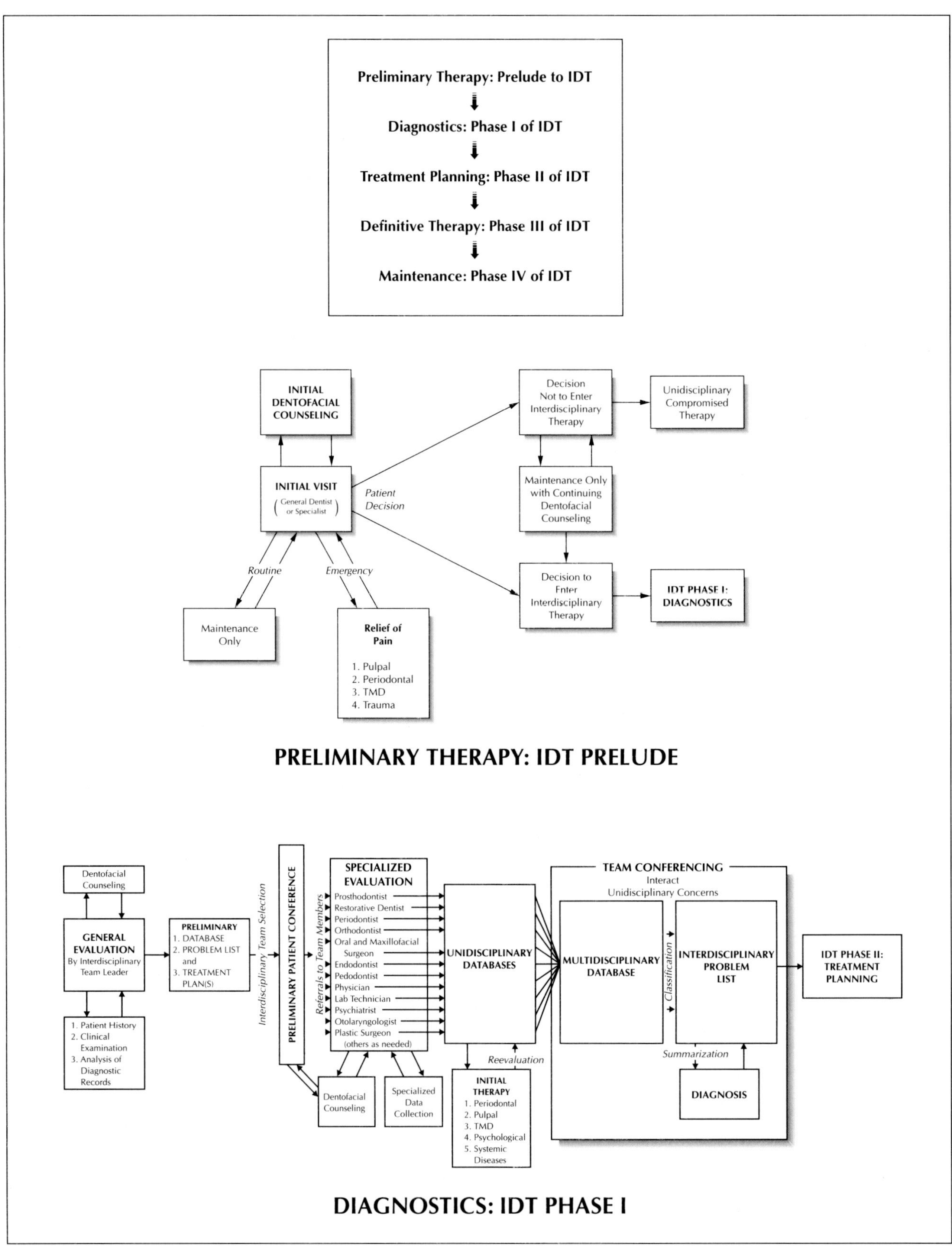

Fig 8-8 IDT flowcharts to be sent with IDT record.

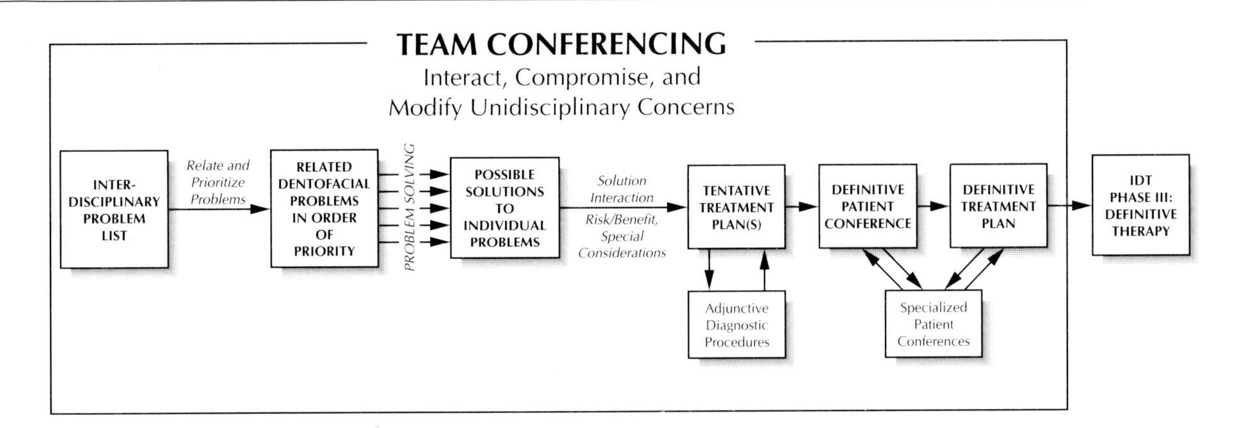

TREATMENT PLANNING: IDT PHASE II

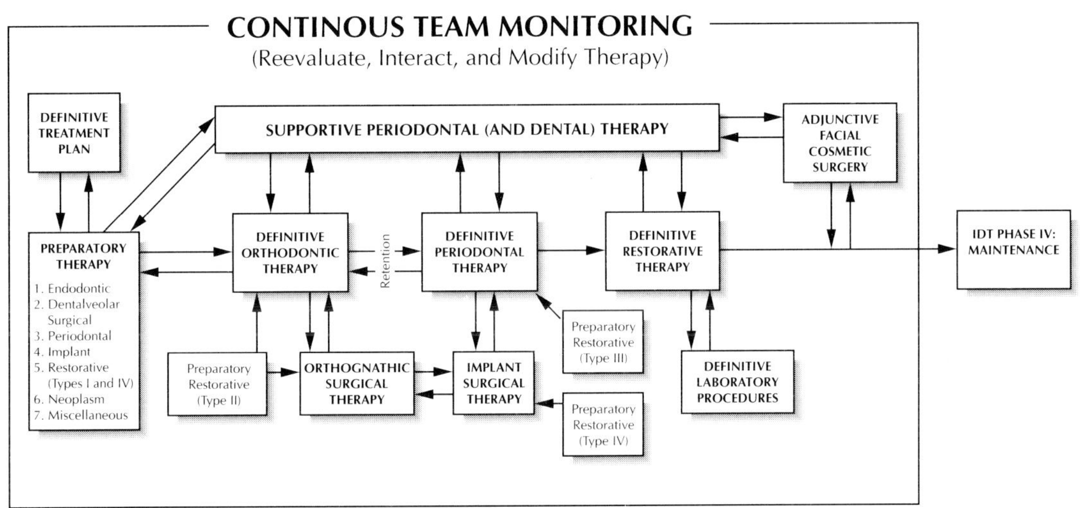

DEFINITIVE THERAPY: IDT PHASE III

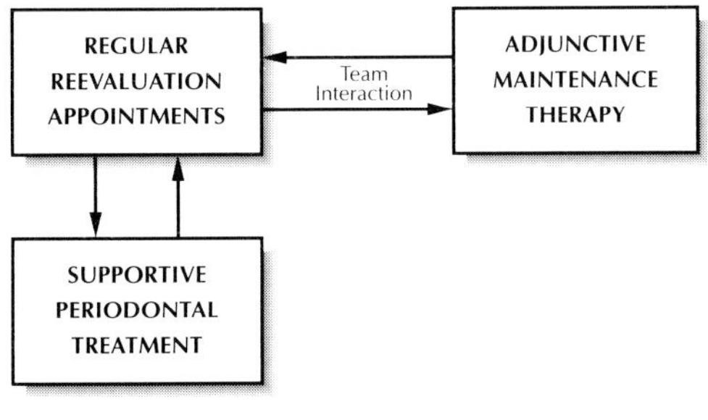

MAINTENANCE: IDT PHASE IV

Fig 8-8 (continued)

IDT Preliminary Problem List Worksheet

Patient: ____________________ Date: __________

I. Chief Concern/Motivation/Expectations/Special Concerns ____________________

II. History (personal, medical, dental and temporomandibular) ____________________

III. Facial/Skeletal ____________________

IV. Temporomandibular ____________________

V. Occlusal (Relationships and function) ____________________

VI. Periodontal ____________________

VII. Dental/Implant ____________________

Specialized Evaluations (**N** = Needed, **C** = Completed, **S** = Screened during general evaluation and <u>not</u> indicated)

Restorative ______	Periodontal ______	Orthodontic ______
Endodontic ______	Implant ______	Medical ______
	Oral and Maxillofacial Surgical ______	Other ______

Fig 8-9 Example of IDT preliminary problem list worksheet.

IDT Preliminary Treatment Planning Worksheet

Patient: ______________________ Date: ____________

I. DIAGNOSTIC AND TREATMENT PLANNING PHASES

- General Evaluation (date completed, areas only screened and records not made)
- Specialized Evaluations by Interdisciplinary Team Members (including date and any records needed)
- Initial Therapy
- Reevaluation after Initial Therapy
- Miscellaneous

II. DEFINITIVE THERAPY PHASE

- Supportive Periodontal and Dental Therapy
- Special Considerations for Team Monitoring
- Preparatory Therapy
- Definitive Therapy
- Miscellaneous

III. MAINTENANCE PHASE

- Supportive Periodontal and Dental Therapy
- Miscellaneous (retention, special considerations, etc.)

Fig 8-10 Example of IDT preliminary treatment planning worksheet.

IDT Dental Treatment Planning Worksheet

Patient: ______________________________ Date: ______________

Individual tooth objectives for restorative, periodontal, surgical, endodontic and orthodontic therapies:

[1]	1(8)	2(7)	3(6)	4(5)	5(4)	6(3)	7(2)	8(1)	9(1)	10(2)	11(3)	12(4)	13(5)	14(6)	15(7)	16(8)	[2]
[5]				A(5)	B(4)	C(3)	D(2)	E(1)	F(1)	G(2)	H(3)	I(4)	J(5)				[6]
MAXILLARY																	
R																	L
MANDIBULAR																	
[8]				T(5)	S(4)	R(3)	Q(2)	P(1)	O(1)	N(2)	M(3)	L(4)	K(5)				[7]
[4]	32(8)	31(7)	30(6)	4(5)	5(4)	6(3)	7(2)	8(1)	9(1)	10(2)	11(3)	12(4)	13(5)	14(6)	15(7)	16(8)	[3]

[1] R↑
(8)1 ______
(7)2 ______
(6)3 ______
(5)4 ______
(4)5 ______
(3)6 ______
(2)7 ______
(1)8 ______

[2] L↑
(1) 9 ______
(2)10 ______
(3)11 ______
(4)12 ______
(5)13 ______
(6)14 ______
(7)15 ______
(8)16 ______

[3] L↓
(8)17 ______
(7)18 ______
(6)19 ______
(5)20 ______
(4)21 ______
(3)22 ______
(2)23 ______
(1)24 ______

[4] R↓
(1)25 ______
(2)26 ______
(3)27 ______
(4)28 ______
(5)29 ______
(6)30 ______
(7)31 ______
(8)32 ______

Primary Dentition or Additional Space ______

Fig 8-11 Example of IDT dental treatment planning worksheet.

IDT Diagnostic and Treatment Planning Summary

IDT Team Members:	
Restorative	Dr. Broyles
Periodontal	Dr. Renegar
Orthodontic (Leader)	Dr. Roblee
O & M Surgical	Dr. Bolding

PATIENT: Johnny IDT Date: ____________

Preliminary Problem List and History

I. CHIEF CONCERN/MOTIVATION/EXPECTATION

- **A.** "Replace poor quality crowns in front top four teeth and underbite condition requires jaw reset"
- **B.** Selfmotivated
- **C.** "More attractive smile and better bite"

II. HISTORY

- **A.** 29 year 7 month old white male
- **B.** Previous full orthodontic therapy

III. FACIAL/SKELETAL

- **A.** Anterior divergent straight profile with nice upper lip, full lower lip and strong chin button
- **B.** Class III skeletal relationship with prognathic mandible and mandibular dentoalveolar protrusion
- **C.** Midface hypoplasia (flat)
- **D.** High mandibular plane angle
- **E.** Increased face height

IV. TEMPOROMANDIBULAR

- **A.** Positive bruxing history
- **B.** Wakes up with "sore jaws"
- **C.** Tenderness during palpation in right and left lateral capsules of TMJ's

V. OCCLUSAL

- **A.** Class III dental malocclusion with mild anterior openbite
- **B.** End to end interincisal relationship
- **C.** Traumatic functional occlusion with severe working and balancing interferences

VI. PERIODONTAL

- **A.** Localized periodontal inflammation with bleeding upon probing around overcontoured crowns #s 7, 8, 9 and 10 with probable "Biologic width" problem
- **B.** Improper gingival relationship in maxillary anterior region

VIIDENTAL/IMPLANT

- **A.** Upright mandibular incisors
- **B.** Relative interarch transverse discrepancy
- **C.** Composite resin veneers #s 5, 6 and 11with no enamel reduction
- **D.** Overcontoured crowns #s 7, 8, 9 and 10
- **E.** Moderate occlusal wear

Preliminary Treatment Plan

I. DIAGNOSTIC AND TREATMENT PLANNING PHASES

- **A.** General Evaluation and Diagnostic Records (Dr. Roblee, completed)
  - ➢ Except full-mouth radiographic survey
  - ➢ Periodontal screening only
- **B.** Specialized Evaluations by INTERDISCIPLINARY TEAM MEMBERS:
  - ➢ Orthodontic evaluation (Dr. Roblee, completed)
    - • Cephalometric analysis
  - ➢ TMJ Tomographic evaluation (Dr. Roblee, completed)
  - ➢ Oral and Maxillofacial Surgical evaluation (Dr. Bolding, date)
  - ➢ Restorative evaluation (Dr. Broyles, date)
    - • Full-mouth radiographic survey
  - ➢ Periodontal evaluation (Dr. Renegar, date)
- **C.** Inital Therapy
  - ➢ Periodondal (Dr. Renegar)
    - • Conservative therapy to control inflamation

The following is a part of the Preliminary Treatment Plan that may be altered during the Diagnostic and Treatment Planning Phases of IDT and should not be initiated until after those phases are completed:

II. DEFINITIVE THERAPY PHASE

- **A.** Supportive Periodontal and Dental Therapy
  - ➢ Alternating 4-month schedules (Drs. Broyles/Renegar)
- **B.** Special Considerations for Team Monitoring
  - ➢ Monitor TMD symptoms and treat if necessary
- **C.** Preparatory Restorative Therapy (Dr. Broyles)
  - ➢ Remove overcontoured crowns #s 7, 8, 9 and 10 and place properly contoured provisional restorations to allow soft tissue healing
  - ➢ Remove direct composite veneers #s 5, 6 and 11
- **D.** Preparatory Dentoalveolar Surgical Therapy (Dr. Bolding)
  - ➢ Extract #s 4, 13, 21 and 28 (Dr. Bolding)
- **E.** Presurgical Orthodontic Therapy (Dr. Roblee)
  - ➢ Selectively close extraction sites with minimum anchorage in maxillary arch and maximum anchorage in mandibular arch to correct mandibular dentoalveolar protrusion and to set up arches for orthognathic surgical procedures
  - ➢ Selectively extrude maxillary anterior teeth to properly align gingival tissues
- **F.** Orthognathic Surgical Procedures (Dr. Bolding)
  - ➢ Segmental maxillary osteotomies to advance and impact the maxilla in a clockwise direction
  - ➢ Autorotate mandible
- **G.** Post-surgical Orthodontic Therapy
  - ➢ Gnathologically finish occlusion in Class I molar relationship
- **H.** Definitive Periodontal Therapy (Dr. Renegar)
  - ➢ Periodontal plastic surgical procedures:
    - • Possible crown lengthening, if necessary, to correct "biologic width" #s 7, 8, 9 and 10 and further enhance gingival alignment
- **I.** Definitive Restorative Therapy (Dr. Broyles)
  - ➢ Bonded all porcelain crowns #s 6, 7, 8, 9, 10 and 11

III. MAINTENANCE PHASE

- **A.** Maintain a 6-month alternating supportive periodontal and dental therapy schedule after Definitive Therapy is completed (Drs. Broyles/Renegar)
- **B.** Maintain result with maxillary centric relation nighttime splint and mandibular bonded lingual retainer (Dr. Roblee)

Fig 8-12 IDT diagnostic and treatment planning summary, containing the preliminary problem list and treatment plan.

RICHARD D. ROBLEE, D.D.S, M.S.
ORTHODONTICS

1915 GREEN ACRES ROAD
FAYETTEVILLE, ARKANSAS 72703
(501) 521-6060
FAX (501) 521-4161

(Date)

(Doctor's name and address)

Re: (Patient's first and last name)

Dear (Doctor's first name):

(Patient's first and last name) has completed the Diagnostic and Treatment Planning Phases of Interdisciplinary Dentofacial Therapy and is ready to proceed with the Definitive Therapy.

Enclosed is a copy of the IDT Summary which contains the Interdisciplinary Problem List and Definitive Treatment Plan dated (date). Please thoroughly review it to make sure that it is complete and correct to your satisfaction. After you have reviewed it, initial the appropriate box at the bottom of the page and return this letter to my office in the enclosed envelope. If you are satisfied with it, keep the Summary for your records. If you are not satisfied with it, make the appropriate corrections and additions and send it back to me with this letter. If you would like to review the IDT Record again, please contact my office to arrange delivery.

This sign-off sheet is solely intended to assure that each team member has maximum input into the Interdisciplinary Dentofacial Therapy diagnostic and treatment planning process. It does not seek to substantiate legal causes, but instead insures that an optimal treatment plan has been formulated from all the different discipline's perspectives. Thank you for completing this form. I appreciate the opportunity to work with you to help (patient's first name).

Sincerely,

Richard D. Roblee, D.D.S., M.S.

Please initial one of the following options and return this letter in the enclosed envelope

- ❑ I agree with the IDT Summary in its current form.
- ❑ I agree with the IDT Summary with the additions/corrections I have indicated on the IDT Summary or this page
- ❑ I cannot agree with the IDT Summary in its present form because of the major corrections/additions I have indicated on the IDT Summary, this page, or an attachment

Comments, corrections or additions:

Fig 8-13 Example of letter sent for team members' approval of definitive treatment plan prior to definitive therapy.

IDT Summary

IDT Team Members:	
Restorative	Dr. Broyles
Periodontal	Dr. Renegar
Orthodontic (Leader)	Dr. Roblee
O & M Surgical	Dr. Bolding
ENT Physician	Dr. Baker

PATIENT: Johnny IDT Date: ______________

Interdisciplinary Problem List and History

I. CHIEF CONCERN/MOTIVATION/EXPECTATION
- **A.** "Replace poor quality crowns in front top four teeth and underbite condition requires jaw reset"
- **B.** Selfmotivated
- **C.** "More attractive smile and better bite"

II. HISTORY
- **A.** 29 year 7 month old white male
- **B.** Previous full orthodontic therapy
- **C.** Partial mouthbreather

III. FACIAL/SKELETAL
- **A.** Anterior divergent straight profile with nice upper lip, full lower lip and strong chin button
- **B.** Class III skeletal relationship with prognathic mandible and mandibular dentoalveolar protrusion
- **C.** Midface hypoplasia (flat)
- **D.** High mandibular plane angle
- **E.** Increased face height
- **F.** Relative interarch transverse discrepancy

IV. TEMPOROMANDIBULAR
- **A.** Positive bruxing history
- **B.** Wakes up with "sore jaws"
- **C.** Tenderness during palpation in right and left lateral capsules of TMJ's

V. OCCLUSAL
- **A.** Class III dental malocclusion with mild anterior openbite
- **B.** End to end interincisal relationship
- **C.** Bilateral end-to-end occlusion
- **D.** Traumatic functional occlusion with severe working and balancing interferences

VI. PERIODONTAL
- **A.** Localized periodontal inflammation with bleeding upon probing around overcontoured crowns #s 7, 8, 9 and 10 with probable "Biologic width" problem
- **B.** Improper gingival relationship in maxillary anterior region
- **C.** Minimal attached tissues facial #s 23, 24, 25 & 26
- **D.** Mild clefting on facial #s 4 & 5

VIIDENTAL/IMPLANT
- **A.** Upright mandibular incisors
- **B.** Composite resin veneers #s 5, 6 and 11with no enamal reduction
- **C.** Overcontoured crowns #s 7, 8, 9 and 10
- **D.** Moderate occlusalwear
- **E.** Large amalgam restorations #s 14 & 30

ADDITIONAL DIAGNOSTIC RECORDS MADE
(Type, Provider, and Date) (Include in IDT Record)

____
____
____
____
____
____

Definitive Treatment Plan

I. DIAGNOSTIC AND TREATMENT PLANNING PHASES
- **A.** General Evaluation and Diagnostic Records (Dr. Roblee, completed)
  - ➢ Except full-mouth radiographic survey
  - ➢ Periodontal screening only
- **B.** Specialized Evaluations by INTERDISCIPLINARY TEAM MEMBERS:
  - ➢ Orthodontic evaluation (Dr. Roblee, completed)
    - • Cephalometric analysis
  - ➢ TMJ Tomographic evaluation (Dr. Roblee, completed)
  - ➢ Oral and Maxillofacial Surgical evaluation (Dr. Bolding, completed)
  - ➢ Restorative evaluation (Dr. Broyles, completed)
    - • Full-mouth radiographic survey
  - ➢ Periodontal evaluation (Dr. Renegar, completed)
  - ➢ Ear, Nose and Throat evaluation (Dr. Baker)
- **C.** Inital Therapy
  - ➢ Periodondal (Dr. Renegar)
    - • Conservative therapy to control inflamation

II. DEFINITIVE THERAPY PHASE
- **A.** Supportive Periodontal and Dental Therapy
  - ➢ Alternating 4-month schedules (Drs. Broyles/Renegar)
- **B.** Special Considerations for Team Monitoring
  - ➢ Monitor TMD symptoms and treat if necessary
  - ➢ Monitor attached gingival #s 4, 5, 24, 25, 26 & 27
- **C.** Preparatory Restorative Therapy (Dr. Broyles)
  - ➢ Remove overcontoured crowns #s 7, 8, 9 and 10 and place properly contoured provisional restorations to allow soft tissue healing
  - ➢ Remove direct composite veneers #s 5, 6 and 11
- **D.** Preparatory Dentoalveolar Surgical Therapy (Dr. Bolding)
  - ➢ Extract #s 4, 13, 21 and 28 (Dr. Bolding)
- **E.** Presurgical Orthodontic Therapy (Dr. Roblee)
  - ➢ Selectively close extraction sites with minimum anchorage in maxillary arch and maximum anchorage in mandibular arch to correct mandibular dentoalveolar protrusion and to set up arches for orthognathic surgical procedures
  - ➢ Selectively extrude maxillary anterior teeth to properly align gingival tissues
- **F.** Orthognathic Surgical Procedures (Dr. Bolding)
  - ➢ Segmental maxillary osteotomies to advance and impact the maxilla in a clockwise direction
  - ➢ Autorotate mandible
  - ➢ Possible reduction genioplasty
- **G.** Post-surgical Orthodontic Therapy
  - ➢ Gnathologically finish occlusion in Class I molar relationship
- **H.** Definitive Periodontal Therapy (Dr. Renegar)
  - ➢ Periodontal plastic surgical procedures:
    - • Possible crown lengthening, if necessary, to correct "biologic width" #s 7, 8, 9 and 10 and further enhance gingival alignment
    - • Possible free gingival grafts on facial #s 4, 5, 24, 25, 26 & 27
- **I.** Definitive Restorative Therapy (Dr. Broyles)
  - ➢ Bonded all porcelain crowns #s 6, 7, 8, 9, 10 and 11
  - ➢ Crowns #s 14 & 30

III. MAINTENANCE PHASE
- **A.** Maintain a 6-month alternating supportive periodontal and dental therapy schedule after Definitive Therapy is completed (Drs. Broyles/Renegar)
- **B.** Maintain result with maxillary centric relation nighttime splint and mandibular bonded lingual retainer (Dr. Roblee)

Fig 8-14 IDT summary, containing the history, final problem list, and definitive treatment plan.

RICHARD D. ROBLEE, D.D.S, M.S.
ORTHODONTICS

1915 GREEN ACRES ROAD
FAYETTEVILLE, ARKANSAS 72703
(501) 521-6060
FAX (501) 521-4161

(Date)

(Patient's name and address)

Dear (Patient's first name):

On behalf of your Interdisciplinary Team, I would like to thank you for allowing us to help you with your dentofacial needs. This letter will summarize your therapy to date and it will also serve as a schedule for your different Specialized Evaluations. Please note that this is a Preliminary Treatment Plan that may change after the Specialized Evaluations are completed.

A complete set of General Dentofacial Diagnostic Records has been made and evaluated. You returned for a preliminary consultation on (date). The following findings and Preliminary Treatment Plan were discussed.

PRELIMINARY PROBLEM LIST AND HISTORY:

PRELIMINARY TREATMENT PLAN:

This format of diagnosing and treatment planning will allow this Diagnostic Phase of Interdisciplinary Dentofacial Therapy to progress as smooth and orderly as possible. More importantly, this format enables full utilization of the expertise of the different team members to formulate the most optimal treatment plan for you. The same care and thoroughness will be provided during your Definitive Therapy Phase to ensure the best results possible.

I am greatly looking forward to working with the other team members to help you. Please do not hesitate to contact me if you have any comments or questions.

Sincerely,

Richard D. Roblee, D.D.S., M.S.

RDR:lhn

Fig 8-15 Example of letter to patient with preliminary treatment plan and problem list, prior to definitive therapy.

IDT Progress Notes

PATIENT NAME: ______________________________

Team Members with Voice Mail # : ______________ # ______ ______________ # ______
______________ # ______ ______________ # ______
______________ # ______ ______________ # ______

Date	Procedures Completed and Misc. Notations	Next Procedures	Team Members Initials

Fig 8-16 Example of IDT progress notes form, to be updated throughout therapy.

RICHARD D. ROBLEE, D.D.S, M.S.
ORTHODONTICS

1915 GREEN ACRES ROAD
FAYETTEVILLE, ARKANSAS 72703
(501) 521-6060
FAX (501) 521-4161

Re: (patient)

Dear Interdisciplinary Team Members:

This package contains (patient's name) IDT Diagnostic and Treatment Record (IDT Record). The purpose of the IDT Record is to help coordinate the Specialized Evaluations so that each team member's expertise can be fully utilized to formulate the most optimal treatment plan. After the Definitive Treatment Plan is completed the IDT Record is used as a concise formatted reference to help ensure optimal definitive therapy and maintenance. The instructions for use during the Diagnostic and Treatment Planning Phases of IDT are #'s 1-10 and the instructions for the Definitive Therapy Phase of IDT are #'s 5, 6 & 7.

1. You should receive this package at least one day prior to your evaluation so that you have time to properly analyze the records.
2. Perform your Specialized Evaluation and make any additional specialized records as you see necessary.
3. If you find additional problems that warrant the expertise of an additional team member, please make that referral and appointment for the patient. Then list the new Specialized Evaluation, team member, date and your initials in the correct place on the Preliminary Treatment Plan to ensure that the new provider will also receive this package in ample time.
4. Utilize the enclosed Specialized Evaluation Summary Sheet with your name on it to list your additions or changes to the Preliminary Problem List and History, and to the Preliminary Treatment Plan. In addition, list any additional evaluations that you may have referred the patient for, and any additional diagnostic records you have made. Also, include the new records in the IDT Record if you think they might be utilized by another team member.
5. After you have completed your evaluation or other procedures, put your initials by the left-hand side of where your procedure is listed on the IDT Diagnostic and Treatment Planning Summary (IDT Summary).
6. Look at the IDT Summary to see who will need the records next. When you are finished, please transfer the records to the next team member so that he or she will have ample time to evaluate them before their appointment. If you have the last evaluation, transfer the records back to my office.
7. Properly document the IDT Progress Notes.
8. If you do not have time to complete the enclosed paperwork before the next evaluation, please transfer this package as needed to the next evaluator and mail your summary to me after you complete it.
9. Initiate any needed Initial Therapy which is appropriate to your area of expertise. After your Initial Therapy is completed, reevaluate the patient and document any changes that need to be made to the original Preliminary Problem List and Treatment Plan. Please notify me of these changes after your Initial Therapy has been completed.
10. The Tentative Treatment Plan(s) cannot be properly formulated until all Evaluations, Initial Therapy and Reevaluations have been completed. When completed the patient will be consulted of his/her treatment option(s) so that the Definitive Treatment Plan can be decided. A IDT Summary will be made at that time and mailed to you for your final approval.

Thank you for following this format - it will help ensure that we give (patient) the best results possible. I look forward to the opportunity to work with you to help her. This should be a very rewarding case for everybody concerned, especially (patient). Please do not hesitate to contact me if you have any comments or questions concerning this case or the IDT Record.

Best personal regards,

Richard D. Roblee, D.D.S., M.S.

Fig 8-17 Letter sent with IDT record to team member who is to perform specialized evaluations and therapy.

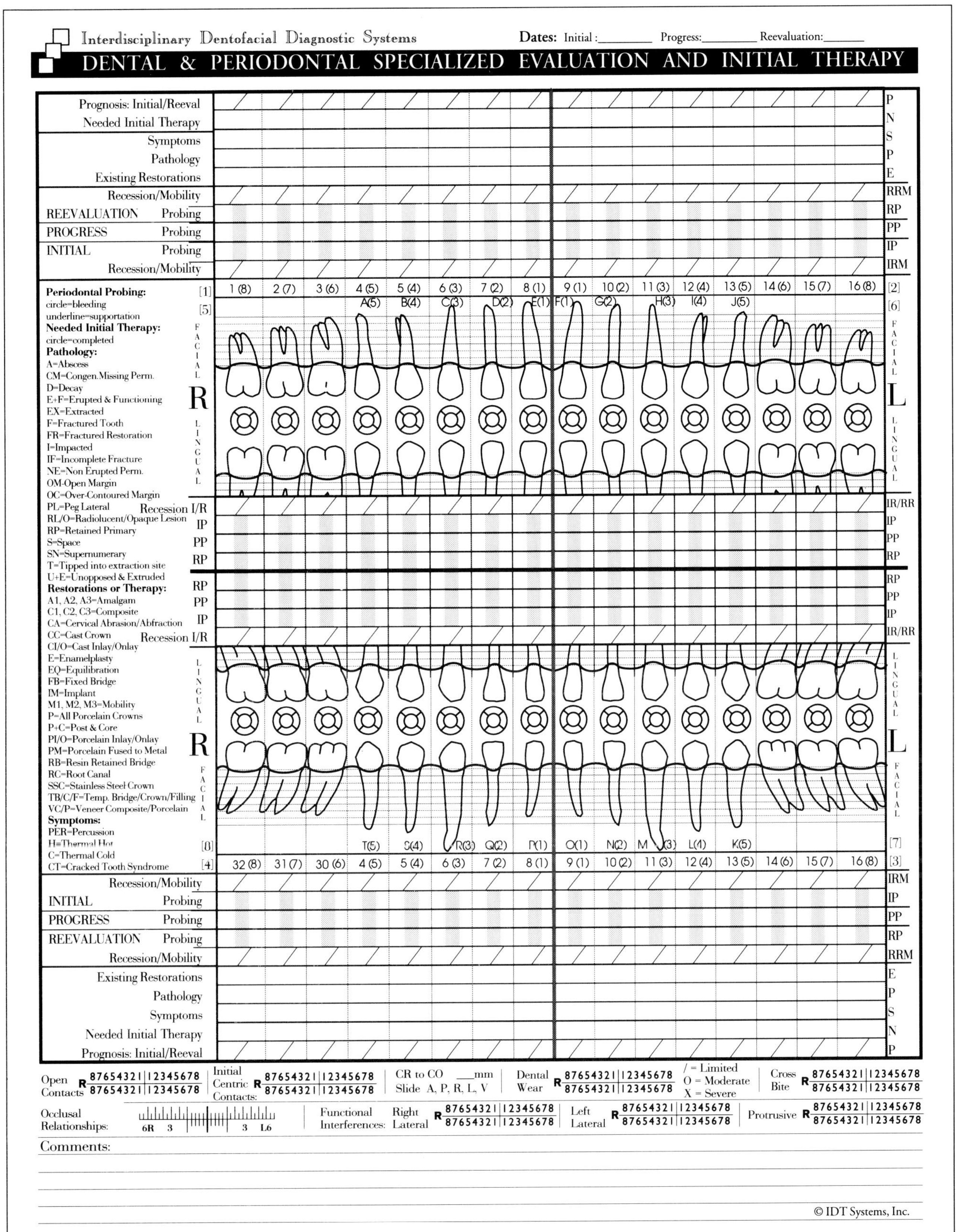

Interdisciplinary Dentofacial Diagnostic Systems

Dates: Initial :________ Progress:________ Reevaluation:______

DENTAL & PERIODONTAL SPECIALIZED EVALUATION AND INITIAL THERAPY

Prognosis: Initial/Reeval	P
Needed Initial Therapy	N
Symptoms	S
Pathology	P
Existing Restorations	E
Recession/Mobility	RRM
REEVALUATION Probing	RP
PROGRESS Probing	PP
INITIAL Probing	IP
Recession/Mobility	IRM

[1] 1 (8) 2 (7) 3 (6) 4 (5) 5 (4) 6 (3) 7 (2) 8 (1) 9 (1) 10 (2) 11 (3) 12 (4) 13 (5) 14 (6) 15 (7) 16 (8) [2]

[5] A(5) B(4) C(3) D(2) E(1) F(1) G(2) H(3) I(4) J(5) [6]

FACIAL R LINGUAL — FACIAL L LINGUAL

Periodontal Probing:
circle=bleeding
underline=supportation
Needed Initial Therapy:
circle=completed
Pathology:
A=Abscess
CM=Congen.Missing Perm.
D=Decay
E+F=Erupted & Functioning
EX=Extracted
F=Fractured Tooth
FR=Fractured Restoration
I=Impacted
IF=Incomplete Fracture
NE=Non Erupted Perm.
OM-Open Margin
OC=Over-Contoured Margin
PL=Peg Lateral
RL/O=Radiolucent/Opaque Lesion
RP=Retained Primary
S=Space
SN=Supernumerary
T=Tipped into extraction site
U+E=Unopposed & Extruded
Restorations or Therapy:
A1, A2, A3=Amalgam
C1, C2, C3=Composite
CA=Cervical Abrasion/Abfraction
CC=Cast Crown
CI/O=Cast Inlay/Onlay
E=Enamelplasty
EQ=Equilibration
FB=Fixed Bridge
IM=Implant
M1, M2, M3=Mobility
P=All Porcelain Crowns
P+C=Post & Core
PI/O=Porcelain Inlay/Onlay
PM=Porcelain Fused to Metal
RB=Resin Retained Bridge
RC=Root Canal
SSC=Stainless Steel Crown
TB/C/F=Temp. Bridge/Crown/Filling
VC/P=Veneer Composite/Porcelain
Symptoms:
PER=Percussion
H=Thermal Hot
C=Thermal Cold
CT=Cracked Tooth Syndrome

Recession I/R	IR/RR
IP	IP
PP	PP
RP	RP
RP	RP
PP	PP
IP	IP
Recession I/R	IR/RR

LINGUAL R FACIAL — LINGUAL L FACIAL

[8] T(5) S(4) R(3) Q(2) P(1) O(1) N(2) M(3) L(4) K(5) [7]

[4] 32 (8) 31 (7) 30 (6) 4 (5) 5 (4) 6 (3) 7 (2) 8 (1) 9 (1) 10 (2) 11 (3) 12 (4) 13 (5) 14 (6) 15 (7) 16 (8) [3]

Recession/Mobility	IRM
INITIAL Probing	IP
PROGRESS Probing	PP
REEVALUATION Probing	RP
Recession/Mobility	RRM
Existing Restorations	E
Pathology	P
Symptoms	S
Needed Initial Therapy	N
Prognosis: Initial/Reeval	P

Open Contacts R 87654321 | 12345678 / 87654321 | 12345678 — Initial Centric Contacts: R 87654321 | 12345678 / 87654321 | 12345678 — CR to CO ___mm Slide A, P, R, L, V — Dental Wear R 87654321 | 12345678 / 87654321 | 12345678 — / = Limited O = Moderate X = Severe — Cross Bite R 87654321 | 12345678 / 87654321 | 12345678

Occlusal Relationships: 6R 3 3 L6 — Functional Interferences: Right Lateral R 87654321 | 12345678 / 87654321 | 12345678 — Left Lateral R 87654321 | 12345678 / 87654321 | 12345678 — Protrusive R 87654321 | 12345678 / 87654321 | 12345678

Comments:

Fig 8-18 Example of IDT dental and periodontal specialized evaluation and initial therapy form.

SPECIALIZED EVALUATION SUMMARY

Patient: ______________________ **Date:** ______________

Evaluation: ______________________

IDT Team Member: ______________________

1. Additions or changes to Preliminary Problem List and History:

2. Suggestions, additions or changes to Preliminary Treatment Plan:

3. Additional diagnostic records made or needed.

4. Additional referrals made or suggested for Specialized Evaluations.

5. Initial therapy needed, initiated, or completed.

______________________ Signature

______________ Date

Fig 8-19 Example of IDT specialized evaluation summary form.

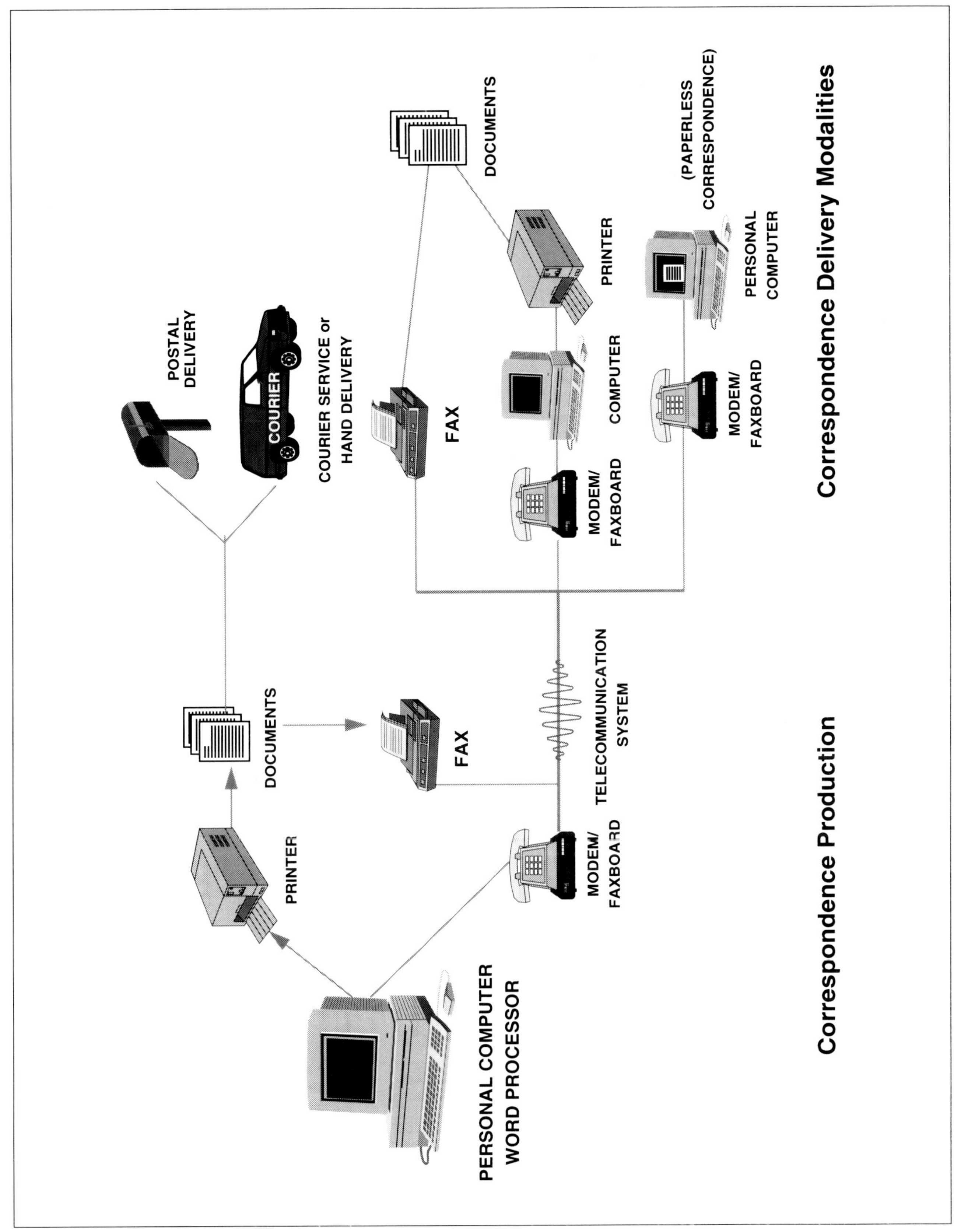

Fig 8-20 IDT correspondence production and delivery using electronic communication.

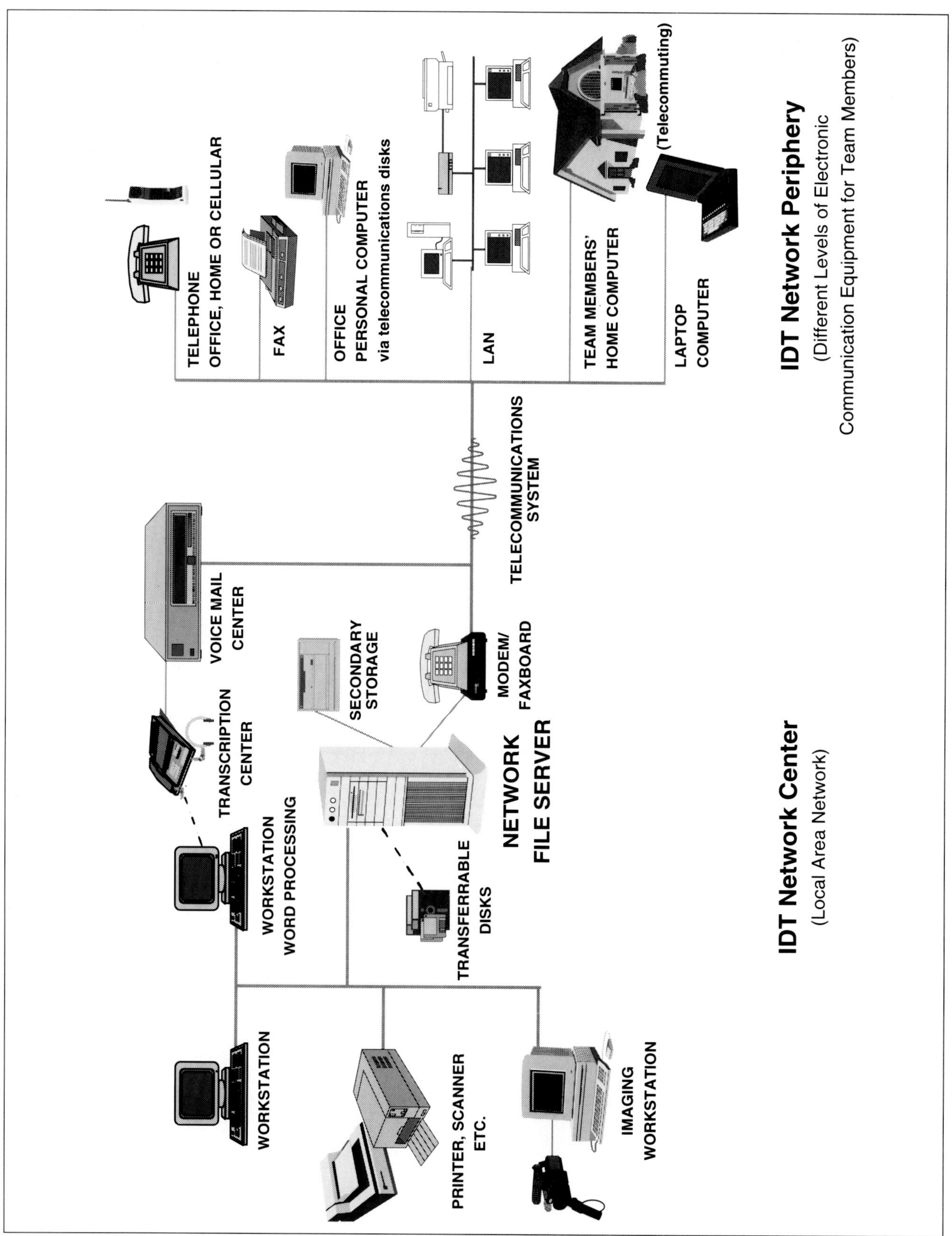

Fig 8-21 Ideal IDT electronic network configuration, consisting of an IDT network center and IDT periphery.